ECONOMICS
AND
HEALTH CARE

ECONOMICS AND HEALTH CARE

By

HIRSCH S. RUCHLIN, Ph.D.

Assistant Professor, Graduate Program in Health Care Administration, Baruch College-Mount Sinai School of Medicine, City University of New York; Assistant Professor, Department of Administrative Medicine, Mount Sinai School of Medicine, City University of New York

and

DANIEL C. ROGERS, Ph.D.

Economist, Agency for International Development

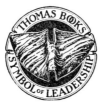

CHARLES C THOMAS · PUBLISHER

Springfield · Illinois · U.S.A.

Published and Distributed Throughout the World by
CHARLES C THOMAS · PUBLISHER
BANNERSTONE HOUSE
301–327 East Lawrence Avenue, Springfield, Illinois, U.S.A.

© 1973, *by* CHARLES C THOMAS · PUBLISHER
ISBN 0–398–02712–9
Library of Congress Catalog Card Number: 72–88468

With THOMAS BOOKS *careful attention is given to all details of manu-
facturing and design. It is the Publisher's desire to present books that are
satisfactory as to their physical qualities and artistic possibilities and
appropriate for their particular use.* THOMAS BOOKS *will be true to
those laws of quality that assure a good name and good will.*

Printed in the United States of America
K–8

To
Ari, Deena, Clifford, and Keith

PREFACE

ECONOMISTS have penetrated into all realms of the health care
industry. The daily agenda of health care administrators and
planners is replete with issues having definite economic connota-
tions. Among these issues are projecting demand, determining
production methods, and choosing among alternative processes intended to accomplish the same goal. In an attempt to cope with
these issues, many health care institutions employ economists on a
permanent or consultive basis. Even at the highest policy levels,
a definite economic input into health-related issues is clearly dis-
cernible. A clear indication of this is the recent selection of four
prominent health economists, Rashi Fein, Martin Feldstein, Victor
Fuchs, and Herbert Klarman, to serve on the Institute of Medicine
formed by the National Academy of Sciences.

The diffusion within the mass of the health establishment of
an elementary understanding of economic analysis, both in the abstract and as related to health care issues, has not kept pace with
the growing importance of economic issues and the increasing
contribution of economics to health administration and public
policy issues. This gap could be at least partially bridged by ac-
quainting members of the health care industry with a select number of economic concepts and tools having a direct bearing on
issues in the health field and illustrating the applicability of these
concepts to specific problems germane to the health field. It is to
this task that this book is addressed.

The presentation begins by introducing the reader to the discipline of economics and to the economics of health. Chapter Two
presents a brief overview of national income accounting and es-

tablishes the relationship between income and the consumption of health services. The following chapter introduces the concept of indices, describes the composition of the Consumer Price Index and the Medical Care Price Index, and notes the structural short-comings of these measures of general price movements in the economy as a whole and in the medical care sector. The next six chapters are sequentially devoted to the exposition of demand, production, and investment theory and the illustration of the applicability of these theories to specific issues in the health field. Chapter Ten focuses on an elementary presentation of the theory of economic growth and the process of economic planning both in the abstract and as related to the health field. Chapter Eleven presents a discussion of the financing of health-related services, an overview of the United States tax structure and its affect on providing health care services, and a brief summary of various alternative financing schemes which attempt to improve both the financial situation and the economic efficiency of the health industry. Finally, two appendices develop the essentials of mathematics and statistics required for an intelligent consumption of the burgeoning health economics literature. All technical terms and definitions appearing in these appendices are italicized thereby permitting, with the aid of the index, the use of the mathematical and statistical material as a glossary. It is recommended that these appendices be read in conjunction with the demand chapters and consulted thereafter as needed.

Incorporated within Chapters Five, Seven, and Nine are research studies undertaken by other health economists. These studies have been specifically selected from the health economics literature for their relative simplicity, their use of analytic tools, and their direct focus on demand, production, and investment theory, respectively.

The approach embodied in this text and some of the basic material contained therein was developed during our tenure at Teachers College, Columbia University, when we illustrated the applicability of economic analysis to educational issues in a previous publications.[1] Major responsibility for adapting the elements

[1] Rogers, Daniel C. and Ruchlin, Hirsch S.: *Economics and Education: Principles and Applications*. New York, Free Press, 1971.

of economic theory presented here to the health field and for the literature search upon which Chapters Five, Seven, and Nine are based was borne by Hirsch S. Ruchlin; Daniel C. Rogers assumed major responsibility for adapting the material contained in Chapter Ten.

H.S.R.

D.C.R.

LIST OF TABLES

I. National Health Expenditures, Selected Years, 1950–
1970 5

II. Health Care Expenditures, by Object, 1950 and 1969 . 5

III. Gross National Product and Gross National Income,
1971 21

IV. Total and Per Capita Personal Income by State and 21
Region, 1970 22

V. Money and Real Gross National Product, Selected
Years, 1930–1971 25

VI. Median Annual Salaries of Public Health Nurses,
1955–1971 26

VII. Percentage Share of Aggregate Income Received by
Each Fifth of Families, 1970 29

VIII. Infant Mortality Rates by Color and Family Income,
1964–1966 30

IX. Average Number of Filled And Decayed Primary And
Permanent Teeth Per Child Aged 6–11 by Family Income, 1963–1965 30

X. Number of Physician Visits Per Person Per Year, by
Sex, Color, and Family Income, July 1965—June
1967 31

XI. Visits Per One-Hundred Families To Selected Types of
Medical Specialists, by Family Income, July 1963—
June 1964 31

XII. Indices of Health and Hospital Expenditures, by State,
1969 36

XIII. Index of Item A   40

XIV. The Construction of a Laspeyeres and Paasche Price
      Index   43

XV. The Consumer Price Index, Annual Average, 1971   .   44

XVI. The Medical Care Price Index, Selected Years, 1935–
      1971   48

XVII. Percentage Increase in Average Cost of Treatment, Se-
      lected Illnesses, 1951–1952 to 1964–1965   52

XVIII. Selected Output Values for Production Function
      $Q = 50 \ C^{1/2}L^{1/2}$ 105

XIX. National Health Expenditures, by Type, Selected
      Years, 1950–1969   232

XX. National Health Expenditures, by Source, Selected
      Years, 1950–1969   234

XXI. Health Care Expenditures As A Percent of Total Social
      Welfare Expenditures, by Level of Government, Se-
      lected Years, 1935–1970   235

XXII. Federal Government Health Care Expenditures, Se-
      lected Years, 1950–1970   236

XXIII. Federal Aid to State and Local Governments for Health
      Care Use, 1965–1971   237

XXIV. Federal Per Capita Grants for Health Purposes to
      State and Local Governments, 1970   238

XXV. State and Local Government Per Capita Health and
      Hospital Expenditures, 1969   239

XXVI. Per Capita Health and Hospital Expenditures,
      Twenty-Five Largest Cities, 1969   240

XXVII. Distribution of Tax Revenue by Source, Selected Years,
      1942–1969   242

XXVIII. Personal Health Care: Third Party Payments and Pri-
      vate Consumer Expenditures, Selected Years, 1950–
      1969   246

LIST OF FIGURES

1. Lorenz Curve of United States Income Inequality, 1970 . . 32
2. Demand Curve 56
3. Derivation of an Aggregate Demand Curve 57
4. Shifts in Demand 59
5. Market Equilibrium 63
6. Diagrammatic Representation of Selected Values of Production Function $Q = 50\ C^{\frac{1}{2}}L^{\frac{1}{2}}$ 106
7. Geometric Determination of Production Efficiency . . . 107
8. Transformation Curve 114
9. Geometric Determination of the Optimal Combination of Two Outputs with Fixed Input Specifications 115
10. Production Expansion Path 117
11. Total Cost Curve 118
12. Average Cost Curve 119
13. Coexisting Interest Rates 162
14. Graphic Determination of the Internal Rate of Return . . 171
15. Neoclassical Production Isoquants 213
16. Demographic Transition 217
17. Diagrammatic Representation of Slope and Tangent . . . 265
18. Graph of Equation $C = 4 + E + E^2$ 267
19. Graph of Equation $C = aS^2 + bS + d$ 271
20. Characteristics of a Distribution 276
21. Symmetry 279
22. Correlation 281
23. Least Squares Line 283

CONTENTS

	Page
Preface	vii
List of Tables	xi
List of Figures	xiii
Chapter 1. Health Economics and Economic	
Analysis: An Introduction	3
The Health Care Industry: An Overview . .	4
Direct Delivery Organizations:	
The Institutional Setting	7
Economics	10
Economic Abstractions	11
Economic Methodology and	
Empirical Research	14
Positive and Normative Issues	17
Chapter 2. National Income and Health Care	18
National Income Accounts	18
Real Versus Monetary Charges	23
Limitations of National Income Accounting .	26
Inequality In The Distribution of Income and	
Health Care Services	28
National Income Accounts and Taxation . .	33
Chapter 3. The Medical Care Price Index	38
Index Numbers	38
The Consumer Price Index	43
The Medical Care Price Index	46
An Alternate Measure of Medical Care Cost .	51

Chapter 4. Demand **54**

   Demand: Definition and Determinants . . . 55

   Price Elasticity of Demand 60

   Demand and Market Equilibrium 62

   Reformulations of Demand Theory 65

   Demand Versus Need 67

   Appendix: Price Elasticity of Demand

   Formulas 68

Chapter 5. Demand Studies 71

   The Demand for General Hospital

   Facilities—Gerald D. Rosenthal 73

Chapter 6. Production and Cost 101

   The Production Process 102

   Production Functions 104

   Diminishing Returns and Returns to Scale . . 110

   Transformation Curves 113

   Derivation of Cost Curves 117

   Appendix: Mathematical Derivation of

   Minimum Cost Solution 120

Chapter 7. Production and Cost Studies 123

   Variations in Cost Among Hospitals of

   Different Sizes—Harold A. Cohen 125

   An Economic and Linear Model of the Hos-

   pital—Helmy H. Baligh and Danny J. Laugh-

   hunn 144

Chapter 8. Investment 158

   Interest: Causes and Functions 160

   Present Value 163

   Benefit-Cost Ratio 168

   Internal Rate of Return 169

   Planning-Programming-Budgeting 171

   Investment in Human Capital 172

Chapter 9. Investment Studies 175

   Costs and Benefits of Medical Research: A Case

   Study of Poliomyelitis—Burton A. Weisbrod . 178

   Cost Effectiveness Analysis Applied to the Treat-

ment of Chronic Renal Disease—Herbert E.
Klarman, John O'S. Francis, and
Gerald D. Rosenthal 196
Chapter 10. Economic Growth and Health 207
Economic Growth 208
The Neoclassical Model 210
Health and Economic Growth 216
Planning 221
Health Planning 226
Chapter 11. Financing Health Care 230
Financing: Macro Aspects 231
Financing: Micro Aspects 245
A Review of Selected Alternate
Reimbursement Plans 251
Appendix I. Mathematical Tools 259
Models and Their Components 259
Equations, Constants, Parameters,
and Variables 259
Consistency 262
Functions 263
Derivatives 264
Simple Derivatives 264
Second Derivatives and Maximization . . 269
Partial Derivatives 271
Appendix II. Statistical Tools 273
Probability and Sampling 273
Characteristics of Distributions 275
Measures of Association 280
Simple Correlation 280
Multiple Correlation 284
Simple Regression 285
Multiple Regression 286
Dummy Variables 288
Selected Bibliography 291
Name Index 297
Index 300

ECONOMICS
AND
HEALTH CARE

Chapter One

HEALTH ECONOMICS AND ECONOMIC ANALYSIS: AN INTRODUCTION

HEALTH ECONOMICS is a relatively new field. As an area of study, it attracted very little attention and interest as late as the 1950's. A major change occurred during the 1960's, typified by a renewed cost consciousness within the health field at large, a shift from an exclusively humanistic approach to health care administration to one incorporating an increasing utilization of managerial techniques and quantitative research methodologies, and by the incorporation of social science inputs into the medical and public health curricula. Most students of the United States health scene expect this development to continue and to increase in importance, at least in the near future.

At the level of the health administration practitioner, an understanding of health economics research is becoming imperative as managerial studies incorporating extensive doses of economic concepts and techniques are being commissioned and published. The economic research being generated today no longer resembles the intuitive or geometric approaches which have long characterized the traditional undergraduate introductory course in economics. As in any dynamic field, change is constantly occurring. In the area of economic research this change is characterized by the diffusion of mathematical and econometric techniques even into the most elementary research contributions and management consulting reports. A correlate of change is a feeling of obsolescence or ignorance among those who received their training in an earlier period.

As the purpose of this book is to acquaint the reader with the theoretical and quantitative foundations of modern research and to introduce the discipline of health economics to those who have chosen a career in the health field, the first chapter attempts to set the stage for the concepts and tools to be developed in subsequent chapters. A general overview of the health field from an economic perspective is provided, stressing those aspects of the industry's institutional environment that are most important to its economic performance. In addition, an overview of economics as a discipline and of economic theory as a tool of analysis is provided.

THE HEALTH CARE INDUSTRY: AN OVERVIEW

The health care industry is among the largest and fastest growing industries in the United States. National expenditures for health care exceeded seventy-five billion dollars in 1971. Average health care expenditures per person in 1971 were 358 dollars. The growth of national health care expenditures, the allocation of the health care dollar between the direct provision of services, research, and facilities construction, and the distribution of expenditures between the private and public (governmental) sectors of the economy is detailed in Table I for the twenty-one-year-period 1950–1970. Not only have national health care expenditures increased more than five-fold during this period, rising from 12,151,000,000 dollars to 67,240,000,000 dollars but they have also accounted for a larger proportion of total national expenditures, rising from 4.6 per cent to 7.0 per cent of Gross National Product.[1] The increases for services were larger than those for research or facility construction, and the source of the largest dollar increase in expenditures was the private sector. In percentage terms, on the other hand, the largest increases were registered in the area of research and in the public expenditures category. Within the public sector, the largest annual increases occurred in the post 1965 period, a period characterized by government's assumption of an increasing responsibility for providing medical care to the elderly and the poor.

[1] See Chapter Two for a definition of Gross National Product.

TABLE I

NATIONAL HEALTH EXPENDITURES, SELECTED YEARS, 1950–1970
(in millions of dollars)

Expenditure Category	1950	1960	1965	1970 [1]
Total Expenditures	12,130	26,367	38,912	67,240
Per cent of Gross National Product	4.6	5.3	5.9	7.0
Expenditures by Use				
Health and Medical Services	11,282	24,673	35,683	61,922
Per cent of Total Expenditures	93.0	93.6	91.7	92.1
Medical Research	111	592	1,391	1,890
Per cent of Total Expenditure	0.9	2.2	3.6	2.8
Medical Facilities Construction	737	1,102	1,838	3,428
Per cent of Total Expenditures	6.1	4.2	4.7	5.1
Expenditures by Source				
Private Expenditures	9,064	19,972	29,366	42,258
Per cent of Total Expenditures	74.7	75.7	75.5	62.8
Public Expenditures	3,065	6,395	9,546	24,982
Per cent of Total Expenditures	25.3	24.3	24.5	37.2

[1] Preliminary estimates.
Source: U.S. Bureau of the Census: *Statistical Abstract of the United States,* 1971 (92nd Edition), Washington, D.C., U.S. Government Printing Office, 1971, p. 62.

TABLE II

NATIONAL HEALTH EXPENDITURES, BY OBJECT, 1950 AND 1969 [1]
(in millions of dollars)

Object of Expenditure	1950 Amount	1950 Per cent	1969 Amount	1969 Per cent	Per cent Increase 1950 to 1969
Hospital Care	3,845	29.9	23,897	37.4	521.5
Physicians' Services	2,755	21.4	12,486	19.6	353.2
Dentists' Services	975	7.6	4,031	6.3	313.4
Drugs and Sundries	1,730	13.4	6,599	10.3	281.4
Eyeglasses and Appliances [2]	490	3.8	1,757	2.8	258.6
Nursing Home Care	142	1.1	2,639	4.1	1,758.5
Research	117	0.9	1,841	2.9	1,473.5
Medical Facilities Construction	840	6.6	3,056	4.8	263.8
Other [3]	1,973	15.3	7,506	11.8	280.4
TOTAL	12,867	100.0	63,812	100.0	395.9

[1] For calendar years; therefore, data differs from those in Table I, which are for fiscal years.
[2] Includes fees of optometrists and expenditures for hearing aids, orthopedic appliances, artificial limbs, crutches, wheelchairs, etc.
[3] Includes the services of registered and practical nurses in private duty, visiting nurses, podiatrists, physical therapists, clinical psychologists, chiropractors, naturopaths, and Christian Science practitioners, and the net cost of insurance and administrative expenses of Federally financed health programs.
Source: U.S. Bureau of the Census: *Statistical Abstract of the United States, 1971* (92nd Edition), Washington, D.C., U.S. Government Printing Office, 1971, p. 63.

Within the health services domain, the increase in expenditures was far from uniform, as can be seen from Table II. The largest expenditure increase occurred in nursing home care, followed by research, hospital care, and physicians' services. In absolute terms, however, hospital care accounts for over 37 per cent of current total health services expenditures and physicians' services account for approximately another 20 per cent. From a short-term perspective the relative rates of increase noted in Table II are likely to continue but hospital care and physicians' services will still remain the dominant expenditure categories. It is for this reason that so much attention within the health economics field is focused on hospitals and physicians.

The health care industry encompasses a myriad of institutions. The categories enumerated in Table II do not give a clear indication of the boundaries of the health care industry, although they do highlight the areas receiving the greatest attention in the health economics literature. Adopting a functional framework, the institutional components of the health care industry can be defined as:

1. *Direct delivery organizations* consisting of short and long-term care hospitals, extended care facilities, private and group medical and dental practices, and laboratories.

2. *Regulatory and planning agencies,* which are primarily governmental, with jurisdiction over facility construction, delivery of care to patients paid for by government funded programs such as Medicare and Medicaid, and the host of general public health programs and projects such as the control of communicable diseases, disease prevention programs, the establishment of sanitation codes, nutritional programs, and environmental control.

3. *Third party payers* consisting of government and private insurance companies providing insurance coverage and payments for the services of direct delivery organizations.

4. *Supportive organizations* consisting of trade associations, foundations, educational institutions, and research organizations.

5. *Suppliers* providing supplies to direct delivery organizations.

It should be clear from the above definitions that institutional categories two through five focus primarily on the activities of institutional category one, direct delivery organizations. They either regulate, reimburse, promote, or support the functioning of direct delivery organizations. Although the tools and concepts to be developed in subsequent chapters are equally applicable to institutional categories two through five, the presentation focuses largely on category one.

By choosing to focus primarily on direct delivery organizations, the analysis of the health care industry becomes reoriented to an analysis of the medical care industry. One must not equate medical care and health care, as the former is but one component of the latter. In addition to medical care, education, sanitation, nutrition, housing, and the quality of the environment are direct contributors to health. In fact, the nonmedical care components may be the prime contributors to a nation's health profile. However, since the medical care sector accounts for the largest proportion of identifiable health care expenditures, has the best developed data sources, and has benefited from the public relations activities of its supporting organizations, it has received the most attention from researchers. To a great extent this attention is justified, as improvements in the economic environment of the health care industry will stem largely from internally or externally induced improvements in direct delivery organizations.

DIRECT DELIVERY ORGANIZATIONS:
THE INSTITUTIONAL SETTING

From an economic perspective, the health care industry functions within a sheltered environment. The profit motive which underlies much of economic activity is absent in a large proportion of the industry. The modal[2] pattern of ownership or control within the dominant health care institution, the hospital, is voluntary (charitable) as opposed to proprietary (profit making). Institutions under voluntary control enjoy special financial

---

[2] Refer to Appendix II for a definition of this term.

privileges and generally enjoy the greatest measure of communal support. Profit maximization or achieving a targeted profit level is not only *not* the prime consideration of voluntary institutions but is usually not a consideration at all. However, economic realities dictate that every institution operate within certain budget restraints, with the precise restraints determined largely by the prevailing reimbursement philosophies and the amount of philanthropic contributions. No health care institution can operate in the *red* (i.e. deficits not covered by total current income from all sources) for prolonged periods of time without remedial action being undertaken. Because of philanthropic contributions, income from services rendered does not always have to cover expenditures. However, once the level of anticipated contributions has been established, economic realities must be taken into consideration.

A second factor differentiating the health industry from other sectors of the economy is the preoccupation with quality. In no other economic sector, with the possible exception of the space exploration program, is quality stressed as strongly. Professional training for the medical, nursing, and allied health occupations practically ignores the fact that quality is not costless, and that cost factors deserve serious consideration. Preoccupation with high quality care may possibly be warranted if society has consciously decided to require only the best in the medical area, with full knowledge that resources will constantly be diverted from other worthwhile endeavors, and if high quality care is available in equal measure to all. Neither condition prevails today nor is likely to prevail in the foreseeable future. As will be seen shortly, scarcity of resources relative to wants and needs is *the* economic fact of life. Unless this is realized, preoccupation with quality can only result in a rationing of quantity.

A third characteristic of the health field is the absence of a competitive climate. Many direct delivery organizations enjoy a virtual monopoly within their geographic area due either to the existing maldistribution of health care resources or to population density factors which preclude the establishment of additional institutions. Where more than one institution providing identical or comparable care exists, competition is barred by the prevailing

and accepted sentiment against any type of individual advertising or public evaluation of the quality of care rendered by
institutions or individuals. An additional impediment to competition is the fact that most professional organizations have been
able to or are attempting to control entry into their respective
professional areas through control over educational programs,
licensing, and accreditation. A taut, disciplined labor supply
does not encourage competition.

The prevalence of health insurance and the nature of the
insurance arrangement is an additional distinguishing characteristic of the health field. Most insurance policies, whether paid for
directly by the individual or received as a fringe benefit, stipulate
specific coverage patterns, often with no deductables or coinsurance payments required. While most insurance policies
stipulate precise benefits to the insured they do not stipulate a
precise payment to the providing institution for the insured
service. Institutions are reimbursed based primarily on their
actual cost of providing care. Once insured, individuals are apt
to regard the consumption of health services within the insured
limits as being free, thus removing a primary economic determinant of demand. The effect of the removal of financial
constraints from certain ranges of demand and the knowledge
that institutions will be reimbursed at almost full cost is not lost
on the decision-making process of the providers of care.

Although these four facets of the health field influence the
economic behavior of health care institutions they do not completely insulate the industry from economic realities and crises.
Budgets have to be balanced, choices have to be made among
competing wants, and attempts at estimating potential demand
must be made in applying for federal funds for facility construction under such programs as the Hill-Burton Act. Directives for
attaining economic efficiency will ultimately be forthcoming
within the industry. Institutional arrangements are subject to
change; arrangements that once appeared sacred are now the
focal point of lively debate. The growing dissatisfaction with
the provision and distribution of health services cannot be sup-
pressed indefinitely. Even without radical change, economic considerations are receiving more and more attention in the health

field. It is our contention that economic concepts and tools *can* be applied to the health industry in its current institutional state and *will* be applied in greater measure in the future. It is the intent of this volume to demonstrate and explain the applicability of economic theory to health administration, planning, and research. Before embarking upon this mission, a brief overview of economics as a discipline and economic theory as a tool of analysis is warranted.

ECONOMICS

Economics is concerned with two primary factors, desires and resources, and economic issues involve a basic confrontation between these two opposing forces. The confrontation is brought into being primarily because desires are infinite whereas resources are finite. The history of civilization is a continuous illustration of man's wants exceeding his means; it appears safe to predict that as affluent as society may yet become there will always be unfulfilled wants.

The *raison d'etre* of economics is man's desire to satisfy as many wants as possible with the existing stock of resources. This is achieved by using the stock of available resources as efficiently as possible so as to derive the greatest benefit from them. Economics does not prejudge society's desires. It is not a discipline concerned with morals. Rather it takes society's wishes as given and attempts to fulfill as many of these desires as possible with a minimum of resource input. Whatever the source of scarcity, be it the limits of nature or the limits of human capacity, the existence of scarcity coupled with unlimited wants sets the stage for an economist.

Economics as a discipline encompasses a broad spectrum of subareas. The American Economic Association has arranged these subareas into ten major groupings: general economics, theory, history, systems; economic growth, development, planning, fluctuations; economic statistics; monetary and fiscal theory and institutions; international economics; administration, business finance, marketing, accounting; industrial organization, technological change, industry studies; agriculture, natural resources;

manpower, labor, population; and welfare programs, consumer economics, urban and regional economics. Economic analysis, which is the term applied to the theoretical tools economists use regardless of their specialty area, is divided into two components: macroeconomics and microeconomics. Macroeconomics deals with aggregate problems affecting the economy at large and microeconomics focuses on disaggregated problems specific to individual units or subsectors of the economy.

On the micro level economists may be concerned with the most minute detail of an individual institution's economic existence, such as the goods or services it buys, the type of labor it hires, its wage and salary scale, its production decisions, and its investment decisions. These same items of economic data may also interest a macro economist from his vantage point. From a macro standpoint interest would focus on factors affecting aggregate industry consumption patterns, wage patterns, production patterns, and investment patterns.

Health economics, which cuts across several of the categories enumerated above, draws upon both macro and micro theory. Some topics in health economics, such as investment and productivity, utilize both macro and micro tools. Others, like the use of national income statistics and the integration of health into economic growth, draw primarily upon the mainstream of macroeconomics; while questions of supply and demand and production have their theoretical foundations in microeconomic theory.

ECONOMIC ABSTRACTIONS

Economists, following in the footsteps of other researchers, have adopted many methodological and theoretical abstractions which reappear time and again in economic writings and research. Three abstractions, *rationality, markets,* and *competition,* merit special clarification.

Economic doctrines, precepts, and theories usually postulate *rationality* on the part of the individual or group empowered to make economic decisions. Rationality simply defined means being reasonable—reasonable in an economic sense. That is, on the accepted assumption that economic goods provide pleasure rather than pain, if A is judged to be more pleasurable than B, and B possesses greater utility than C, then A must be preferred to C. Rationality further implies that individuals and groups adopt measures which lead to a given goal with the use of a minimum of resources. Hence, directly following from the assumption of rationality are maximization of gain given a set of resources, or minimization of resource use or cost given a goal.

Economists refer to *markets* in analyses of a wide variety of problems. To an economist, a market does not refer to a fixed structure in which trading takes place, although such a structure may house participants in the market. The members of the New York and American Stock Exchanges in the Wall Street area of Manhattan are part of the securities market, but do not constitute it in its entirety. Rather a market is a concept that incorporates all individuals or institutions that remain in contact concerning any economic good or service.

The only criteria for inclusion in a market are the ability and willingness to participate. Markets do not have fixed boundaries. Rather, they are delineated by time, distance, personal, and financial constraints. The market for a surgeon's services may be confined to a particular hospital in a city or may be international depending on whether the patient is in need of an immediate operation or can wait a few days. This is an example of a variable time constraint. Eligibility for nonemergency services at municipal health clinics is circumscribed by geographic constraints. Personal factors determine the preference of admission to health institutions under religious or nondenominational control; while financial factors have a greater affect on the decision to demand private or public health services.

It is not necessary to have purchased or sold an item to be part of the potential market for that item. An individual could be part of the potential market for public health services even if he has never used a public health facility because it is physically available to him and he has the right to utilize its services. However, he will not be part of the potential market if only people below a designated income level were eligible for the services of the institution and his income exceeded that level. It is simple to describe a potential market, but for most markets it is often quite difficult to specify exactly who will be and who will not be part of that market.

Economists conceive of the market as the supreme regulator of economic desires. Within the context of a market, demanders and suppliers make their respective desires known, and based on these data economic activity occurs. Consumers' demands, as registered in the market by purchases, prompt production and supply, while the availability of goods and services satisfies demand. The market, if unimpeded by institutional or legal constraints, becomes the unbiased arbitrator of desires and resources, signaling the need for an increase (when there is a shortage) or curtailment (when there is a surplus) in production and/or price in any specified area. An additional characteristic of the market is that it automatically adapts to changes in tastes, technology, and government policy. The following example of the engineering market illustrates the mechanics of the market mechanism for engineering manpower.

When the Soviet Union launched its first orbital satellite (Sputnik) in 1957, and the United States discovered itself lagging behind in the space race, the United States' demand for engineers and scientists increased dramatically. Demand, however, exceeded the available supply. In response to this imbalance, firms offered higher starting salaries to graduates with degees in these areas and attempted to bid qualified engineers and scientists away from their competitors. Government funding for science education and space research increased significantly. Within a matter of years, the number of engineers and scientists increased dramatically as students responded to the improved opportunities in these fields. By the late 1960's, as military and domestic needs began to take precedence over science research and as the United States achieved a dominant position in the space race by being the first nation to land men on the moon, the need for additional engineers and scientists declined. The output of engineers and scientists did not decline proportionately; a surplus of engineers and scientists existed by 1969–1970; and the financial attractiveness of these professions declined. Consequently, a smaller proportion of college students are currently entering these fields, and unemployed engineers and scientists are seeking employment in other spheres. Entry and exit from these professional groups were accomplished automatically by the invisible hand of economic rationality guiding each person in the market to do that which will benefit him the most.[3]

Many types of markets are conceivable ranging from those which are highly monopolistic (few sellers) to those which are highly competitive (many sellers). Economists, while noting the existence of many market structures, consistently refer to one basic type, the *perfectly competitive market*. This type, by definition, includes so many buyers and sellers that no participant can influence the overall outcome of the market by his offer or failure to offer to purchase or supply goods or services. It is the market as symbolized by the totality of all its participants, rather than any individual, which determines the price and quantity of goods and services. Realizing that perfectly competitive markets may never exist, because of financial and legislative barriers to entry or population density considerations which can not support more than one institution of any type within a designated geographic area, economists still lobby for the development of a *competitive atmosphere* to the extent that it is feasible. It is only under a competitive atmosphere that economic efficiency will be motivated. The absence of competition is an open invitation to inefficient behavior as institutions are not prompted to improve their performance by their competitors or consumers, and society at large must tolerate the results of inefficient performance (higher prices, lower quantity, and inferior quality), if they need the goods or services produced by the institution under consideration and no acceptable substitutes are available. While a competitive atmosphere may not benefit the labor force participants or directors of any particular institution as it forces them to eliminate all types of pleasantries, it does benefit society at large by contributing to lower prices, increased quantity, and higher quality.

ECONOMIC METHODOLOGY AND EMPIRICAL RESEARCH

The goals of economics, as well as most other sciences, are explanation and prediction. These goals are achieved by com-

[3] The operation of an economic market and the determinants of market activity will be dealt with at greater length in Chapter Four.

bining theoretical and empirical research. Theorizing is based primarily on deductive reasoning and conceptualizations. Implications are then drawn based on the assumptions and the economic arguments of the theory. Empirical research is primarily inductive, since particular research findings are used to generalize about a larger group or population. The two research techniques are complementary in that theory provides a framework for conducting empirical research and empirical research tests the explanatory and predictive power of a given theory.

Theory represents simplifications and generalizations of the real world. Theory never describes any particular situation or event completely, nor does it attempt to. To preserve its power of generalization and applicability to a host of situations, theory must concentrate on one, or a few, crucial characteristics which a broad group of events seem to have in common. By highlighting these crucial or pivotal characteristics, theory becomes a useful framework for analyzing and interpreting events. Theories cannot and should not be judged on the basis of whether individuals assert that they act as a theory states they do. If the end result of their behavior conforms to the theoretical expectation, the theory is validated and useful. The crucial test of any theory's validity is not what people say they do but rather what they actually do.

Theoretical arguments are formulated as models. Gardner Ackley captured the essence of models and theories in the following statement:

> A model . . . uses what we know or think we know about economic behavior patterns, technology, or institutions to permit us to make predictions—more or less specifically depending on how much or little we know . . .
>
> Economic models . . . are succinct statements of economic theory. Theory, in turn, is simply a generalization or abstraction of experience and observation. We see thousands of farmers producing and supplying wheat. We can observe many things about these farmers and their productive activities: the color of their eyes, the number of their children, their various productive techniques, the number of acres they farm, and millions of further details. We choose, however, to make one significant abstraction about their behavior. We select from among all of our observations one relationship which we think is most relevant and significant—that they tend to grow more wheat at a higher than at a lower price. We throw away all the rest of our information (we could not, in any case, remember or record very much of it), and

summarize our knowledge about the supply of wheat in a single function. Frequently, perhaps, our abstractions and generalizations from experience and observation are erroneous, or unnecessarily incomplete. But that is simply the difference between bad or inadequate and better or more complete theory.[4]

The function shown in the following equation

$$S_z = f(P_z)$$

is a simplified model of the theory of supply, and is read as the supply of Z is a function of the price of Z, where Z can represent any good or service. A model can be specified either verbally or mathematically, although the latter technique is both more concise and readily amenable to empirical research. Once the elementary economic relationships are understood, it is possible to broaden the analysis by both adding variables to any one equation and additional equations to incorporate larger and larger sectors of economic activity into a model.

Since economics is a social science, dealing with human beings, it is extremely difficult to undertake controlled experiments. A controlled experiment is one in which only one factor or variable is allowed to change so that the effect of that one factor can be determined. To approximate controlled experiments, social scientists employ the *ceteris paribus* (other things equal) assumption. That is, the effect of changes in one variable are determined assuming that all other variables are held constant. This process can then be repeated to determine the effects of each of the other variables being considered. In theoretical work, this is accomplished simply by thinking through the effects of the one variable on all other variables. In empirical work, the effect of one variable alone is typically determined by statistical devices.[5] Thus, a multi-faceted problem can be investigated in the absence of controlled experiments through the *ceteris paribus* assumption.

---

[4] Ackley, Gardner: *Macroeconomic Theory.* New York, Macmillan, 1961, pp. 14–15. Refer to Appendix I for further discussion of models, theories, and functions.

[5] Refer to Appendix II for a discussion of regression analysis, a statistical technique employed in economic research to isolate the effect of one variable, among a host of variables, on another variable.

POSITIVE AND NORMATIVE ISSUES

A fundamental distinction must be made between normative and positive issues. Normative issues are those that involve value judgments and, as a result of this factor, there is room for disagreement on these issues between men of reason.[6] Positive issues involve an analysis of what is, as opposed to what ought to be, and as such leave no room for disagreement. Unemployment either is or is not, for example, 4 per cent; the demand for physician care is or is not increasing; the geographic distribution of medical services is or is not unequal. In such instances economic theory and accepted and proven statistical tools should lead to uniform conclusions regardless of the political persuasion or ideology of the economist studying the problem.

To the extent that economic theory and statistical sources are not complete and statistics are not perfectly gathered, there may be differences even within positive economics. One area of research that illustrates such differences is the question of whether economies of size exist in hospital operations.[7] As data sources improve and as research tools become even more refined, these differences should disappear.

[6] For an interesting illustration of conflicting views on the functioning of competitive markets and the subsequent role to be assigned to government, see, Freidman, Milton: *Capitalism and Freedom.* Chicago, University of Chicago Press, 1962, and Galbraith, John K.: *The Affluent Society.* Boston, Houghton Mifflin, 1958, and Galbraith, John K.: *The New Industrial State.* Boston, Houghton Mifflin, 1967.

[7] For a discussion of what initially appears to be conflicting research findings, see, Mann, Judith K., and Yett, Donald E.: The analysis of hospital costs: A review article. *Journal of Business, 41,*:191, 1968.

Chapter Two

NATIONAL INCOME
AND HEALTH CARE

NATIONAL INCOME accounts are a frequently used reference frame in health economics research. Analysis of health expenditures by category are frequently reported as a proportion of national income, and income categories are often used as a base for indicating inequalities in both the consumption of various health care services and in indices of health. In addition to its frequent use in research, national income accounts are of interest to health administrators and planners as they constitute the basic framework for measuring and evaluating the performance of any economy in terms of how rapidly it is growing, how stable it is, how its internal structure is changing over time, and how it allocates resources among its various sectors. As aggregate economic trends largely determine the climate within which health care institutions operate, an understanding of trends in the economy at large, as represented in the national income accounts, is of vital importance.

The first part of this chapter is devoted to a presentation of the construction, interpretation, and limitations of the national income accounts and includes a brief discussion of price indices and their uses in conjunction with national income accounts data. The second part of the chapter focuses on using selected elements of the national income accounts to measure interpersonal and interregional inequalities in health related services.

NATIONAL INCOME ACCOUNTS

Economic well-being can be measured in many different ways. One indicator of economic well-being, the one most often utilized, is the annual total of goods and services produced by an economy. The basic national income account category used to measure annual total production of goods and services is called *Gross National Product* (GNP). It is defined as *the total money value of final production of goods and services in an economy in any one year.* The national income accounts are expressed in monetary units because money serves as the common denominator for an economic system. Simple addition of actual units of various products would pose severe problems, especially for comparative purposes. If a firm produces 40,000 units of drug A and 10,000 units of drug B in one year and in another year produces 10,000 units of drug A and 40,000 units of drug B, in which year is the production greater? Converting the number of units of drug A and drug B into their monetary values provides a ready-made comparative and additive device.

A distinction between final products and intermediate products is required in any national income tally. Final products are those that are sold directly to consumers, while intermediate products are those used in the production of other goods or services. To include the value of goods or services used as intermediate products would entail double counting. For example, when the metal is produced which is to be incorporated into a hospital bed, it is considered an intermediate product. In the computation of GNP, the value of the hospital bed is directly included, but the value of the metal used to manufacture the bed is not separately included. The value of the latter is already included in the cost (price) of the bed since the producer of the bed paid the producer of the metal for this material and included its costs in the price of the bed.[1] However, if metal is a final product in the sense that it is sold directly to consumers and not used as an intermediate product in the production process of another good, it is included in the national income accounts.

A second methodological convention adopted in calculating the national income accounts is the exclusion of the dollar value

---

[1] One method of calculating GNP in the industrial sector of the economy where goods are produced through the joint effort of many firms and industries is to include only the *value added* at each stage of production, that is, the extent that the value of the output is greater than the value of the material put into it.

of items that are sold secondhand. Such sales entail only a *transfer* and not a production of goods. One hospital sells another hospital a used x-ray machine and receives the money value of the used x-ray machine as payment. This transaction does not reflect an addition to economic production, as additional output was not created. However, the services of an agent or middleman who may have arranged this transaction are considered a productive activity, in that both the buyer and the seller consider themselves better off as a result of their trade. Thus while the proceeds from the sale of a used item are omitted from the national income accounts, the earnings of people engaged in selling such items are included.

GNP statistics can be derived in two alternate ways, either by summing the value of final output, or by summing the income generated at each stage in the production process. These two methods are referred to as Gross National Product (GNP), and as Gross National Income (GNI), respectively. Both approaches yield identical estimates of aggregate production.

The tally of final output, GNP, is usually divided into four major component groups: consumption, investment, government, and net exports. This breakdown is based on the use to which the final production is put. GNI is based on the summation of the payments to the factors of production (traditionally classified as land, labor, and capital) and includes wages and salaries, rent, interest, depreciation, taxes, and profit. Profit is a balancing item for any activity in the sense that after the factors of production are remunerated, any remaining amount (which could be either positive or negative) is designated as profit and payable to the owners of the enterprise. Although a target profit rate may be set for any activity, its realization depends on the final outcome of the productive endeavor, not on initial expectations.

Table III details the 1971 GNP and GNI estimates and illustrates the two alternative calculating approaches. It further lists some of the subdivisions of the major categories as illustrations of the relative importance of federal versus state and local units, and goods versus services in overall consumption patterns. In addition to Gross National Product, the United States Department of Commerce publishes four other major national in-

TABLE III

GROSS NATIONAL PRODUCT AND GROSS
NATIONAL INCOME, 1971 [1]
(in billions of dollars)

Gross National Product			Gross National Income		
Personal Consumption		662.2	Compensation of Employees		641.8
Goods	379.2		Wages and Salaries	574.3	
Services	283.0		Supplements to Wages		
Gross Domestic			and Salaries	67.7	
Investment		150.8	Proprietor's Income		68.3
Fixed Investment	148.7		Rental Income		24.3
Changes in Business			Corporate Profits		80.7
Inventories	2.1		Interest		35.6
Net Exports		0.7	Depreciation		94.0
Exports	65.5		Indirect Business Taxes [2]		102.1
Imports	64.8				
Government Purchases		233.1			
Federal	97.6				
State and Local	135.5				
TOTAL		1,046.8	TOTAL		1,046.8

[1] Preliminary
[2] This category consists primarily of sales taxes.
Source: Federal Reserve Bulletin, 58, A-70/A-71, 1972.

come accounts statistics. They are Net National Product (NNP),
National Income (NI), Personal Income (PI), and Disposable
Income (DI). Each of these statistics are related to the GNP
measure.[2]

As the personal income statistic is widely utilized in discussions
of the demand for and the financing of health care services, it
merits discription in greater length. *Personal income* is defined
as payments to the population from all sources: from businesses,
government, households, and institutions. All forms of income
from these sources are included in personal income: wages and
salaries, other labor income, income of owners of unincorporated
business (proprietors' income), rental income, dividends, interest,
and transfer payments.[3]

Because the financing of health care services provided at the
public expense is primarily derived from the taxes raised by
state and local governments, and taxes are dependent on income

[2] For a discussion of these national income accounts, and their relationship to
Gross National Product, see, Samuelson, Paul A.: *Economics,* 8th ed. New York,
McGraw-Hill, 1970, pp. 185–190.

[3] Transfer payments are payments to individuals for which no services are
currently rendered. They can be payments from the government (for example,
interest on government debt, veterans payments, and welfare) or from business
firms (for example, workers' compensation).

TABLE IV

TOTAL AND PER CAPITA PERSONAL INCOME
BY STATE AND REGION, 1970

State and Region	Total Personal Income (in millions of dollars)	Per Capita Personal Income
United States	798,949	3,921
New England	50,788	4,277
Maine	3,235	3,257
New Hampshire	2,660	3,590
Vermont	1,545	3,465
Massachusetts	24,851	4,360
Rhode Island	3,711	3,902
Connecticut	14,786	4,856
Mideast	189,763	4,464
New York	87,111	4,769
New Jersey	33,085	4,598
Pennsylvania	46,329	3,927
Delaware	2,383	4,324
Maryland	16,789	4,255
Great Lakes	164,667	4,082
Michigan	36,124	4,059
Ohio	42,382	3,972
Indiana	19,679	3,781
Illinois	50,131	4,502
Wisconsin	16,351	3,693
Plains	60,471	3,701
Minnesota	14,580	3,824
Iowa	10,418	3,688
Missouri	17,350	3,704
North Dakota	1,848	2,995
South Dakota	2,108	3,165
Nebraska	5,570	3,751
Kansas	8,598	3,823
Southeast	140,391	3,195
Virginia	16,827	3,607
West Virginia	5,259	3,021
Kentucky	9,901	3,073
Tennessee	12,128	3,085
North Carolina	16,331	3,207
South Carolina	7,616	2,936
Georgia	15,345	3,332
Florida	24,938	3,642
Alabama	9,832	2,853
Mississippi	5,706	2,575
Louisiana	11,130	3,049
Arkansas	5,376	2,791
Southwest	57,761	3,479
Oklahoma	8,488	3,312
Texas	39,671	3,531
New Mexico	3,185	3,131
Arizona	6,418	3,591
Rocky Mountain	17,723	3,529
Montana	2,349	3,379
Idaho	2,310	3,240

TABLE IV (continued)

State and Region	Total Personal Income (in millions of dollars)	Per Capita Personal Income
Wyoming	1,181	3,556
Colorado	8,468	3,816
Utah	3,416	3,213
Far West	112,540	4,313
Washington	13,671	3,993
Oregon	7,777	3,705
Nevada	2,267	4,562
California	88,825	4,426
Alaska	1,400	4,592
Hawaii	3,445	4,527

Source: U.S. Department of Commerce, Office of Business Statistics: *Commerce News* OBE 71–55 (August 31, 1971).

and wealth (wealth being accumulated income), the income level of the population residing in these governmental units is of importance. The income of a state or locality is conventionally defined as the sum of the personal income of its inhabitants. To adjust for the differing population sizes of various geographic units, per capita personal income is utilized. Per capita personal income is calculated by dividing total personal income by population size. Table IV details total personal income and total personal income per capita by region and state for 1970. Two features of this table merit special attention. First, the per capita measure yields an entirely different ranking of states than the total personal income measure. Connecticut, which on a total basis ranks eighteenth, ranks first on a per capita basis. Second, the per capita personal income measure clearly highlights the wide differences in income levels between regions and states. Per capita personal income not only accounts for some of the variation in public health expenditures, but is also a prime determinant of an area's *ability* to finance health care expenditures, a concept that will be discussed in greater detail in the concluding section of this chapter.

REAL VERSUS MONETARY CHANGES

Changes in the value of any economic index measured in monetary terms can be the result of two factors. The first is changes in consumers' preferences among goods or services

and/or changes in the quantity of resources utilized in production. Price changes resulting from these factors mirror shortages or surpluses and the activity of a market to correct this
imbalance.[4] The second is changes in the value of the monetary
unit, the dollar. Such changes only reflect changes in the value of
the common denominator used to measure economic activity as
opposed to real changes in total production.

Since the national income accounts are measured in money
terms, one may be interested in deflating or inflating these data
to remove the effect of price changes that are solely due to
changes in the value of the monetary unit. This is particularly
important in a time series (longitudinal) analysis, since what is
to be investigated is real economic changes, changes net of the
size of the measuring unit. For example, in comparing GNP
measures for any two years, the apparent change in GNP may
not be due to increases or decreases in production but rather to
changes in the purchasing power of the dollar resulting from
inflation or deflation. Therefore, researchers often utilize national
income accounts expressed in *real* terms, that is, in dollar units
adjusted for changes in the value of the monetary unit. These
adjusted dollar units are often referred to as *constant dollars,*
indicating that the value of the dollar is being kept constant at a
particular value. The adjustment technique relies on the utilization of price indices.[5]

Published price indices are readily available. The three major
types are the *Consumer Price Index,* the *Wholesale Price Index,*
and the *GNP-deflator.* Although the principles underlying the
construction of these indices are similar, the items included in
them differ as their names indicate. The Consumer Price Index
is constructed to reflect changes in the prices of goods and services
bought by a typical family. The Wholesale Price Index focuses
on the consumption of goods and services relevant to business
firms as opposed to households. The GNP-deflator includes elements of both of the other two and is constructed to reflect the
aggregate composition of Gross National Product. Due to the

---

[4] For a more detailed discussion of the rationing function of prices within markets
refer to Chapter Four.

[5] Refer to Chapter Three for a general discussion of indices.

different combinations of goods and services from which these indices are calculated, it is not uncommon to observe different rates of increase or decline among them.

The process of converting monetary measures into real measures entails the division of the monetary measure by an appropriate index. Frequently the quotient resulting from this division is multiplied by 100 to convert the quotient into the same dollar magnitude as the original monetary measure. Table V lists actual

TABLE V

MONEY AND REAL GROSS NATIONAL PRODUCT,
SELECTED YEARS, 1930–1971

Year	(1) *GNP* *Current Dollars* *(in billions* *of dollars)*	(2) *GNP-Deflator* *(1958 = base year)*	$(3) = \frac{(1)}{(2)} \times 100$ *Real GNP* *(in billions of* *1958 dollars)*
1930	90.4	49.3	183.5
1935	72.2	42.6	169.5
1940	99.7	43.9	227.2
1945	211.9	59.7	355.2
1950	284.8	80.2	355.3
1955	398.0	90.9	438.0
1958	447.3	100.0	447.3
1960	503.7	103.3	487.7
1965	684.9	110.9	617.8
1970	976.8	135.3	729.3
1971 [1]	1,046.8	141.6	739.3

[1] Preliminary

Source: Economic Report of the President, 1972, Washington, D.C., U.S. Government Printing Office, 1972, pp. 195, 198.

GNP, the GNP-deflator, and real GNP for selected years over the period 1930–1971. Dividing GNP in current dollars by the GNP-deflator index and multiplying the quotient by 100 yields real GNP. More specifically, since the GNP-deflator index uses 1958 as the base from which price changes are measured, the derived real GNP values are shown in constant (1958) dollars. Thus prior to the base year, 1958, the GNP-deflator index inflates rather than deflates because a dollar purchased more prior to 1958 than in 1958. As the dollar purchased less in the post-1958 period than in 1958, the GNP-deflator index deflates the actual Gross National Product values reported subsequent to the base year.

An analysis of changes in nurses' salaries over time provides another example of how price indices are used. As nurses' salaries are reported in current dollars, and as the purchasing power of the dollar has declined in recent years, the real increase in nurses' salaries is less than a simplistic view of the salary schedules would indicate. Table VI lists current and real average salaries paid to public health nurses in local health units from 1955 to

TABLE VI

MEDIAN ANNUAL SALARIES OF PUBLIC
HEALTH NURSES, 1955–1971

Year	Annual Median Salary, Staff Nurse, Local Health Units	Consumer Price Index (1967 = 100)	Annual Median Salary (in constant 1967 dollars)
1955	$3,662	80.2	$4,566
1956	3,828	81.4	4,703
1957	4,107	84.3	4,872
1958	4,301	86.6	4,967
1959	4,408	87.3	5,049
1960	4,540	88.7	5,118
1961	4,652	89.6	5,192
1962	4,902	90.6	5,411
1963	5,079	91.7	5,539
1964	5,313	92.9	5,719
1965	5,603	94.5	5,929
1966	5,811	97.2	6,149
1967	6,460	100.0	6,460
1968	7,225	104.2	6,934
1969	7,712	109.8	7,024
1970	8,477	116.3	7,301
1971	8,895	121.3	7,333

Source: Salary Data: American Nurses Association: *Facts About Nursing.* New York, American Nurses' Association, Annual
Price Index: *Economic Report of the President, 1972.* Washington, D.C., U.S. Government Printing Office, 1971, p. 247

1971. Current salary data were adjusted for changes in the Consumer Price Index, as this index best reflects changes in the overall cost of living. Thus, for example, what initially appeared to be a 142.9 per cent increase (5,233 dollars) from 1955 to 1971, actually was only a 69 per cent increase (2,767 dollars) after the general cost of living increase is taken into account.

LIMITATIONS OF NATIONAL INCOME ACCOUNTING

The national income accounts as they are currently constructed are imperfect indicators of economic activity or well-being in that they do not take account of certain economic attributes and transactions which materially affect society's well-being. Five major limitations are noteworthy.

The national income statistics are overestimates of economic well-being to the extent that they do not take account of certain major disutilities that result from the production and consumption processes themselves. While air and water pollution result directly from production and the utilization of modern transportation media, no adjustment is made for these negative attributes. Similarly, to the extent that urban overcrowding and crime result from industrialization, economic well-being is overstated by omitting an adjustment for these occurrences.

On the other side of the ledger the amount of leisure consumed by members of society has increased significantly during the last few decades. The reduction of the standard work week from sixty hours at the turn of the century, to forty-eight, forty, and now thirty-seven hours has vastly increased the leisure time enjoyed by the average member of society. Leisure is definitely a part of economic well-being but it is not accounted for in the national income accounts.

Second, national income statistics give no indication of the composition or distribution of total output. A distributional change away from military research to research oriented to allieviating poverty may make society either better or worse off, yet national income data do not and can not reflect this; nor do they reflect the distribution of income among the members of society. While many people would agree that society's well-being increases as the inequality in the income distribution is lessened, national income accounts as currently constructed do not show this.

A third limitation is the lack of a comprehensive quality adjustment. The quality of goods and services has not remained uniform over time. While some quality adjustments have been made, many others have not, due to the great difficulty of evaluating them. Two examples where quality adjustments are lacking illustrate this point. The quality of medical care has increased tremendously during the last half century while the quality (as judged by durability) of automobiles and homes has declined. Unless one assumes that overall quality changes are offsetting, with improvements equal in weight to deteriorations, the national income accounts are deficient because of this fact.

Fourth, the national income accounts do not include most nonmarket activities such as the productive services of housewives, and all types of do-it-yourself work such as healthy members of a family caring for sick members. If workers (nurses or housekeepers) were hired to perform these tasks, their earnings would be included in the national income accounts.

Finally, the national income accounts are an arbitrary system. Classifications and criteria for including or excluding certain types of economic activities are based on value judgments. The four major categories of Gross National Product—consumption, investment, government spending, and net exports—could easily be subdivided or replaced. These four categories occupied economists' thinking in the 1930's when the national income accounts system was formulated and were consequently emphasized. One could argue that if society adopts the goal of eradicating poverty, a new category emphasizing expenditures in this area should be explicitly included in the national income accounts. The realization that education and health care are important determinants of both poverty and economic growth supports the argument that such expenditures should be netted out from existing categories and highlighted by a separate category rather than included in the consumption and government categories, as is current practice.

All the imperfections in the current composition of the national income accounts notwithstanding, it should be recognized that these data do represent a major step forward in our stock of economic knowledge. They do provide a fairly comprehensive view of the economy which greatly facilitates empirical research.

INEQUALITY IN THE DISTRIBUTION OF INCOME AND HEALTH CARE SERVICES

The inequality in the income distribution referred to earlier has important implications for health economics. In the derivation of per capita personal income, total personal income was divided by the population size. The resulting per capita figures may give the mistaken impression that the income generated by an economy is divided equally among all the members of the economy. This, of course, is not the case; income is distributed far from equally. That is, the lowest *x* per cent of population in terms of income commands less than *x* per cent of total income. For example, the lowest 50 per cent of the population in terms of income, commands less than 50 per cent of total income, and the lowest 99 per cent of the population commands less than 99 per cent of the income. Perfect income equality would imply that any *x* per cent of the population receives *x* per cent of the income. Table VII depicts the income inequality prevailing in

TABLE VII

PERCENTAGE SHARE OF AGGREGATE
INCOME RECEIVED BY EACH
FIFTH OF FAMILIES, 1970

Income Rank	Percentage
Total Families	
Per cent	100.0
Lowest 20 per cent	5.5
Second 20 per cent	12.0
Middle 20 per cent	17.4
Fourth 20 per cent	23.5
Highest 20 per cent	41.6
Top 5 per cent	14.4
White	
Per cent	100.0
Lowest 20 per cent	5.8
Second 20 per cent	12.3
Middle 20 per cent	17.4
Fourth 20 per cent	23.4
Highest 20 per cent	41.1
Top 5 per cent	14.2
Negro and Other Races	
Per cent	100.0
Lowest 20 per cent	4.5
Second 20 per cent	10.4
Middle 20 per cent	16.5
Fourth 20 per cent	24.5
Highest 20 per cent	44.0
Top 5 per cent	15.4

Source: U.S. Bureau of the Census: *Current Population Reports*, Series P-60, No. 8, Income in 1970 of families and persons in the United States, Washington, D.C., U.S. Government Printing Office, 1971, p. 28.

the United States during 1970. In all the groupings the top 5 per cent of the population received more than 14 per cent of the income, and the lowest 20 per cent received less than 6 per cent of the income.

The distribution of health care services in the United States is also unequal, as seen by the data reported in Tables VIII through XI. The inequality is evident in breakdowns both by race and income. Infant mortality is higher among nonwhites than whites, and higher among lower income than higher income groups. Dental care for youngsters is positively related

TABLE VIII

INFANT MORTALITY RATES BY RACE
AND FAMILY INCOME, 1964–1966

Color	*Rate per 1,000* *Legitimate Live Births*
White	20.5
All Other	37.1
Income Class	
Under 3,000	31.8
3,000–4,999	24.9
5,000–6,999	17.9
7,000–9,999	19.6
10,000 and over	19.6

Source: U.S. Department of Health, Education, and Welfare, Public Health Service: *The Health of Children—1970.* Washington, D.C., U.S. Government Printing Office, 1970, p. 5.

with income, while dental decay is inversely related with income. Thus children born into wealthier families receive more dental care and, partially as a result, have less dental decay.[6] Physicians' visits are directly related to income, signifying that more medical

TABLE IX

AVERAGE NUMBER OF FILLED AND
DECAYED PRIMARY AND PERMANENT
TEETH PER CHILD AGED 6–11, BY
FAMILY INCOME, 1963–1965

Income Class	*Number of Teeth*	
	Filled	*Decayed*
Under 3,000	0.7	3.4
3,000–4,999	1.3	3.0
5,000–6,999	2.1	2.2
7,000–9,999	2.7	1.7
10,000–14,999	3.3	1.4
15,000 and over	3.6	0.7

Source: U.S. Department of Health, Education and Welfare, Public Health Service: *The Health of Children—1970.* Washington, D.C., U.S. Government Printing Office, 1970, p. 37.

[6] Income is associated with other factors that also influence decay, such as a family's diet.

TABLE X

NUMBER OF PHYSICIAN VISITS PER PERSON PER YEAR,
BY SEX, COLOR, AND FAMILY INCOME,
JULY 1965—JUNE 1967

	Both Sexes		Male		Female	
Income Class	*White*	*Nonwhite*	*White*	*Nonwhite*	*White*	*Nonwhite*
Under 3,000	4.3	3.5	3.9	2.9	3.7	3.9
3,000–6,999	4.3	3.0	3.9	2.8	4.8	3.3
7,000 and over	4.7	3.4	4.2	3.3	5.1	3.5

Source: U.S. Department of Health, Education and Welfare, Public Health Service: *Differentials in Health Characteristics by Color, United States, July 1965—June 1967*, Public Health Service Publication No. 1,000—Series 10—No. 56. Washington, D.C., U.S. Government Printing Office, 1969, p. 18.

attention is received by higher income groups [7] and at any income level, whites display a greater utilization of physicians' visits than nonwhites regardless of sex. Similarly, a direct relationship exists between the use of medical specialists and income class.

Inequality can also be portrayed diagrammatically through the use of a Lorenz curve. A *Lorenz curve* is a diagrammatic plotting of the two variables being compared, with the comparison base plotted in percentage terms on the horizontal axis and the variable for which the inequality is being investigated plotted in

TABLE XI

VISITS PER ONE HUNDRED FAMILIES TO SELECTED TYPES OF
MEDICAL SPECIALISTS, BY FAMILY INCOME,
JULY 1963—JUNE 1964

Income Class	*Pediatrician*	*Obstetrician-Gynecologist*	*Opthalmologist*	*Otolarynogologist*
All income	59.6	52.4	34.0	18.9
under 3,000	14.4	19.5	23.0	9.7
3,000–4,999	49.1	50.9	25.1	15.6
5,000–6,999	79.1	71.5	31.5	21.1
7,000–9,999	92.8	77.0	42.4	24.9
10,000 and over	106.6	79.4	62.9	32.9
	Orthopedist	*Dermatologist*	*Psychiatrist*	
All income	17.6	15.3	7.3	
under 3,000	9.7	7.6	4.3	
3,000–4,999	13.6	10.0	6.1	
5,000–6,999	19.3	14.1	7.2	
7,000–9,999	24.2	21.0	9.0	
10,000 and over	30.7	34.7	13.7	

Source: U.S. Department of Health, Education, and Welfare, Public Health Service: *Family Use of Health Services, United States, July 1963—June 1964*. Public Health Service, Publication No. 1,000—Series 10—No. 55. Washington, D.C., U.S. Government Printing Office, 1969, pp. 24–25.

[7] At the lowest levels of income, the cost of physicians' visits may be subsidized by governmental payments thereby removing the effect of income on the consumption of physicians' services.

percentage terms on the vertical axis. The Lorenz curve appearing in Figure 1 depicts graphically the inequality in income distribution in the United States during 1970 based on the data presented in Table VII. Per cent of the population is plotted along the horizontal axis and per cent of income along the vertical axis. The graph is bisected by a diagonal which is the locus of points where the percentages of the two factors are equal. Thus the diagonal represents a state of total equality. Inequality is represented by a curve (Lorenz curve) divergent from the diagonal. The more unequal the distribution, the

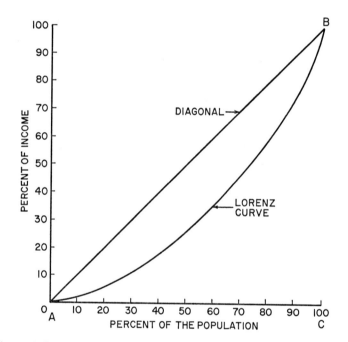

Figure 1. Lorenz curve of the United States income inequality, 1970.

greater the disparity between the diagonal and the Lorenz curve. At the extreme, total inequality would be represented by a Lorenz curve following the right angle A C B.[8]

The inequality in the distribution of health care services is both affected by and effects the distribution of income and wealth. Members of poor families cannot afford to purchase

[8] Such a situation would imply that all the income is available to only one person.

health care services and in many cases cannot even afford to consume those services provided at reduced or no direct cost.[9] With the passage of time, the limited opportunities for consuming health care services perpetuates and accentuates the inequality in income and wealth, as poorer health leads to a greater degree of worker absenteeism, unemployment, and lower earnings.

NATIONAL INCOME ACCOUNTS AND TAXATION

National income accounts are a basic data source for measures of state and local fiscal capacity and tax effort, two concepts with extremely important implications for financing public health care services. One aspect of economic analyses of state and local financing of health care services is the question of how much an area spends for health care services as opposed to how much an area *could* spend. Implicit in such discussions is the assumption that greater expenditures mean better health care services, *ceteris paribus*. The question of how much an area could spend hinges on its *fiscal capacity* and *tax effort*. The concept of fiscal capacity reflects the resources embodied within an area which could be taxed to raise revenue. Thus, the fiscal capacity of an area is determined by the total resources of the area's population: its income, wealth, and business activity. Tax effort is simply the extent to which an area makes use of its fiscal capacity.[10]

There are two approaches to measuring fiscal capacity. The first approach focuses on income and analyzes indices of an area's income out of which taxes can be paid. The second approach focuses on an area's wealth and seeks to measure the taxable resources embodied within an area in order to estimate the amount of revenue that could be raised under various levels of wealth. The ideal approach would be a measure including both wealth and income, but the available national income data report only income and thus dictate the use of the first approach.

Per capita health care expenditures are a good measure of an area's effort in financing health care services, as the data indicate

[9] For an elaboration of this point see Chapter Four.

[10] For a detailed discussion of these concepts see, The Advisory Commission on Intergovernmental Relations: *Measures of State and Local Fiscal Capacity and Tax Effort*. Washington, D.C., U.S. Government Printing Office, 1962.

the aggregate amount being spent relative to the population of the area at which the expenditures are directed. However, such per capita expenditures do not perfectly reflect or adjust for the ability of an area to finance such expenditures. Two obvious adjustments for ability (fiscal capacity) are a measure of an area's economic capacity to provide the service and the relative size of any population groups requiring greater health care expenditures than the norm. The greater an area's economic capacity, the greater its ability to finance public services, as a larger base is available for taxation. Similarly, the greater the number of very young and old inhabitants relative to the area's total population, the greater the health needs. Therefore, a given expenditure level in an area with a high proportion of the population requiring greater care represents a lower level of effort, where effort is interpreted as expenditure adjusted for need. Additional adjustments can be proposed, such as taking account of the relative cost of providing health care services in any area, or utilizing an area's morbidity rate as an additional measure of need.

As the current discussion is primarily indicative of how to adjust effort for ability, and as the precise nature of any adjustment must stem from the thrust of the analysis being undertaken, the ensuing presentation is confined solely to illustrating a method of adjusting a gross effort measure for income and population considerations. The precise adjustments entail dividing the effort measure (per capita health expenditures), where health expenditures are measured by state expenditures on health services and hospitals, by personal income per capita, since the larger this ratio the greater an area's effort. This quotient is then divided by the proportion of the population requiring more health care services than the norm, this group being defined as all those in age groups 0 to 5 and 65 and over. The adjusted effort measure can be represented as:

$$\text{Adjusted Effort} = \frac{\text{Per Capita Health Expenditures}}{\text{Per Capita Income}} \div \begin{array}{l}\text{Proportion of the} \\ \text{Population in Age} \\ \text{Categories 0–5} \\ \text{and 65 and Over}\end{array}$$

Table XII presents indices of effort and adjusted effort by state, utilizing 1969 data. To enable interstate comparisons, the effort and adjusted effort measures were converted into indices, with the United States average serving as the base. The effort and adjusted effort indices were then ranked to simplify comparisons. The results of this exercise indicate that differences do exist between what various states are spending on health care services and their ability to provide these services. In eighteen states the two indices were within five rank points of each other,[11] while in sixteen states the rankings were at least ten rank points apart.[12] In only twenty-three states did the adjusted effort measure exceed the effort index; in twenty-five states the reverse was true; and in two states both measures were equal. In almost every large, major, industrial state adjusted effort was less than actual effort. On a geographic basis, southern states displayed much higher expenditure patterns relative to their ability than northern and middle atlantic states. These findings are contrary to what one would have expected based on the prevailing hypothesis that large industrial states and states located in the eastern part of the country are the most liberal in providing public services.

While one should be reluctant to draw conclusions from an analysis which excludes private and federal government expenditures,[13] is based on data for only one year, and does not incorporate adjustments for factors other than income and size of the population requiring greater care than the norm, comparisons of the type inherent in effort and adjusted effort discussions can be important considerations in allocating federal funds earmarked for health care among states. The amount of the federal contribution could be related either to the size of the differential

[11] Those states are as follows: New York, Delaware, Hawaii, Rhode Island, Alaska, Maryland, Virginia, Colorado, New Hampshire, Oklahoma, North Dakota, Maine, Montana, Nevada, Texas, Ohio, South Dakota, and Arizona.

[12] Those states are as follows: Wisconsin, Illinois, Missouri, Nebraska, South Carolina, Washington, North Carolina, West Virginia, Indiana, California, New Jersey, Arkansas, Alabama, Tennessee, New Mexico, and Mississippi.

[13] The Public Health Service provides a significant proportion of the health services in Arizona, a state which ranked last in the above analysis. The inclusion of Public Health Services expenditures would undoubtedly improve Arizona's rankings under both effort measures. Analagous conditions undoubtedly exist in other states.

TABLE XII

INDICES OF HEALTH AND HOSPITAL
EXPENDITURES BY STATE, 1969

State	Effort		Adjusted Effort	
	Index	Rank [1]	Index	Rank [1]
New York	185.4	1	146.9	6
Delaware	166.9	2	158.2	3
Hawaii	156.8	3	167.8	2
Rhode Island	150.8	4	140.3	8
Connecticut	150.3	5	124.4	11
Alaska	137.0	6	153.8	4
Maryland	134.6	7	137.2	9
Massachusetts	131.9	8	112.3	16
Louisiana	127.3	9	169.3	1
Virginia	116.8	10	144.9	7
Colorado	116.5	11	130.5	10
Michigan	111.6	12	107.2	19
Minnesota	111.4	13	107.1	20
Wisconsin	102.4	14	100.8	26
New Hampshire	101.8	15	115.2	15
Illinois	101.4	16	86.6	40
Pennsylvania	101.1	17	101.2	25
Missouri	97.9	18	96.0	31
Vermont	97.8	19	100.0	28
Nebraska	97.7	20	90.1	34
South Carolina	95.7	21	147.5	5
Georgia	94.4	22	119.3	13
Kansas	94.3	23	91.3	32
Wyoming	93.9	24	109.5	17
Washington	89.6	25	88.9	37
Oklahoma	88.6	26	102.3	23
North Carolina	88.3	27	121.3	12
West Virginia	87.3	28	117.9	14
Indiana	87.2	29	87.4	39
North Dakota	83.8	30	100.2	27
California	83.6	31	76.4	42
Maine	83.4	32	91.1	33
Oregon	82.4	33	84.8	41
Iowa	81.8	34	76.0	43
Florida	79.7	35	75.1	44
New Jersey	78.1	36	71.1	46
Utah	78.0	37	98.7	30
Arkansas	77.4	38	101.6	24
Alabama	75.4	39	108.8	18
Tennessee	74.3	40	98.9	29
Montana	74.2	41	88.2	38
New Mexico	73.4	42	102.7	22
Idaho	71.7	43	89.5	36
Kentucky	71.7	43	89.8	35
Mississippi	67.3	45	96.1	31
Nevada	65.8	46	65.5	48
Texas	64.1	47	73.9	45
Ohio	59.2	48	58.5	49
South Dakota	58.6	49	65.6	47
Arizona	43.1	50	49.3	50
U.S.	100.0		100.0	

[1] In case of a tie the same rank was assigned to both states and
the succeeding rank was skipped.

between effort and effort adjusted for ability or directly to the adjusted effort measure. In these ways federal funds would complement rather than supplant state expenditures and thus provide the states with an economic incentive to increase their expenditures on health care services and other public services whose supply society wishes to increase.

Chapter Three

THE MEDICAL CARE PRICE INDEX

I N THE previous chapter the concept of price indices was briefly
introduced and their use as deflators and as convenient tools
in measuring relative performance in regard to financing health
care services was illustrated. In this chapter, the construction and
utilization of index numbers is analyzed in greater detail and
attention is focused on the Consumer Price Index and particularly
on one of its components, the Medical Care Price Index. The
construction and components of these indices are reviewed, the
basic changes that have occurred in the medical care area as
reflected in the Medical Care Price Index are noted, and the
limitations of this measure of medical care cost and cost changes
are discussed. The concluding section of the chapter reports and
discusses an alternate measure that has been proposed as an
indicator of cost behavior in the medical care area.

INDEX NUMBERS

An *index number* is a *statistic used to obtain an overall picture
of change or relative value*. Indices are often used to transform
data from absolute to relative values to facilitate comparisons. An
illustration of this use is the interstate comparison of health and
hospital financing presented in Chapter Two. It is much simpler
to compare units (states, time periods, etc.) when all figures are
transformed into relative terms through the device of index
numbers. For example, it is simpler to compare different states
by noting how they compare to a national average than by trying
to analyze how they compare with each other.

Indices can also be constructed to reflect change in either an individual item or in a group of items representative of a particular market. In constructing a series of index numbers, the object is to combine the pertinent information on a large number of different commodities, services, or activities into one meaningful summary figure that will accurately reflect the average change from time to time, or place to place. Individual goods and services are subject to many influences which cause their price and supply to vary from time to time. Some of the influences are peculiar to a particular item; others stem from powerful forces that bear on all markets for goods and services, such as changes in population, tastes, and technology. Thus the price and supply characteristics of individual items will pursue a somewhat individualistic course and no one of them, or subgroup of them, can be expected to reflect changes in the general pervasive forces affecting the total economy or the broad market of which the item under consideration is a component. General indices are therefore constructed in an attempt to describe the typical behavior of a large population of goods or services.

The construction of general indices require the assigning of weights to each item within the composite. The purpose of the weights is to reflect the relative importance of each item within the market represented by the composite index, thereby assuring that changes in attributes of important and minor items are not counted equally. A frequently used weight in any composite index is the proportion of a budget accounted for by the designated item.

Not only do index numbers simplify the understanding of the typical movement of individual and mass data, but the simple summary form in which index numbers are stated facilitates the performance of additional computations. New studies may be executed and conclusions may be reached which would have been impossible or extremely time consuming if each individual data series had to be considered separately. For example, real wages are defined as actual (money) wages adjusted for changes in the cost-of-living. Thus if wages increased 10 per cent while the cost-of-living rose 20 per cent, the real wage, that is, the quantity of goods and services the person can purchase, has gone down. Rather than attempt to piece together changes in the cost-of-living by estimating changes in a host of items, one can use one of the published indices compiled by the Bureau of Labor Statistics of the United States Department of Labor. The index most often used for this purpose is the Consumer Price Index.

Indices are constructed by first selecting one year or one observation as the *base,* the benchmark to which all others will be compared.[1] A division of the values for all the other observations by the value of the base yields an *index.* Such an index would have a value of 1 for the base observation. In practice, most indices utilize a value of 100 for the base; indices having 100 as their base are constructed in the same manner as indices with 1 as their base except that the quotients are multiplied by 100.

The construction of an index number series for a single hypothetical item, item A, is illustrated in Table XIII. Column 2 contains time series (longitudinal) values for item A, and columns 3 and 4 contain indices of item A constructed by choosing year 5 as

TABLE XIII

DERIVATION OF AN INDEX
Base = *Year 5*

Year	*Item A*	*Index of Item A* (*yr 5 = 1*)	*Index of Item A* (*yr 5 = 100*)
1	186	0.47	47
3	291	0.74	74
5	392	1.00	100
7	499	1.27	127
9	685	1.75	175

Base = *Year 1*

Year	*Item A*	*Index of Item A* (*yr 1 = 1*)	*Index of Item A* (*yr 1 = 100*)
1	186	1.00	100
3	291	1.56	156
5	392	2.12	212
7	499	2.68	268
9	685	3.68	368

the base. The value of item A in the base year becomes 1 or 100 (392 = 1 or 100) and all other values are then adjusted by the factor $\frac{1}{392}$ or $\frac{1}{392} \times 100$, yielding the index reported in columns 3 and 4. The difference between the two indices reported in columns

[1] The base observation can be selected either arbitrarily or based on any systematic criteria such as cycles of data generation or major events which are hypothesized to affect the activity under consideration.

3 and 4 is that the former has a base value of 1 and the latter a base value of 100. A comparison of the value of item A in year 5 and year 7 indicates that the value of item A in year 7 was 27 per cent greater than in year 5. Similarly, a comparison between years 5 and 1 indicated that the value for item A in year 5 was 212.77 per cent of the value of year 1 $\left(\dfrac{100}{47} \times 100\right)$, or 112.77 per cent greater than the value of year 1.

It is important to distinguish between the *percentage increase over* the base value and the *percentage of* the base value. The difference between the two is that the *percentage of* the base value is always greater by 100 percentage points than the *percentage increase over* the base since it includes the base amount whose value is 100.

Another year could be chosen as the base year without changing the relative values of the indices. For example, if year 1 were chosen as the base year, each value would be multiplied by the factor 1/186 or 100/186 yielding the index set shown in the lower half of Table XIII. As in the previous case the increase in the value of item A from year 1 to year 5 was 112 per cent; and from year 5 to year 7, 27 per cent $\left(\dfrac{268 - 212}{212}\right)$.

Within the health care field, and within the economy at large, index numbers are used primarily to measure price changes in a designated bundle of goods or services over time. Two major types of indices are used to study price movements over time: the *Laspeyeres Index* and the *Paasche Index*.

The Laspeyeres Index measures price changes associated with a designated bundle of goods and services whose quantities consumed remain or are assumed to remain invariant over the period of study. The formula for its computation is as follows:

$$L = \frac{\sum_{j=1}^{n} P_{ij} Q_{oj}}{\sum_{j=1}^{n} P_{oj} Q_{oj}}$$

where L is the Laspeyeres index; P, price; Q, quantity utilized of any item included in the overall composite index; i, the current time period; o, the base time period; and the symbol $\sum_{j=1}^{n}$ represents the sum of the expression following it for all values of j beginning at the lower limit of 1 to the upper limit of n (see the example in Table XIV). Thus the Laspeyeres Index measures the cost in year i of the bundle of goods and services purchased in the base year relative to the cost of that bundle in the base year.

The Paasche Index measures price changes associated with a designated bundle of goods and services where the perspective is the present so that today's bundle of goods and services is priced today and in the past. The Paasche Index is calculated as:

$$P = \frac{\sum_{j=1}^{n} P_{ij} Q_{ij}}{\sum_{j=1}^{n} P_{oj} Q_{ij}}$$

where P is the Paasche Index. Therefore the Paasche Index measures the relative cost of the bundle of goods and services purchased in year i, that is, the cost of the goods and services in year i relative to what that same bundle would have cost in the base year.

Table XIV contains hypothetical price and quantity data for three items representative of a market over two time periods. Utilizing the Laspeyeres formula, the increase between the two time periods is 5.77 per cent, whereas the use of the Paasche formula yields an increase of 0.49 per cent. Thus the choice of base or current period mixture of goods and services can lead to significant differences in the value of the index measure calculated.

There is no perfect index number when prices and quantities are both changing. The Paasche and Laspeyeres indices can be thought of as forming limits within which the truth lies. As it

TABLE XIV

THE CONSTRUCTION OF A LASPEYERES
AND PAASCHE PRICE INDEX

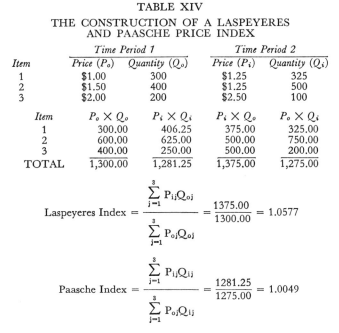

	Time Period 1		Time Period 2	
Item	*Price (P_o)*	*Quantity (Q_o)*	*Price (P_i)*	*Quantity (Q_i)*
1	$1.00	300	$1.25	325
2	$1.50	400	$1.25	500
3	$2.00	200	$2.50	100

Item	$P_o \times Q_o$	$P_i \times Q_i$	$P_i \times Q_o$	$P_o \times Q_i$
1	300.00	406.25	375.00	325.00
2	600.00	625.00	500.00	750.00
3	400.00	250.00	500.00	200.00
TOTAL	1,300.00	1,281.25	1,375.00	1,275.00

$$\text{Laspeyeres Index} = \frac{\sum_{j=1}^{3} P_{ij}Q_{oj}}{\sum_{j=1}^{3} P_{oj}Q_{oj}} = \frac{1375.00}{1300.00} = 1.0577$$

$$\text{Paasche Index} = \frac{\sum_{j=1}^{3} P_{ij}Q_{ij}}{\sum_{j=1}^{3} P_{oj}Q_{ij}} = \frac{1281.25}{1275.00} = 1.0049$$

is quite costly to calculate two indices, the Laspeyeres formula is the most frequently used in constructing general indices. It is the cheaper index to construct for longitudinal analyses because new weights do not have to be calculated each year since the same bundle of goods and services is used for all years.

THE CONSUMER PRICE INDEX

The Consumer Price Index measures changes in prices of goods and services customarily bought by *urban wage earners,* both families and single persons living alone. The index is based on approximately 400 items which were specifically selected by the Labor Department as representative of the entire bundle of goods and services purchased by wage earners and clerical workers. These four hundred items are grouped into five major categories, which are detailed in Table XV together with the major components of each category and the index value for 1971.

The Consumer Price Index is computed based on a Laspeyeres

price index formula. The base period weights are derived from data gathered in the 1960–1961 Survey of Consumer Expenditures conducted by the United States Department of Commerce, which details how consumers spent their income over the entire

TABLE XV

THE CONSUMER PRICE INDEX, 1971

	1971 *(1967 = 100)*
1. Food	118.4
Food at home	116.4
Cereals and bakery products	113.9
Meats, poultry, and fish	116.9
Dairy products	115.3
Fruits and vegetables	119.1
Other foods at home	115.9
Food away from home	126.1
2. Housing	124.3
Shelter [1]	128.8
Rent	115.2
Homeownership [2]	133.7
Fuel and utilities [3]	115.1
Fuel oil and coal	117.5
Gas and electricity	114.7
Household furnishings and operation	118.1
3. Apparel and upkeep [4]	119.8
Men's and boys'	120.3
Women's and girls'	120.1
Footwear	121.5
4. Transportation	118.6
Private	116.6
New Cars	112.0
Used Cars	110.2
Gasoline	106.3
Public	137.7
5. Health and Recreation	122.2
Medical care	128.4
Personal care	116.8
Reading and recreation	119.3
Other goods and services	120.9
All items	121.3

[1] Also includes hotel and motel rates not shown separately.
[2] Includes home purchase, mortgage interest, taxes, insurance, and maintenance and repairs.
[3] Also includes telephone, water, and sewerage service not shown separately.
[4] Also includes infants' wear, sewing materials, jewelry, and apparel upkeep services not shown separately.
Source: Monthly Labor Review, 95 (3), 97–101, 1972.

spectrum of goods and services. The relative importance (weights) of the major items included in the Consumer Price Index are as follows: food—22.4 per cent, housing—33.2 per cent, apparel—10.6 per cent, transportation—13.9 per cent, health and recreation—19.8 per cent.[2] The base period for measuring price changes curently in use in 1967.[3]

Price quotations used in calculating the Consumer Price Index are collected periodically in fifty-six major cities consisting of the twelve largest cities in the country, sixteen other large cities, eleven medium size cities, and seventeen small cities, chosen to represent all urban areas in the United States.[4] Within each city price quotations are obtained from a sample of providers of the goods and services included in the index. Prices of food, fuels, and a few other items are obtained monthly in every city included in the survey. Prices of most other items are collected monthly in the five largest cities and quarterly in all other cities. Mail questionnaires are used to obtain price changes in items whose prices change infrequently, such as local transit fares, public utility rates, and newspaper prices. Price quotations for all other items are solicited through personal visits conducted by representatives of the Bureau of Labor Statistics. To insure that the same item is priced during each survey, descriptions of both quality and quantity are specified. The quantity description is straightforward, while quality is based solely on recognizable, measurable, physical characteristics of an item which are thought to influence its price.

Four points about the use and interpretation of the Consumer Price Index merit special attention. First, the actual cost-of-living, as mirrored by the total amount of money a consuming unit spends, is determined by the prices of items *and* the quantity of items purchased. The Consumer Price Index measures only price changes; it contains no information about changes in the quantity of goods and services purchased resulting from changes in family

---

[2] German, Jeremiah J.: Some uses and limitations of the Consumer Price Index, *Inquiry*, 1:140, 1964.

[3] The lack of consistency between the price and quantity base years is attributable to the complex, yet fragmented nature of data collection at the federal level. Prior to 1971, the base for price comparison was an average of a three-year period, 1957–1959. Within the near future, the Survey of Consumer Expenditures will be updated and the overall Consumer Price Index revised to incorporate this change.

[4] For a listing of these cities see, U.S. Department of Labor, Bureau of Labor Statistics: *The Consumer Price Index for May 1971*. Washington, D.C., U.S. Department of Labor, August 1971.

income, size, or tastes. Second, quality changes which are not of a physical or tangible nature remain unaccounted. Third, the index does not and can not indicate whether any particular price or group of prices is too high or too low. All it indicates is the pattern of price change from a designated base period. Fourth, the index is unrepresentative of price changes occurring in rural areas and of the consuming patterns of select population groups, such as the retired, professional workers, and managerial workers. These limitations notwithstanding, the Consumer Price Index does provide a fairly comprehensive picture of price movements in the United States economy.

THE MEDICAL CARE PRICE INDEX

The Medical Care Price Index is one component of the larger, more comprehensive, Consumer Price Index. As can be seen from Table XV, it is one component of the health and recreation category. Medical care expenditures account for 5.7 per cent of the total Consumer Price Index and 28.8 per cent (5.7/19.8) of the health and recreation component of the aggregate index. The medical care component of the Consumer Price Index, or the Medical Care Price Index, is a measure of the change in the prices paid for a sample of typical medical care goods and services consumed by urban wage earners and clerical workers. Since the Medical Care Price Index is the only overall measure of change in the price of medical care that is published regularly, it is commonly used as an index for the total population.

Prices have been collected on medical care items since 1918, the birth date of the Consumer Price Index. However, it is only since 1935 that prices were collected based on precise specifications rather than a brief description of each item. The items included in the Medical Care Price Index and their values for selected years from 1935 to 1971 are recorded in Table XVI. A cursory glance at Table XVI indicates that price quotations are not available, on a continuous basis, for every item included in the index, as the index is changed and updated periodically to reflect changes in the consumption of medical care services. However, in most instances, historical price quotations are secured in an attempt to preserve continuity and comprehensiveness.[5]

On an aggregate basis, the price of medical care services increased significantly over the period 1935 to 1971. Prices in 1935 were 32 per cent of 1967 prices, indicating a general price increase to 314.46 per cent of the original price $\left(\frac{100}{31.8} \times 100\right)$, or 214.46 per cent over this thirty-three-year period. In the four years comprising the post-1967 period, medical care prices rose 28.4 per cent. The Consumer Price Index increased from a value of 41.1 in 1935 to 121.3 in 1971 (1967 = 100) indicating a 143.3 per cent general price increase in the pre-1967 period and a 21.3 per cent price increase from 1967 to 1971. In both the pre-1967 and post-1967 period medical care prices increased at a greater rate than prices of the aggregate of the four hundred items constituting the Consumer Price Index.

Within the medical care sector proper, the greatest price increases in both the pre-1967 and post-1967 periods were registered by hospital daily service charges and operating room charges. A 740.3 per cent increase occurred from 1935 to 1967 (daily service charges only) and a 60.8 per cent increase from 1967 to 1971.[6] Physicians' and dentists' fees increased approximately 50 per cent from 1935 to 1967 and 28 per cent from 1967 to 1971. Price trends for the drug and prescription component of the Medical Care Price Index display an atypical trend. Not only did they display a smaller rate of increase than

[5] For a discussion of the changes in the composition and sampling procedures used to solicit price quotations for the Medical Care Price Index, see, Langford, Elizabeth A.: Medical care in the Consumer Price Index, 1936–1956, *Monthly Labor Review, 80*:1053, 1957; American Medical Association, Commission on the Cost of Medical Care: *General Report,* Volume 1, Chicago, American Medical Association, 1964, Chapter 3; and Berry, William F. and Dougherty, James C.: A closer look at rising medical costs, *Monthly Labor Review, 91* (11) :1, 1968.

[6] The hospital services component of the Medical Care Price Index was revised in February 1972. Prior to this date, hospital services were represented in the index by daily service charges for private and semiprivate hospital rooms. Effective February 1972 this component will now be represented by a sample of 10 specifications, 7 of which are new to the index. The 10 specifications are as follows: semi-private room; operating room charges; x-ray, diagnostic series, and upper G.I.; laboratory fees; electrocardiogram; tetracycline; intravenous solution; oxygen; tranquilizer; and physical therapy. Annual price quotations for these specifications will not be available until the beginning of 1973; consequently the material presented here is based on the old version of the index.

TABLE XVI

THE MEDICAL CARE PRICE INDEX, SELECTED YEARS, 1935–1971
(1967 = 100)

	1935	1940	1945	1950	1955	1960	1965	1967	1968	1969	1970	1971
Medical Care Services	31.8	32.5	37.9	49.2	60.4	74.4	87.3	100.0	107.3	116.0	124.2	128.4
Professional Services:												
Physicians' fees												
General physician office visits	39.2	39.6	46.0	55.2	65.4	77.0	88.3	100.0	105.6	112.9	121.4	129.8
General physician house visits	38.8	39.1	45.7	54.9	65.4	75.9	87.3	100.0	105.8	113.3	122.6	131.4
Herniorrhapy (adult)	39.1	39.6	44.7	52.9	61.2	75.0	87.6	100.0	106.5	114.5	122.4	131.0
Tonsillectomy and adenoidectomy (adult)	—	—	—	—	—	—	91.3	100.0	104.6	108.8	115.0	123.4
Obstetrical cases	41.8	41.5	48.8	60.7	69.0	80.3	91.0	100.0	104.9	110.3	117.1	125.2
	32.1	33.0	41.0	51.2	68.6	79.4	89.0	100.0	105.2	113.5	121.8	129.0
Pediatric care, office visits	—	—	—	—	—	—	85.8	100.0	104.9	114.4	122.7	132.0
Psychiatrist, office visits	—	—	—	—	—	—	88.0	100.0	105.3	113.5	119.4	124.8
Dentists' fees	40.8	42.0	49.6	63.9	73.0	82.1	92.2	100.0	105.5	112.9	119.4	127.0
Filling, adult, amalgam, one surface	40.4	42.1	49.2	63.9	72.5	81.9	91.3	100.0	105.4	113.1	120.3	128.0
Extractions (adult)	39.5	40.3	48.6	62.8	73.8	82.0	93.9	100.0	105.2	112.9	118.6	126.9
Dentures, full upper	—	—	—	—	—	—	92.2	100.0	106.1	112.3	118.3	124.9
Other Professional Services:												
Examination, prescription, and dispensing of eyeglasses	56.7	58.1	63.9	73.5	77.0	85.1	92.8	100.0	103.2	107.6	113.5	120.3
Routine laboratory tests	—	—	—	—	—	—	94.8	100.0	103.5	107.5	111.4	116.1

TABLE XVI (continued)

	1935	1940	1945	1950	1955	1960	1965	1967	1968	1969	1970	1971
Hospital Service Charges:												
Daily service charges	11.9	12.7	16.2	28.9	41.5	56.3	76.6	100.0	113.2	127.9	143.9	160.8
Semiprivate rooms	12.8	13.7	17.6	30.3	42.3	57.3	75.9	100.0	113.6	112.8	145.4	163.1
Private rooms	14.2	15.1	18.9	31.3	44.1	57.8	77.7	100.0	112.7	126.7	141.7	157.5
Operating room charges	—	—	—	—	—	—	82.9	100.0	111.5	128.7	142.4	156.2
X-ray, diagnostic series, upper G.I.	—	—	—	—	—	—	90.9	100.0	104.3	109.3	116.3	124.9
Drugs and Prescriptions	70.7	70.8	74.8	88.5	94.7	104.5	100.2	100.0	100.2	101.3	103.6	105.4
Prescriptions	65.4	66.2	71.5	92.6	101.6	115.3	102.0	100.0	98.3	99.6	101.2	101.3
Anti-infectives	—	—	—	—	—	135.1	113.2	100.0	92.4	91.8	89.9	80.2
Sedatives and hypnotics	—	—	—	—	—	101.3	97.2	100.0	102.7	108.8	116.2	122.9
Ataractics	—	—	—	—	—	107.4	101.2	100.0	99.7	99.7	100.4	101.7
Anti-spasmodics	—	—	—	—	—	99.7	98.0	100.0	100.9	101.4	103.1	107.1
Cough preparations	—	—	—	—	—	99.1	96.4	100.0	103.4	110.2	119.0	126.0
Cardiovasculars and anti-hypertensives	—	—	—	—	—	103.9	99.3	100.0	100.6	103.2	106.6	111.1
Analgesics, internal	—	—	—	—	—	—	—	100.0	—	102.5	105.3	107.8
Anti-obesity	—	—	—	—	—	—	—	100.0	99.4	103.0	107.8	114.9
Hormones	—	—	—	—	—	—	98.0	100.0	96.0	94.8	94.8	94.9
Over-the-counter items	—	—	—	—	—	—	98.0	100.0	102.5	103.2	106.2	110.2
Multiple vitamin concentrates	—	—	—	—	—	—	103.8	100.0	99.8	98.4	98.0	96.6
Aspirin compounds	—	—	—	—	—	—	96.2	100.0	101.6	102.3	106.8	114.1
Liquid tonics	—	—	—	—	—	—	98.0	100.0	100.1	100.1	101.0	101.3
Adhesive bandages, package	—	—	—	—	—	—	94.8	100.0	105.8	108.2	113.8	122.6
Cold tablets or capsules	—	—	—	—	—	—	99.8	100.0	102.6	104.5	107.8	111.3
Cough syrup	—	—	—	—	—	—	96.1	100.0	104.7	105.6	107.8	112.4

Source: 1935–1970: U.S. Department of Labor, Bureau of Labor Statistics. (worksheets); 1971: *Monthly Labor Review*, 95(3):100–101, 1972.

the parent index, rising by only 41.4 per cent from 1935 to 1967 and by 5.4 per cent from 1967 to 1971, but in some specific instances such as anti-infectives and multiple vitamin concentrates prices actually declined from 1960 to 1971.[7]

As was noted in the section on the Consumer Price Index, the price trends reflected by the index are influenced by the methodology used in constructing the index. Three attributes of the Medical Care Price Index deserve special attention, even at the risk of being repetitive. First, the index focuses on a select population group. The major omission in this regard is the elderly, a group which accounts for a greater utilization of medical services than indicated by their numerical size. Second, whereas changes in the composition of the index and in the weights attached to the price of each item occur infrequently, medical techniques change quite frequently. Consequently, significant time lags occur before both the introduction of new products and services into the index and the relative weighting of items used in providing medical care is updated to reflect current medical practice. For example, operating room charges, laboratory tests, and x-rays were first included in the index in 1963 although their use predates that year by a sizeable period.

A third shortcoming, and one of major proportion, is the failure to correct adequately for quality changes. The factors underlining this omission are of a dual nature. On one hand, quality changes are hard to discern and identify as they result from a process of continual change. There have been few quality changes which have had an immediate and major effect on, for example, the nature of a physician's visit. Improvements in quality stem largely from research and the increased education and skill of physicians, phenomena which by their very nature are continuous rather than discrete. On the other hand, quality changes in the medical field are largely confined to improving the probability of disease prevention or cure, comfort and satisfaction of the patient, changes in the average length of a hospital stay, and the number of physician

---

[7] One explanation for price decreases is that the high costs of pharmaceutical research are usually incorporated into a drug's price during its first marketing years. Mass production, plus competition from competing drug companies usually leads to a price cut in succeeding marketing periods.

visits per illness. None of these occurrences fall within the definition of quality change used in constructing the index. As noted previously, quality changes are confined to those features which are physical, easily recognizable, and have a direct relation to price. The reduction in the average length of stay in a short-term hospital from approximately 9 days in 1946 to approximately 7.5 days in 1971 with the concomitant concentration of services provided has undoubtedly contributed to the large increases in hospital daily service charges registered in the Medical Care Price Index. If this component of the index were the average cost of a hospital *stay* rather than of a hospital *day*, the component would be 83 per cent $\left(\frac{7.5}{9}\right)$ of the value currently reported.

AN ALTERNATE MEASURE OF MEDICAL CARE COST

Realizing the shortcomings of the current Medical Care Price Index, health economists have been engaged in attempts to construct an alternate measure of medical care costs which would more accurately depict developments in the medical care sector. One such attempt is Ann Scitovsky's proposed *Cost of Selected Illness Index*.[8] Scitovsky proposes abandoning the current practice of pricing individual commodities such as drugs, hospital days, and physicians' services and focusing instead on the cost of treating a group of illnesses. Illness episodes rather than physicians' fees, hospital charges, and drug costs would be the *bundle* of goods and services to be priced periodically. Scitovsky notes that once it is determined which illnesses loomed especially large in consumers' medical care budgets, a sample of illnesses could be chosen as the basis of the proposed index, and the pricing of the cost of treatment can be based on data contained in physicians' records.

Three features of the proposed Cost of Selected Illness Index are noteworthy. First, people are concerned with medical care,

[8] Scitovsky, Anne A.: An index of the cost of medical care—A proposed new approach, in S. Axelrod (ed.). *The Economics of Health and Medical Care.* Ann Arbor, Bureau of Public Health Economics, The University of Michigan, 1964, pp. 128–147.

not items such as antibiotics, physicians' fees, and drug costs. Therefore, on a conceptual basis, it is more realistic to treat the service purchased as the treatment of an illness rather than a series of individual items. If the method of treatment of the illnesses selected changes, it would be reflected in the proposed index although it would not be in the index currently in use. Second, given that the components of an index are changed infrequently, the choice of illnesses in the sample would be outdated less frequently than the choice of inputs currently priced for the Medical Care Price Index. A final consideration is that one could easily select the sample of illnesses to be surveyed so as to enable separate sub-indices to be computed for different age, occupational, racial, income, and geographic groups, if such a fine breakdown were desired.

Scitovsky selected five illnesses as a pilot study for the Cost of Selected Illness Index and gathered data from physicians' records kept at the Palo Alto Medical Clinic in Palo Alto, California for

TABLE XVII

PERCENTAGE INCREASE IN AVERAGE COSTS
OF TREATMENT, SELECTED ILLNESSES,
1951–1952 to 1964–1965

Illness	*Percentage Increase*
Acute Appendicitis	87
Maternity care	72
Otitis media (ear infection) in children	68
Cancer of the breast	106
Fracture of the forearm [1]	
a. Splint only	75
b. Cast only	55
c. Closed reduction, physician's office	110
d. Closed reduction, hospital	167
or	
c. Closed reduction, local or no anesthetic	87
d. Closed reduction, general anesthetic	315

[1] The cases are grouped by degree of severity as indicated by type of treatment. The second grouping of the cases in categories c and d is more meaningful because in 1951–1952 category c, "closed reduction, physician's office," included some cases severe enough to require a general anesthetic which was, however, given in the physician's office, a practice no longer followed in 1964–1965.

Source: Scitovsky, Anne A.: Changes in the costs of treatment of selected illnesses, 1951–1965, *American Economic Review*, 57:1184, 1967.

the period 1951–1952 to 1964–1965. The illnesses selected and the percentage increase in average cost over the study period are listed in Table XVII. Whereas the Medical Care Price Index displays an average price increase of approximately 74 per cent for the fifteen-year period 1951–1965, the use of Scitovsky's index yields an average increase for some illnesses in excess of 100 per cent.[9]

Although the Scitovsky proposal has intuitive appeal, its calculation would entail much greater expenditures than those involved in constructing the current Medical Care Price Index. Furthermore, it would have to be considered a separate entity and could not be included in the parent Consumer Price Index. One could, as Scitovsky proposes, calculate both indices (the Medical Care Price Index and the Cost of Selected Illness Index) ; the availability of a cost of illnesses index would be of great value for insurance and other reimbursement uses.

[9] For a detailed discussion of Scitovsky's findings see, Scitovsky, Anne A.: Changes in the costs of treatment of selected illnesses, 1951–1965, *American Economic Review, 57*:1182, 1967.

Chapter Four

DEMAND

THE CONCEPT of demand is one of the most elementary and crucial concepts of economic theory; it provides a systematic framework for interpreting the behavior of any consumer or consuming group. While the factors that motivate consumption are many, and while they may differ among individuals, the elements of demand theory provide a useful guide for interpreting and explaining individual and aggregate behavior. In addition, demand theory is used to facilitate prediction. Once the factors contributing to any event are identified and understood, one is in a good position to predict future events by hypothesizing or extrapolating specific behavior patterns for the causal factors— the factors that determine demand.

Within the health field an understanding of demand is especially important. The resources available to meet health needs are usually determined directly or indirectly by government or other third party action. The construction and funding of health related facilities and the training of health manpower, at all skill levels, are highly susceptible to financing policies adopted by agencies serving as the representative of the public. Before a commitment is made to expend scarce resources on supplying health facilities or services, it is important to understand the factors influencing demand in order to determine, and if necessary create, the appropriate conditions to insure that the services supplied will be wanted.

This chapter begins with a definition of the concept of demand and a discussion of demand determinants. The concept of elasticity is introduced and related to demand theory. In addition two new reformulations of conventional demand theory are briefly reviewed. The chapter concludes with a discussion of the relationship between two concepts that are often erroneously used as equivalents in the health literature: demand and need.

DEMAND: DEFINITION AND DETERMINANTS

Demand is a concept indicating the *amount of a particular good or service that a consumer is willing and able to purchase at each possible price during a specified time period.* Operationally, demand is discussed in terms of a demand schedule or demand curve. A typical demand schedule resembles the following hypothetical illustration:

Point	Price	Quantity Demanded
1	$150	0
2	100	2
3	75	3
4	50	5
5	25	7
6	10	11

A demand curve is a graphic representation of a demand schedule, as can be seen in Figure 2. By convention, price is indicated on the vertical axis and quantity on the horizontal axis. Aggregate demand for any group of consumers for a specific good or service is obtained by summing the quantities demanded by each of the individuals at each of the prices in turn. In constructing demand curves, the summation is of a horizontal nature.[1] That is, at each price the quantity demanded (the horizontal distance from the vertical axis) is added for all individuals to determine the horizontal distance at the given price on the aggregate demand curve ($D_c = D_a + D_b$, as seen in Fig. 3).

From an economic perspective the concept of demand is limited

---

[1] When the good or service under consideration is such that its provision to one person or group automatically provides this same item to another person or group and consumption of the item by one party does not reduce the amount available to the other, e.g. cancer research or swamp spraying, the derivation of the market demand curve requires a *vertical* rather than a *horizontal* summation of individual demand curves. For a rigorous analysis of such cases see, Samuelson, Paul A.: Diagrammatic exposition of a theory of public expenditures, *Review of Economics and Statistics, 37:*350, 1955.

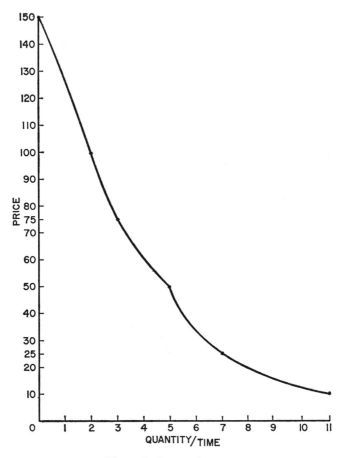

Figure 2. Demand curve.

to effective demand only. While the consuming unit (or units) may want to purchase the item under consideration, they may not possess the financial resources (or have access to credit sources) to do so. Willingness alone does not create demand; only those who both *want* and are *able* to make a purchase are considered relevant demanders. The time element is another factor in demand discussions. The number of items demanded at a given price is much greater during a year than during a week or month. Consequently, whenever reference is made to demand, a specific time dimension is explicitly stated or implicitly assumed.

A fundamental characteristic of demand is the inverse relationship between price and quantity; as price increases, quantity demanded decreases; and as price decreases, quantity demanded increases. This relationship can be explained on intuitive grounds and has been verified by many empirical studies. Intuitively, the higher the price of a good or service the fewer the number of units that will be desired and can be purchased with a fixed budget. For example, a hospital may have earmarked a sum of 5,000 dollars a year for wheelchairs. If the cost of wheelchairs increases and the funds earmarked for this item do not, the hospital can no longer buy the same number of wheelchairs as previously planned. The resultant decline in ability to purchase wheelchairs is a decrease in real income known as an *income effect,* and prompts the purchasing of fewer units of the good or service. The reduction in consumption will depend on the severity of the decline in real income and on the degree to which

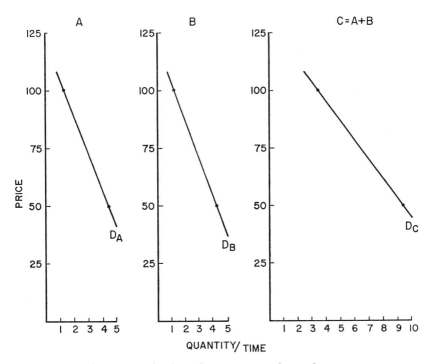

Figure 3. Derivation of an aggregate demand curve.

the item under consideration is a necessity. In practice the effect of this decline in real income will probably not be entirely compensated for by the reduction in the purchase of the item whose price increased, but rather be apportioned over the entire range of goods and services bought, i.e. not only will fewer wheelchairs be purchased but also less of the other items will be purchased.

The decline in purchases may also result from the substitution of now relatively cheaper items for the one whose price rose, i.e. a *substitution effect.* Referring back to the previous example, prior to the price increase the purchasing department of the hospital may have initially planned to buy fifty brand A wheelchairs at a cost of 100 dollars a wheelchair. If the price of brand A wheelchairs increases to 125 dollars, fifty brand B wheelchairs which are cheaper and less durable but cost only 75 dollars may now be purchased.[2] Thus, both the income and substitution effect lead to a smaller quantity demanded of a particular good at higher prices. Similarly, were the price to fall, a greater quantity would be demanded. To obtain this result the nature of the income and substitution effects are reversed. A lower price for one good or service means that if the same bundle of goods and services is purchased some money will now be left over. Consequently the consumption of the item whose price declined, and possibly other items whose price did not change, can increase. Furthermore, this item is now a better competitor with other items and may be substituted for any or all of them.

Demand theory emphasizes the importance of price as a determinant of quantity demanded. However, other factors such as tastes and preferences, money income, and prices of substitute or complementary goods or services also influence demand. While changes in the price of the good or service determine the corresponding changes in quantity demanded, represented diagrammatically by movements along demand curve DD (from points 1 to 2 in Fig. 4), changes in the remaining factors determine shifts in demand, represented diagrammatically by a change

---

[2] Fifty brand B wheelchairs cost only 3,750 dollars. The purchasing department may now recommend the purchase of more than 50 units as the substitute items are less durable or may suggest that the 1,250 dollar surplus be used for other items.

in the position of the demand curve from DD to D'D' or D"D".
The following hypothetical example illustrates this point.

Assume a given demand schedule for preventive medical care.
Demand theory postulates that quantity demanded (number of
visits) is inversely related to price (cost of a visit). Now exogenous changes in tastes, income, or other prices are introduced.
The sudden illness, and possibly death, of a relative or friend

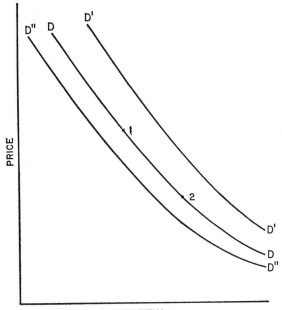

Figure 4. Shifts in demand.

may shift the entire demand schedule for preventive care, i.e.
more will be demanded at each price. This is represented by a
shift of the demand curve to the right (a shift from DD to D'D'
in Fig. 4). Similarly a significant increase in family income may
have an analogous effect, more checkups will now be demanded
at each price when family income increases. Finally, a change in
the relative prices of the provision of care (for example, physicians and chiropractors) may lead to a shift in demand. If the
price of a chiropractor's visit declines relative to that of a
physician's visit, the demand for medical care by physicians may

decline. This decline would be portrayed by a shift in the demand curve for physician visits to the left (a shift from DD to D″D″ in Fig. 4).[3]

A change in demand must not be confused with a change in quantity demanded. Mistakenly calling these two by the same name is one of the most common errors in the popular usage of economics. *A change in demand refers to shifts in the demand curve resulting from changes in tastes and preferences, income, and prices of related goods. A change in quantity demanded refers to a movement along a given demand curve, and results from a change in the price of the good under discussion with all other factors held constant.*

PRICE ELASTICITY OF DEMAND

Price elasticity of demand, defined as the percentage change in quantity divided by the percentage change in price, is a measure of the responsiveness of quantity changes to price changes. A price inelastic demand relationship is said to exist if, in percentage terms, the price change exceeds the resultant quantity change. If the percentage price change is less than the resultant percentage quantity change, a price elastic demand relationship exists. Percentage changes in price and quantity being equal defines a relationship of unitary price elasticity of demand. The formulas used for calculating price elasticity of demand coefficients appear in an Appendix to this chapter; the numerical ranges of any elasticity relationships are as follows:

Elasticity	*Elasticity Value*
Inelastic	Less than one
Elastic	Greater than one
Unitary elasticity	One

The significance of the price elasticity of demand concept lies in its relationship to the total revenue obtainable in any endeavor. Total revenue (TR) for any transaction is defined as

[3] Alternately in the case of complementary goods, defined as goods consumed in some fixed proportion (e.g. sugar cubes and doses of oral polio vaccine), a price increase in one good will lead to a reduction in the demand for the second good, as the consumption of the entire activity (where the activity is defined by the use of both sugar cubes and doses of polio vaccine) is now more expensive.

the price charged per unit (P), times the quantity sold (Q); that is $TR = P \cdot Q$. For any given price change the following relationship between price elasticity of demand and total revenue prevails:

Elasticity	*Total Revenue Resulting From*	
	Price Increase	*Price Decrease*
Inelastic	Increases	Decreases
Elastic	Decreases	Increases
Unitary elasticity	Remains the same	Remains the same

The nature of the changes in total revenue stems from the inverse price-quantity relationship inherent in any demand relationship. An inelastic demand relationship connotes greater percentage change in price than in quantity. Thus a price increase results in greater total revenue as the price increase exceeds, in percentage terms, the quantity decline; and a reduction in price nets a reduction in total revenue as the price reduction exceeds, in percentage terms, the quantity increase. The reverse is true for an elastic demand relationship. As the price and quantity changes are of equal magnitude in percentage terms for a case exhibiting unitary elasticity, total revenue remains unchanged as the price change is offset by a similar but opposite quantity change.

Price increases yield increases in total revenue only when the nature of the demand for the services provided by that enterprise is inelastic. Inelastic demand in turn results from the degree of necessity surrounding the consumption of that service and the range of substitutes. To the extent that the service under consideration is viewed as a necessity, and the availability of substitutes are limited by legal restrictions to entry of additional practitioners or professional ethics which frown on advertising, the supplier of the service is able to increase his total revenue by increasing his price. Most of the services associated with medical care are characterized by inelastic demand relationships.

Elasticity measures can be applied to practically any type of economic data. The discussion up to this point focused on price elasticity of demand, the response in quantity demanded to a change in price. An additional elasticity measure, income elasticity of demand is frequently reported in the health economics literature. *Income elasticity* of demand measures, in percentage terms, the change in demand associated with a change in income. From a public policy viewpoint, a knowledge of the income elasticity of demand associated with various health care services would provide valuable insight in projecting the impact of any income supplement program on the demand for health care services.

DEMAND AND MARKET EQUILIBRIUM

Economic activity is guided by the interaction of the desires of consumers and producers (within the milieu established by legislative, regulatory, and reimbursing agencies) as expressed in the economic concepts of demand and supply. Before one can enter into a descriptive analysis of this interaction, a brief diversion into the realm of supply is required.

The concept of supply closely resembles that of demand, except that it reflects the desires of producers, the second party to any economic activity. *Supply* is defined as the *schedule of amounts of a good or service that producers are willing and able to sell at each possible price, during a specified time period.* The responsiveness of quantity changes to price changes can be represented by measures of price elasticity of supply analogous to price elasticity of demand. The unique characteristic of a supply schedule or curve is a direct (positive) relationship between price and quantity. At a higher price more will be supplied; at a lower price less will be supplied. (A typical supply curve is presented in Figure 5). Although sales price is emphasized as the primary determinant of the quantity supplied, three additional factors influence supply: technology, prices of the factors of production, and prices of related goods.

Technology refers to the state of the arts in production and represents the various ways of combining factors of production to produce a good or service. However, technological (engineering) factors by themselves do not determine the choice of the method of production adopted; cost estimates for each alternative production technique are required to determine which alternative is the most economic. Thus technology and the prices of the factors of production jointly determine supply. If technological advances lead to the adaptation of cheaper productive techniques, and/or if the price of the factors of production decline, more will be supplied at each price; the supply curve shifts to the right. An increase in the price of a good or service to which the current resources of any supplier can be easily adopted will cause a decrease in the supply of the item originally produced; a shift of the supply curve to the left. Whereas changes in the price of the item determine *movements along* a supply curve (changes in quantity supplied), changes in technology, prices of the factors of production, and prices of related goods or services determine shifts in the supply curve (changes in supply).

Assume that the hypothetical demand and supply curves reproduced in Figure 5 represent the respective desires and

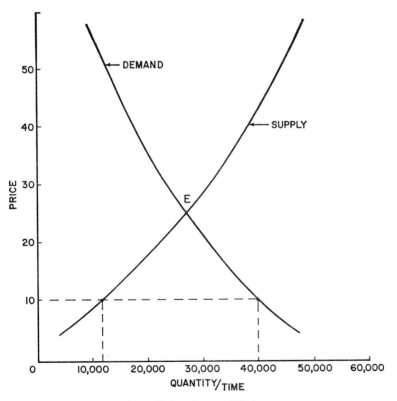

Figure 5. Market equilibrium.

capabilities of all consumers and producers for a good or service, and that this information is known by all the potential participants in this market.[4] Further asume that an initial price of 10 dollars prevails. At this price demanders are willing and able to purchase 40,000 units while suppliers are willing and able to produce 11,000 units. Demand exceeds supply by 29,000 units; such a situation is commonly referred to as a seller's market. Confronted with a shortage at the going price, either one of two things will happen: the item will have to be rationed or the price will have to increase. Rationing involves the adoption of legal or institutional arrangements for allocating the item in short supply; it is not entirely viable as the development of "black markets" attest. On the other hand, if price increases are permitted they will reduce the number of demanders and increase the number of suppliers until a equilibrium point (point E) is reached where demand equals supply. While price rationing, as opposed to nonprice rationing, in the health field *may* be deemed unsatisfactory by society as the health needs of the poor would quickly be subsumed by those of the wealthy, nevertheless, it does exist and has been used to a significant extent.

Had a price of 50 dollars prevailed in our hypothetical market, supply would exceed demand. A surplus of units would exist; such a situation is commonly referred to as a buyer's market. This situation is corrected by either destroying or freely distributing the surplus items or, more likely, by reducing the price. Such a reduction serves to increase the quantity demanded and simultaneously reduce the quantity supplied. Price can be continually lowered until an equilibrium situation is achieved.

Market equilibrium via price rationing has been described as an iterative process with one final market clearing price, i.e. an auction situation. In actuality, equilibrium will be achieved through a succession of nonclearing prices each prompting further price changes in the direction of equilibrium.[5] An equi-

[4] Refer to Chapter One for a discussion of markets.

[5] In a dynamic economy, change is constantly occurring, demand and supply are constantly shifting, and an equilibrium situation as described here may never be attained. However, the forces propelling the market toward an equilibrium are still active under a dynamic environment and do, to a great extent, guide economic activity.

librium price, once established, prevails for the entire market. Those consumers who would have been willing to pay a higher price and those producers who would have been willing to sell the item at a lower price benefit from the equilibrium price. Conversely, consumers who are not willing to pay a price as high as the equilibrium price and producers not willing to sell at a price as low as the equilibrium price are excluded from the market.

The health sector of the United States economy is often characterized by shortages of personnel and facilities rather than surpluses. Of the two methods described for adjusting to a shortage, a combination of price and nonprice rationing appears to have been chosen. The decision as to which of these two alternatives is socially preferable or what should be the optional combination of price and nonprice rationing is a normative one. Rational men can and do differ markedly on this issue. The presentation of the operation of the market mechanism is not intended to imply specific values on this social issue but rather to provide a framework for analyzing the ultimate effects of different courses of social action. Policies that affect demand and not supply, or vice versa, can easily aggravate imbalances that already exist in the market for health care services.

REFORMULATIONS OF DEMAND THEORY

Classical demand theory focuses primarily on individual tangible goods, or the products of a service. Recently economists have reformulated the concept of demand to take account of the nontangible or nonproduct component of an item and of the fact that the demand for a particular good or service is in fact derived from a more basic demand for utility or satisfaction stemming from recognized needs. These reformulations have special significance for the area of health economics.

The traditional price/quantity relationship focuses on the price (direct cost) of the item. If the charge for a clinic visit is 3 dollars, that is often considered to be its cost. In reality, the cost of any good or service is composed of its price (direct cost) plus the cost of the time required and additional out-of-pocket expenses (indirect cost) to obtain the good or service.[6] The time and out-of-pocket components of obtaining many health care services are far from minimal. If a clinic visit entails a wait of, for example, two hours, and if the patient must miss work or forego other gainful activities, hire a babysitter, and bear large carfare expenditures, these costs should be included in the total cost of a clinic visit. The time component of indirect costs is designated as an *opportunity cost* to reflect that time is not a costless commodity. Its use in one endeavor entails sacrificing alternate opportunities.

Ignoring the important indirect costs of physician and clinic visits, and hospital stays could easily lead to erroneous demand projections. Free clinics are not free if crowded waiting rooms are part of the process of attaining health care and if babysitting fees and carfare must be incurred. Complete insurance coverage of hospital and physician charges does not result in free hospitalization as the individual is not compensated for his loss of time and out-of-pocket expenses associated with providing for a substitute to perform household responsibilities. The inclusion of indirect costs helps explain why the actual use of many health facilities is below the estimates of health planners, and why length of stay is inversely associated with income.[7]

Economists have also recently begun to view the demand for particular goods and services as derived from a more basic demand for the satisfaction of specified desires.[8] This view of demand theory has special relevance to the health field as consumer demand for physican visits, hospitalization, medication, etc. is

---

[6] For a rigorous and complete presentation of this reformulation of demand theory, which stresses the time costs entailed in purchasing and/or utilizing any good or service see, Becker, Gary S.: A theory of the allocation of time, *Economic Journal*, 75:493, 1965.

[7] The higher a person's income, the greater his opportunity costs (foregone earnings), and the higher the real cost of hospitalization. Even though no salary loss may accompany a hospitalization, higher income people feel that their *time is too valuable to be wasted* in a hospital bed.

[8] For a rigorous exposition of this view see, Lancaster, Kelvin J.: Change and innovations in the technology of consumption, *American Economic Review*, 56 (2) :14, 1966.

derived (stems) from a more basic demand for preventive and curative health care. Although the consumer (patient) may exercise little control over his utilization of physician time and hospital utilization, he does control his own entry into the health care system. He can choose whether to go to a physician or not. Once he chooses to go, his subsequent lack of control is partly due to his lack of knowledge and partly to legal arrangements surrounding hospital admission and the prescribing of medications.[9] Demand as perceived under this reformulation highlights a commonly ignored fact that it is a mistake to fail to recognize that the patient's (consumer's) basic demand for health care, in the vast majority of cases, is susceptible to price, income, and taste factors.

DEMAND VERSUS NEED

The health literature is replete with prestigious studies outlining the health needs of various population groups. The underlying philosophy of these studies derives from the respective authors' views that health care is a right not a privilege. Having explicitly or implicitly adopted this viewpoint, the authors present respected professional medical judgments as to the nature of the medical and other health related requirements of a given population base. These requirements are translated into projected needs by the application of fixed population/need ratios and public policy prescriptions are based on them.[10]

The estimates contained in such reports merit criticism on two counts: they assume a static production technique implying the absence of productivity increases which could lead to

[9] The prevailing arrangement in the health field which puts the physician in the position of being the consumer's contractor has definite implications on the financing of health care and on the inflation in health care costs. These issues will be analyzed in detail in Chapter Eleven.

[10] See for example, America's health status, needs, and resources, in President's Commission on the Health Needs of the Nation, *Building America's Health,* Volume II, Washington, D.C., U.S. Government Printing Office, 1953; and Report of the Surgeon General's Consultant Group on Medical Education: *Physicians For A Growing America,* Washington, D.C., U.S. Goverment Printing Office, 1959.

greater output from a given labor and captial input,[11] and they
confuse need with demand. In a limited number of instances
involving life or death, acute pain, or permanent disability, need
and demand may be synonymous. In the majority of medical
cases need and demand are two distinct concepts.

A gap between need and demand exists because the quantity
of care people want (in the sense of being willing to buy) and
the quantity of care professionals believe they should want rarely
coincide. Consumer ignorance and the different relative value
schemes of consumers-at-large and elite professional groups, account for part of this gap. The remaining divergence is attributed
to the fact that needs are perceived both absolutely and in a
climate devoid of economic reality while wants (demands) must
be backed up by economic ability. Those deciding needs are
usually so convinced of the absolute merit of the item under consideration that they fail to remember the basic economic fact of
life, the existence of limited resources. Consumers, who must
possess adequate resources (time and money or credit) to convert
potential demand into effective demand, cannot escape economic
reality. Whereas demand is influenced by prices, tastes, and income, need is invariant (it is represented by a demand curve
perpendicular to the quantity axis on a conventional demand
diagram, indicating the total absence of price effects).

Unless the target population group for whom the need is
projected possess both the ability and willingness to translate this
perceived need into effective demand, resources that are allocated
to health areas based on need alone will be underutilized.

Appendix—Price Elasticity of Demand Formulas

Price elasticity of demand (e) is calculated by the use of the
following formula:

$$e = \frac{\text{percentage change in quantity}}{\text{percentage change in price}}$$

$$= \frac{\text{change in quantity}}{\text{original quantity}} \div \frac{\text{change in price}}{\text{original price}}$$

[11] Refer to Chapter Six for a discussion of production techniques (production
functions) and productivity.

Substituting the symbol Δ for the term "change in," Q for quantity, and P for price, the price elasticity of demand formula can be written as: [12]

$$e = \frac{\Delta Q}{Q} \div \frac{\Delta P}{P}$$

or

$$e = \frac{\Delta Q}{\Delta P} \cdot \frac{P}{Q}$$

The price elasticity of demand coefficient can be calculated in one of two ways, depending on the data available. If an equation describing a demand schedule or curve is known, and one wants to calculate a price elasticity of demand coefficient at a given price-quantity combination, *point* price elasticity of demand is the appropriate measure. The formula for point price elasticity of demand (e_p) is:

$$e_p = \frac{dQ}{dP} \cdot \frac{P}{Q}$$

where d is a notation representing differentiation.[13] Given the following demand equation

$$Q = 200 - 20P$$

the point price elasticity of demand at any given price or quantity can be calculated. For example, at a quantity of 100 units, price elasticity of demand is 1.[14]

[12] As economic convention decrees that price elasticity of demand values be positive, a minus sign is introduced in the elasticity calculations, i.e. $e = -\frac{\Delta Q}{\Delta P} \cdot \frac{P}{Q}$. In the absence of such an adjustment the inverse relationship between price and quantity which is characteristic of demand would yield a negative price elasticity of demand value.

[13] Refer to Appendix I for a discussion of this mathematical concept.

[14] Solve for P: $100 = 200 - 20P$
$$-100 = -20P$$
$$-100/-20 = P$$
$$5 = P$$

Calculate $\frac{dQ}{dP}$: $\frac{dQ}{dP} = 0 + 1(-20)P^{1-1}$
$$= -20P^0$$
$$= -20(1)$$
$$= -20$$

→

If an equation for the demand curve or schedule is unknown, and one only has information on two price-quantity combinations, an *arc* price elasticity of demand coefficient can be calculated. The formula for calculating arc price elasticity of demand (e_a) is as follows:

$$e_a = \frac{\dfrac{\Delta Q}{\frac{1}{2}(Q_1 + Q_2)}}{\dfrac{\Delta P}{\frac{1}{2}(P_1 + P_2)}}$$

Considering the following two price-quantity combinations extracted from the hypothetical demand schedule:

Point	Price	Quantity
3	75	3
4	50	5

the arc price elasticity of demand is found to be 1.25, indicating an elastic demand relationship over this range.[15]

In calculating arc elasticities neither point 3 nor point 4 was used as the base from which a price and quantity change occurred. If point 3 were chosen, e_a would equal 2[16] and if point 4 were chosen, e_a would be 0.8.[17] This problem is overcome by using an average of these two points as the base.

Substitute values for $\dfrac{dQ}{dP}$, P, and Q into the formula:

$$e_p = -(-20) \cdot \frac{5}{100} = \frac{100}{100} = 1$$

[15] $\dfrac{-2}{\frac{1}{2}(3+5)} \div \dfrac{-25}{\frac{1}{2}(75+50)} = \dfrac{2}{4} \cdot \dfrac{62.5}{25} = 1.25$

[16] $e_a = \dfrac{-2}{3} \div \dfrac{-25}{75} = \dfrac{2}{3} \cdot \dfrac{3}{1} = 2$

[17] $e_a = \dfrac{-2}{5} \div \dfrac{25}{50} = \dfrac{2}{5} \cdot \dfrac{2}{1} = 0.8$

Chapter Five

DEMAND STUDIES

THE THEORY of demand developed in Chapter Four has wide applicability in the health field. Demand models have been used to explain and predict the utilization of health care facilities and services [1] and to isolate the major determinants affecting the demand for various health professionals.[2] The monograph excerpted here illustrates a conceptual and empirical approach to applying demand theory to research a question of crucial importance to both health administrators and planners: what are the determinants of hospital utilization (defined as the number of patient days per 1,000 population) and of two component elements of hospital utilization—the number of admissions per 1,000 population and average length of stay per admission.[3]

Gerald Rosenthal's monograph, *The Demand For General*

[1] See for example, Weisbrod, Burton: Anticipating the health needs of Americans: Some economic projections, *Annals of the American Academy of Political and Social Sciences, 337*:137, 1961; Feldstein, Paul: The demand for medical care, in Commission on the Cost of Medical Care, *General Report*, Vol. I, Chicago, American Medical Association, 1964; Rosenthal, Gerald: *The Demand for General Hospital Facilities*, Chicago, American Hospital Association, 1964; and Fuchs, Victor and Kramer, Marcia: Expenditures for Physicians' Services in the United States, 1948–1968, New York, National Bureau of Economic Research, (mimeo), 1971.

[2] See for example, Jones, Norman, *et al.*: Health manpower in 1975—Demand, supply, and price, in, *Report of the National Advisory Commission on Health Manpower*, Vol. II, Washington, D.C., U.S. Government Printing Office, 1967; and Fein, Rashi: *The Doctor Shortage: An Economic Analysis*, Washington, D.C., Brookings Institution, 1967.

[3] The current demand model and other demand for health care services models are often criticized for the use of utilization data as a proxy for demand. Utilization appears to be a market equilibrium datum since it is determined by the interaction of demand and supply forces. However, since pure demand data are nonexistent in published form, indicators of utilization are used as *second best* measures.

Hospital Facilities focuses on explaining and predicting the utilization of short-term general and special nonfederal hospital facilities. Whereas utilization estimates have frequently been based on a uniform bed-population ratio (such as 50 beds per 1,000 population), Rosenthal presents an alternate conceptual model based on conventional demand theory for estimating hospital utilization. Chapter Three of the monograph presents the analytical demand model and the scope of the study; Chapter Four lists the twelve explanatory variables used in the analysis and presents hypotheses on the direction of the relationships between each explanatory variable and the measures of utilization; and Chapter Five and Appendix C present and discuss the empirical results. The presentation in Chapter Four of the monograph is of particular interest as it illustrates both a sound methodological technique for choosing explanatory variables for any demand study and the difficulties of obtaining refined empirical measures for a given variable specification. Illustrative of the latter difficulty is the fact that the insurance variable had to be specified in a gross form (the per cent with coverage) rather than in a more refined manner (per cent with coverage adjusted for the scope of the coverage). As data sources are constantly improving, subsequent studies may not encounter similar specification problems.

Linear multiple regression analysis [4] is employed in Chapter Five of the monograph to test a demand model incorporating 2 price variables, 2 income variables, and 8 sociodemographic variables representing aspects of consumer tastes and preferences. The regression coefficients reported represent the *absolute* effect of a one-unit change in any independent variable on the dependent variable—utilization. For example, the coefficient of the price variable (charges for 2-bed room) with respect to patient days per 1,000 population in 1950 is found to be −30.99. Therefore a one *unit* change in price in 1950 led to a 30.99 *unit* decline in patient days per 1,000 population. [5]

The regression results reported in Appendix C of the mono-

---

[4] Refer to Appendix II for a discussion of this statistical technique.

[5] The units in terms of which each variable is specified often differ and must be kept in mind.

graph represent the percentage change in the dependent variable resulting from a 1 per cent change in any of the independent variables. These proportional rather than absolute relationships stem from a logarithmic transformation of the linear regression model.[6] As absolute numerical changes yield percentage changes when converted into logarithms, the logarithmic regression coefficients are also elasticity coefficients since elasticity is defined as the percentage change in one variable for a given percentage change in another variable. Thus the regression coefficient of the price variable in the 1950 logarithmic equation, −0.15, connotes that a 1 per cent change in price results in a 0.15 per cent decline in the number of patients per 1,000 population, and that the price elasticity of demand for one aspect of hospital utilization (number of patients per 1,000 population) is inelastic.

The utilization of the demand estimates in generating projections of short-term hospital utilization is the subject of the remainder of the Rosenthal monograph. The entire monograph deserves the serious attention of all those concerned with improving the efficiency of health delivery at both the administrative and policy levels.

* * *

THE DEMAND FOR GENERAL HOSPITAL FACILITIES [7]

GERALD D. ROSENTHAL

Chapter 3—The Analytical Model

The purpose of this section is to present a new set of estimates of utilization of hospital facilities which will not be subject to some of the difficulties inherent in previous techniques of estimation. These estimates will be derived from the analytical model described in this chapter.

---

[6] See Appendix II for a discussion of this type of transformation.

[7] Reprinted, with permission from Gerald D. Rosenthal: *The Demand For General Hospital Facilities*. Hospital Monograph Series No. 14, Chicago, American Hospital Association, 1964, Chapters 3–5 and pp. 94–95. Copyright © by the American Hospital Association, 1964.

The results of previous estimates of need took the form of numerically uniform bed-population ratios (e.g. 4.5 beds per 1000 population), which could be applied to a particular area with some adjustments for such specific area characteristics as occupancy rate or degree of urbanization. The estimates presented [8] were generated by a process that relates the specific characteristics of each area to its utilization of hospital facilities, without reference to an overall uniform bed-population standard.

SCOPE OF STUDY

For the purposes of this study, utilization will be defined as patient days per 1000 population in institutions classified by the American Hospital Association as short-term general and special nonfederal hospitals. The components of utilization—admissions per 1000 population and average length of stay per admission—will be examined separately. In the final section of the study [9] some of the implications of dealing with utilization in only a single type of hospital will be examined. The total area to be analyzed will be the continental United States, with each of the individual states representing a single unit of observation, with the exception of the District of Columbia, Maryland, and Virginia, which will be considered as a single unit.

The reason for aggregating these last-mentioned areas into a larger unit is worthy of some further discussion. Since one object of this section is to develop a relationship between particular characteristics of the states and the utilization of hospital facilities within the states, it is essential that the utilization attributed to the area reflect primarily the population residing within it. This assumption is obviously unsatisfactory for the area surrounding the District of Columbia. A very large proportion of those receiving care within the District reside in Maryland or Virginia. If this fact is ignored, then the high utilization of the District of Columbia would be attributed to a set of characteristics that did not really reflect the total population drawing on the facilities. With respect to some variables, the data can be misleading. For example, in 1960 the number of persons with some form of hospital insurance in the District of Columbia was 175.3 per cent of the total population. The obvious explanation for this statistic is

---

[8] *Editors' note:* This chapter of the monograph is not reproduced here as it is not directly related to the development of the demand model.

[9] *Editors' note:* See pages 82–91 of Rosenthal's monograph for this discussion.

that many persons who do not reside in the District purchase their insurance within that area.

This "border crossing" problem may also be of some significance with respect to the exchange between Rhode Island and Massachusetts or New York and New Jersey, but the proportion of total utilization attributable to "border crossers" in these states is small. In addition, "border crossing" may take place in both directions between these states, but most of the flow between Washington, D.C., and the two surrounding states is into the District.

For the level of aggregation chosen for this study, combining the District of Columbia with Maryland and Virginia avoids the major source of potential "border crossing" difficulty. It should be noted, however, that the significance of this problem increases as the level of aggregation diminishes. At the smallest political unit, the town, it is possible to find that a particular area will have no hospital facilities and therefore no utilization within its borders. This, quite obviously, would simply mean that whatever utilization had been generated by this area was recorded as consumed within some other area.

THE DEMAND MODEL

The demand model, which is expressed in the formula that follows, provides an analytical framework for estimating utilization for an area from a combination of sociodemographic and economic characteristics. In economic terms, what is desired is an estimate of the demand for hospital facilities in which tastes and preferences as well as price and income are specifically considered. It is assumed that the sociodemographic characteristics of an area reflect most of these tastes and preferences in some systematic way.

The criteria by which the adequacy of the model was measured were primarily those suggested by Theil, i.e. prediction, plausibility, and simplicity.

While the basic criterion for a model that is to be used for allocative or policy purposes is that it "predict" well, the use of this criterion is neither always conclusive nor always feasible. Inasmuch as most, if not all, of the observations are used in the estimation of the parameters, or measures of the true relationships, of the model, ". . . the econometrician is forced to retreat from the prediction criterion, and he can do no more than choose his model in such a way as to maximize the chance that it predicts well." The criteria for this subjective procedure are plausibility and simplicity, which are usually contradictory influences. While plausibility may lead to the inclusion of many variables, the end result may be a model too complicated for fruitful use. On the other hand, too simple a model may require implausible assumptions. The end result, therefore, is in the nature of a compromise.

The model which will be used to estimate the demand for hospital facilities is a least-squares linear multiple regression:

$$Y^i = a + b_1 x_1^i + \ldots + b_n x_n^i + e$$

Where: Y^i = utilization of hospital facilities in state area i,

x^i = characteristic variables of state area i (with subscripts designating specific variable)

a and b = parameters [10] of the demand relationship, and

e = some error variable.

The use of the least-squares model for the analysis of demand has been well justified by Wold. In particular, the nature of the hypothesized "causal" relationship must be understood. The use of this model is an implicit test of the hypothesis that the characteristic variables are related in a "causal" way to utilization in some systematic manner. If they are not so related, the results of the estimation process should yield values for the b's (the measures of the true relationships of the x variables to utilization) that do not differ significantly from zero. In this case, the end result would be the observation that Y equals a, which is tantamount to saying that a equals the mean value of the observed Y's.

In this respect, the process of estimation is twofold. First, the model is used to demonstrate to what extent and in what manner (positive or negative) each of the x, or independent, variables relates to utilization, the dependent variable.[11] If no particular association is found, the end product would be that fact, and, with respect to these variables, no differences in utilization would be anticipated among the states.

However, if the independent variables, or area characteristics, can be related to utilization in some systematic way, the next step is to use this relationship to calculate estimates of bed needs for each area. Such estimates, although derived identically, would specifically reflect the characteristics of each particular area. In simpler terms, if differences in characteristics are associated in some predictable way

---

[10] *Editors' note:* Refer to Appendix I for a definition of parameters.

[11] *Editors' note:* Refer to Appendix I for a definition of the terms independent and dependent variables.

with differences in utilization, then these associations can be used to calculate estimates of utilization from the characteristics.

If the relationship does hold, then it can be said that, for a given combination of characteristics, a particular utilization may be expected. This is a normative relationship in that it expresses the general relation between the specific characteristic variables and utilization. The degree to which factors exogenous to the model are associated with utilization are reflected in the error term in the formula, and in this analysis these errors will be considered deviations from the "normal" pattern described by the model.

Wold emphasizes that "as regards demand analysis, in particular, the regression analysis has to be directed by economic arguments . . . [and that] in each and every application the hypothesis of a causal dependence has to be indicated and supported by nonstatistical considerations." While the regression model is used here to describe an interrelationship, the inference-testing aspects of the technique must be acknowledged. The nonstatistical bases for selecting the variables used in this analysis will be presented in Chapter 4 of this section.

The use of a linear model merits some comment. Although theoretical considerations imply that the demand relationship is curvilinear, over any narrow range of observations the curve is slight and may be reasonably approximated by a linear model. In this case, the choice of the linear model seemed desirable for simplicity, and the empirical results show that the choice was satisfactory. (See Appendix C, which shows and discusses estimates based on a curvilinear model.)

In a sense, both of the two main purposes of regression analysis, to demonstrate causal relationships and to obtain forecasts, are of interest here. The major objective is to design a formula for allocation of hospital facilities in accordance with expected demand, and a model with better "predictive" ability will yield a better allocation. However, the regression estimates may also yield some insights into the relative impact of the particular variables included in the analysis—the extent to which utilization is "caused," in some sense, by the characteristics of the area in which it occurs.

SELECTION OF VARIABLES

One other source of difficulty must be acknowledged. Implicit in the process of selection of variables is the likelihood of imperfect specification: certain variables that are, in fact, related to the dependent variables are not specifically included in the model. In this study the selection of the particular variables to be used is, to some extent, arbitrary. The reasons for their selection must, therefore, be stated.

The decision as to which variables will be examined in any model is the resultant of two pressures. On the one hand, there are many variables that might affect the dependent variable and whose omission from the analysis yields some specification error. On the other hand, if one uses an unlimited number of variables, even if they are selected from a random digit table, ultimately the degree of association will be very high; however, the large number of variables would tend to make the estimation of the impact of any individual variable difficult. Therefore, as previously observed, any final model must be in the nature of a compromise.

In this study the particular variables were selected on the basis of their popularity in the literature. That is, the process of selecting variables was delegated to those who have been in this area of research over the years. Those attributes, of individuals or groups, that are generally considered to have an important effect on hospital utilization were included. It is nevertheless possible that variables that were omitted may actually be closely related to utilization. The present model represents a balance between the value that might result from an additional variable and the difficulties that accompany the inclusion of an excessive number of variables.

The next chapter in this section discusses the effect of the variables on the demand for hospital facilities.

REFERENCES

Theil, H.: *Economic Forecasts and Policy.* Voorburgwal, Amsterdam, North-Holland Publishing Co., 1961, Chapter 6.

Wold, H. and L. Jureen: *Demand Analysis.* New York, John Wiley and Sons, Inc., 1953, pp. 28–59.

Chapter 4—Factors Affecting Demand for Hospital Facilities

Before the specific variables are discussed, an important point must be raised. Much of the empirical evidence in previous studies suggesting that a particular variable is related to utilization, or "causal" in some sense, has been presented without specific acknowledgment that the association may arise from their joint association with some third variable. Although many published studies present data divided into groups of similar characteristics, thereby removing the influence of these characteristics within groups, attempts to account for the influence of unacknowledged variables have been rather limited. It is easy to see that estimates of utilization based on a single characteristic, or even on a few, may produce a good "fit" without actually explaining the relationship. In fact, the relationship observed may be the result not of a "causal" association between these variables but rather of their joint association with another variable which was not included in the model.

In the previous chapter it was emphasized that the nature of the regression technique, and indeed of all econometric models, makes it essential to select, on nonstatistical grounds, the factors that are related to utilization. This chapter will describe the factors to be used in the succeeding analysis. The criteria for selection of these variables were as follows: the frequency of their inclusion in the literature, and a logical expectation of association between each variable and utilization. This logical basis then becomes the hypothesis that the process of estimation tests.

In no case was a variable included solely on the basis that it "worked." Thus, variables were included that do not "help" the analysis in the statistical sense; that is, the empirical results would not be significantly different had the variables been excluded from the model. While there is a temptation to simplify statistically, the result of such simplification may be the creation of a statistical model that, although empirically satisfactory, may not yield the understanding of the relationships among these variables that is desired from the analysis.

It is important to ascertain which of the variables remain independently significant when other variables are also specifically acknowledged, and which of them cease to manifest any independent relationship under the same conditions. Previous research on this problem has taken one of two approaches. One major point of view is that all differences in utilization are directly related to level of income, and that the observed associations of insurance, education, race, and sometimes even age are really the result of their relation to the income variable. Those who subscribe to this viewpoint would maintain that the only "true" determinant of use is income level.

The other approach takes the position that the high degree of association between utilization and each of these other characteristics taken individually implies that there is some causal influence stemming from each of them. For example, the low utilization by nonwhites is taken to imply that there is something peculiar to "nonwhiteness" that causes low utilization, and the possibility that some other variable, not specifically considered, may be responsible for the observed association is not acknowledged.

The techniques that will be applied in this study permit estimation of the simple correlations between each variable and utilization. They also permit the estimation of the partial correlations [12] between utilization and each individual variable, which makes possible an assessment of the independent contribution of each variable to the total utilization. In cases in which the partial correlation is insignificant, the variable contributes little to the process of estimation. However, the development of that information is considered sufficiently important in itself to merit the inclusion of the variable.

Table 1, which follows, lists the dependent variables (measures of utilization) and the independent variables (sociodemographic and

TABLE 1

OBSERVED RANGES AMONG STATES AND THE MEAN FOR ALL STATES FOR VARIABLES INCLUDED IN ANALYSIS: 1950 AND 1960

	1950			1960		
Variables	*High*	*Mean*	*Low*	*High*	*Mean*	*Low*
Measures of Utilization:						
Patient days per 1000 population	1,202.8	870.5	434.4	1,333.7	950.9	657.0
Admissions per 1000 population	230.8	115.2	58.6	181.4	132.9	108.9
Average length of stay (days)	12.9	7.7	3.8	9.7	7.2	5.1
Sociodemographic Variables:						
Per cent over age 64	10.8	8.1	5.4	11.9	9.3	5.4
Per cent under age 15	34.8	28.2	22.6	38.0	32.0	27.6
Per cent of females married	73.3	66.7	58.6	72.2	66.5	62.5
Per cent male	53.9	49.4	47.9	52.2	49.0	47.5
Per cent urban	86.6	55.6	27.9	88.3	62.0	35.2
Per cent over 12 years education	21.0	13.6	8.3	25.2	16.7	11.0
Per cent nonwhite	45.4	9.8	0.1	42.3	10.0	0.2
Population per dwelling unit	4.0	3.4	3.0	3.8	3.3	3.0
Economic Variables:						
Charges for 2-bed room	$12.23	$8.12	$5.72	$24.30	$16.35	$9.70
Per cent over $5999 income	15.3	8.8	3.1	50.2	33.9	16.6
Per cent under $2000 income	72.5	41.5	26.1	45.9	24.9	14.8
Per cent hospital coverage	73.5	37.1	8.9	89.6	66.8	39.4

[12] *Editors' note:* Refer to Appendix II for a discussion of correlation and partial correlation.

economic characteristics) used in the analysis. For each variable, this table presents the observed ranges among the states, as well as the mean for all states. The remainder of this chapter will describe only the hypothesized association between the variables and utilization; the empirical results of the regression analysis will be discussed in Chapter 5.

THE SOCIODEMOGRAPHIC VARIABLES

Age Distribution

The influence of age on the utilization of hospital facilities has been the subject of much recent discussion. In general, the association between age and hospital utilization is a positive one: as individuals age, the likelihood of morbidity increases. The illnesses characteristic of older people are the chronic diseases. These are typically of longer duration and require more hospitalization than the acute diseases found more often among younger age groups. It was expected that this association would manifest itself at the state level of aggregation being considered here. The expectation was that areas with a higher proportion of older people would tend to have higher utilization. Conversely, it was expected that a lower utilization would be associated with a greater proportion of younger population.

There is no reason to expect this association to be uniform over all ages; that is, the relationship may not be linear. Since the incidence of hospitalizable morbidity is much lower among the very young (one to fifteen years of age) than among the middle age groups, the influences of higher proportions of younger people or of older people ought to be considered separately. For these reasons, the age factor will be divided into two variables: the proportion of population over sixty-four years of age and the proportion of population under fifteen years of age. This treatment of the age variable prevents the mistaken inference that two areas with identical proportions of population within one age group have identical age distributions. In dealing with the states as aggregate units, it is necessary to consider specifically the distribution by age within each state. For instance, it would be quite possible for two states to have the same median age, but one state might have the great bulk of its population in the twenty-to-fifty-five age group and the other most of its population in the over sixty-four and under twenty age groups. Unless the associations between utilization and the proportion of population in each of the extreme age groups offset one another, one would expect a different utilization in these two states, other things being equal. The median age measure would obscure this relationship, as would any measure that did not specifically consider those aspects of the age distribution hypothesized to be associated with hospital utilization.

Marital Status

Studies that have examined this characteristic conclude that there is a negative relationship between utilization and marriage. In Great Britain it has been reported that, proportionately, single, widowed, and divorced people used almost twice as much medical care as the married. In the United States, the results of the National Health Survey indicate that, although married people of both sexes account for more discharges in proportion to their numbers than do the other segments of the population, their average length of stay is shorter. The higher proportion of discharges for married females might be explained by maternity cases, but no such ready explanation is available for married males.

Thus it is believed that the aspect of utilization on which marital status has its greatest impact is length of stay, since persons without homes or families are likely to remain longer in the hospital. It may be that the household acts as a substitute facility, so that married persons can obtain more care without hospitalization. This conclusion is supported by the studies of the Saskatchewan Hospital Services Plan.

With regard to the model developed here, the expectation was that those areas with a greater proportion of married persons would have a lower utilization rate. The specific measure to be used is the proportion of females aged fourteen and over who are married. This eliminates the influence of sex distribution, which will be examined separately.

Sex Distribution

The relationship between sex distribution and utilization has been examined under many conditions. In general, the admissions rate for women tends to be higher during the child-bearing ages. This is offset, however, by the longer length of stay noted for males. Over the whole population, it would be expected that a higher proportion of males would result in a greater utilization of hospitals, although the association between admissions per one thousand population and proportion male might show a negative relationship. The measure to be used is the proportion of the population fourteen years old and over that is male.

Degree of Urbanization

The differences in utilization that have been observed with respect to the "ruralness" of an area were expected to emerge in this study. In general, the average length of stay in the hospital is significantly longer in less densely populated areas. This may reflect difficulty of traveling in those areas—for both patients and physicians—and a shortage of physicians in most rural areas. The travel difficulty tends to reduce the number of short stays and, at the same time, encourages a longer first stay for the purpose of avoiding additional trips to the hospital. The physician shortage in rural areas makes it necessary or at least desirable to centralize the location of patients and may result in increases in both length of stay and admissions rate.

The variable that will be used in this study is the proportion of population in each state residing in areas classed as urban by the United States Department of Commerce, Bureau of the Census. It was expected that the relationship between utilization and the proportion of population in urban areas would be positive if other characteristics were not considered. However, the experience in Saskatchewan suggests that, when other characteristics are specifically accounted for, the relationship is negative.

Distribution by Race

The relationship between race and hospital utilization is difficult to ascertain. There is much evidence to support the view that the incidence of disease among nonwhites in the United States is much higher than among whites; the mortality data also support this view. But the association of race with other variables, such as income level, education, and quality of housing, makes the estimation of the specific impact of race difficult. The variable to be used in this study is the proportion of population nonwhite. It was expected that, when the influence of other variables was removed, the higher morbidity among this group would be reflected in a positive relationship between "nonwhiteness" and utilization.

Educational Level

The observed association between educational level and utilization of hospital services reflects two relationships. The Health Information Foundation has observed a high degree of association between educational level, income level, and expenditures for health care. It is difficult to ascertain how much of the association between educational

level and expenditures for health care arises solely from the education factor. Considering hospitalized population only, other studies
have indicated a longer stay for those with less than nine years of
schooling, which more than offsets the lower admissions rate of this
group. This greater utilization by the less well-educated occurs in
spite of the fact that a higher level of education is associated with a
greater awareness of health needs, both preventive and curative.

It was believed that a simple estimate, by state, of median school
years would be unlikely to reveal the educational differences relevant
to utilization. Therefore, the variable used in this study is the proportion of population over twenty-five with thirteen or more years of
school. It was hoped by this means to distinguish between those states
with similar high school completion rates and differing post-high
school education rates. The influence of this variable on hospital
utilization could be in either the positive or the negative direction,
since the greater awareness of health needs tends toward both the prevention of illness and its early treatment.

Population per Dwelling Unit

This variable reflects the size of families in the state. At first it was
thought that this variable would provide a measure of the "degree of
crowdedness" of housing, but the data did not lend themselves to this
type of interpretation. The association between population per dwelling unit and utilization was expected to be similar to the relationship hypothesized for marital status. The existence of a greater number of multiperson family units not only offers alternative facilities
for the treatment of illness but also implies family responsibilities, and
may therefore act as a force tending to reduce length of stay and perhaps elective admissions as well. These factors led to the expectation
that a greater population per dwelling unit would be associated with
a lesser utilization of hospital facilities.

THE ECONOMIC VARIABLES

Price Variations

In general, the role of hospital charges in determining the utilization of hospitals has been ignored except in discussions relating to insurance, which is an implicit price variable. The nonprofit nature of
most of the general hospitals, coupled with the myth that all who
need hospital care will receive it, has precluded any serious examination of the effect of price on the demand for care. Despite this fact,

economic theory dictates the inclusion of price in any study of demand. It was presumed that, given taste and preferences (that is, after acknowledging the sociodemographic variables), the relationship between price and utilization would be negative. The price variable used will be the mean of the most frequent charges for a two-bed room.

Income Distribution

The relationship between income and hospital utilization has received a great deal of attention. Income, as mentioned earlier, is considered by many to be the greatest single determinant of the level of hospital utilization. It was noted in a recent study that one of the most significant characteristics of high-expenditure families (those spending over 300 dollars per year on medical care) was the high level of their annual income. These families were also characterized by a high level of education and greater than average health insurance coverage.

The implication is that there is a positive relationship between income level and hospital utilization. However, there is evidence that the opposite effect might well be considered. A number of studies have pointed out that public assistance recipients receive more medical care than the population as a whole. They also point out that, given identical diagnoses, the length of stay is longer in the ward than in private or semiprivate accommodations. This suggests that the income variable, like the age variable, should be treated in two segments to acknowledge the potential nonlinearity. The income variables will be the proportion of families and unrelated individuals with annual incomes over 5999 dollars and the proportion of families and unrelated individuals with annual incomes under 2000 dollars.

It was anticipated that the relationship between higher income and utilization would be positive while the relationship between lower income and utilization would be negative. However, if the old adage that only the very rich and the very poor get good medical care is true, both the relationships could be positive. If, as was anticipated, lowness of income is a real constraint on use, the states with the highest proportions of families and unrelated individuals with annual incomes under 2000 dollars would have the lowest utilization rates.

Proportion with Insurance

No other single characteristic related to hospital utilization has created the stir of discussion and controversy that has accompanied the growth of health insurance in the United States. There are those who attribute much of the increase in utilization to changes in demand generated by increasing insurance coverage, while others hold that insurance itself does not affect the utilization of hospitals. The latter groups argue that insurance is associated with income, education, and other variables which are themselves associated with utilization and that this fact accounts for the observed association between insurance and utilization.

The important aspect of insurance coverage that influences hospital utilization seems to be the scope of benefits. Comprehensive coverage, which effectively lowers the price of care to the cost of premiums, might be expected to have a strong influence on hospital utilization. However, if a policy pays only 12 dollars per day toward a four-day hospital bill of 300 dollars, the impact of the insurance will be much less. In general, it can be expected that, when the average benefits are reasonably broad, greater insurance enrollment will be associated positively with utilization. In addition, purchasers of insurance tend to be those who are more "medical care conscious" and those in higher income ranges.

When the coverage extends to out-patient benefits and other non-hospital services, there is some evidence that other types of care are substituted for hospitalization. If this were generally so, greater coverage might be associated with a lesser use of hospitals. However, this type of comprehensive coverage is provided by only a small fraction of the health insurance currently in effect. The prevailing type of coverage requires admission to the hospital with a specific preadmission diagnosis. For such admissions, more than 50 per cent of hospital bills are more than 50 per cent covered. It is, therefore, frequently to the patient's advantage to shift from out-patient and physicians' services to hospital in-patient care. In addition, it is believed exceedingly common for patients to be admitted actually for diagnostic work-up but with a specific illness or impairment recorded in order to bring the admission under the scope of the insurance.

In this study, hospitalization insurance is the only type of coverage that will be considered, and no differentiation by breadth of benefit coverage has been made. The measure used is the proportion of population covered by some type of hospital insurance. It was expected that states with a higher proportion of population covered by hospital insurance would have a higher utilization rate, though the relationship between insurance and other variables such as income might invalidate this association.

SUMMARY

It has been the object of this chapter to examine the variables that will be used to estimate the utilization of hospital facilities. In Chapter 5 the demand for hospital facilities will be estimated and the results of this process will be compared with the expectations outlined in this chapter. A procedure for translating demand into estimates of needed beds will be described and the estimates presented in Chapter 6.

REFERENCES

Falk, I. S. and Brewster, A. W.: Hospitalization insurance and hospital utilization among aged persons: March 1952 survey. *Soc. Secur. Bull.,* Nov. 1952.

Health Information Foundation: Use of health services by the aged. *Progress in Health Services,* April 1959.

Odoroff, M. E. and L. M. Abbe: Use of general hospitals: demographic and ecologic factors. *Pub. Health Reports, 72:*397–403, May 1957.

Shanas, E.: *Medical Care Among Those Aged 65 and Over.* Research Series No. 16, New York: Health Information Foundation, 1960.

U.S. Senate, Committee on Labor and Public Welfare: *The Aged and Aging in the United States: A National Problem.* A Report by the Subcommittee on Problems of the Aged and Aging to the Committee on Labor and Public Welfare. Washington, D.C., U.S. Government Printing Office, 1960.

Abel-Smith, B. and Titmuss, R. M.: *The Cost of the National Health Service in England and Wales.* Cambridge, Cambridge University Press, 1956.

Health Information Foundation. Health and the changing American family. *Progress in Health Services,* Sept. 1958.

Saskatchewan Hospital Services Plan: *Annual Report,* 1956, Saskatoon: Saskatchewan Department of Public Health, 1957, pp. 16–17.

Health Information Foundatiion: The changing pattern of hospital use. *Progress in Health Services,* May 1958.

Dickinson, F. G.: *Age and Sex Distribution of Hospital Patients.* Bureau of Medical Economics Bul. 97, Chicago, American Medical Association, 1955.

U.S. Public Health Service: *National Health Survey. Hospitalization: Patients Discharged from Short-Stay Hospitals, United States, July 1957—June 1958.* Public Health Service Pub. No. 584-B7, Washington, D.C., U.S. Department of Health, Education, and Welfare, 1958.

Roth, F. B., *et al.:* Some factors influencing hospital utilization in Saskatchewan. *Canad. J. Pub. Health, 46:*303–23, Aug. 1955.

Health Information Foundation: The health of the non-white population. *Progress in Health Services,* April 1958.

Health Information Foundation: Families with high expenditures for health. *Progress in Health Services,* Nov. 1960.

The Commonwealth Fund: *Health and Medical Care in New York City.* A report for the Special Research Project in the Health Insurance Plan of Greater New York, Cambridge, Harvard University Press, 1957.

Deasy, L. C.: Socio-economic status and participation in the poliomyelitis vaccine trial. *Sociological Studies of Health and Sickness,* Dorrian Apple (Ed.) New York, McGraw-Hill Book Co., Inc., 1960, pp. 15–25.

Koos, E. L.: Illness in regionville. *Sociological Studies of Health and Sickness, op. cit.,* pp. 9–14.

Health Information Foundation: Families with high expenditures for health. *Progress in Health Services,* Nov. 1960.

Roemer, M. I., *et al.:* Medical care for the indigent in Saskatchewan. *Canad. J. Pub. Health,* 45:460–70 Nov. 1954 and 502–8 Dec. 1954.

Anderson, O. W. and Feldman, J. J.: *Family Medical Costs and Voluntary Health Insurance: A Nationwide Survey.* New York, Blakiston Division of McGraw-Hill Book Co., Inc., 1956.

Densen, P. M., *et al.: Prepaid Medical Care and Hospital Utilization.* Hospital Monograph Series No. 3, Chicago, American Hospital Association, 1958.

Health Information Foundation: Families with high expenditures for health, *Progress in Health Services,* Nov. 1960.

U.S. Public Health Service. *National Health Survey. Proportion of Hospital Bill Paid by Insurance, Patients Discharged from Short-Stay Hospitals, United States July 1958—June 1960.* Public Health Service Pub. No. 584-B30, Washington, D.C., U.S. Dept. of Health, Education, and Welfare, Nov. 1961.

Health Information Foundation: Health insurance benefits and the American family. *Progress in Health Services.* Feb. 1957.

Roemer, M. I. and M. Shain: *Hospital Utilization Under Insurance.* Hospital Monograph Series No. 6, Chicago, American Hospital Association, 1959.

Chapter 5—The Parameters of Demand

In the preceding chapter, the relationships that might be expected between the demand for hospital facilities and area characteristics were stated; in this chapter the relationships found through the use of the demand model are presented. In addition to the total demand relationship (patient days per one thousand population, the dependent variable), the components of demand, admissions per one thousand and average length of stay, also dependent variables, were individually regressed against the same set of independent variables, the area sociodemographic and economic characteristics.

The estimates of the relationships between utilization of hospital facilities and the characteristics considered in the model are presented in Table 2 for 1950 and 1960. In terms of descriptive ability, the results indicate a high degree of association. The rather high corrected [13] multiple correlation coefficients shown in the table imply that

---

[13] *Editors' note:* A statistical correction was made to account for degrees of freedom. For a discussion of this statistical adjustment see Appendix II.

TABLE 2

DEMAND RELATIONSHIPS FOR 1950 AND 1960

Independent Variables	1950 Regression Coefficients and (Standard Errors)			1960 Regression Coefficients and (Standard Errors)		
	Patient Days per 1000 Population	Admissions per 1000 Population	Average Length of Stay	Patient Days per 1000 Population	Admissions per 1000 Population	Average Length of Stay
Constant	11,578.49	−514.40	115.57	110.14	186.49	−3.43
Charges for 2-bed room	− 30.99 (19.19)	0.63 (3.85)	−0.22 (0.17)	− 39.09 (8.72)	− 3.58 (1.06)	−0.12 (0.05)
Per cent over $5999 income	11.96 (19.95)	− 1.37 (4.00)	.03 (.17)	5.43 (5.79)	.21 (.70)	.02 (.03)
Per cent under $2000 income	− 21.22 (7.34)	− 1.94 (1.47)	− .06 (.06)	− 14.24 (6.82)	− 2.03 (.83)	− .02 (.04)
Per cent hospital coverage	− .76 (2.12)	.52 (.43)	− .03 (.02)	5.83 (2.13)	.34 (.26)	.03 (.01)
Per cent over age 64	− 41.07 (40.86)	12.04 (8.19)	−1.05 (.35)	22.83 (25.28)	1.26 (3.06)	.10 (.14)
Per cent under age 15	− 13.38 (23.50)	2.96 (4.71)	− .10 (.20)	23.69 (21.11)	6.48 (2.56)	− .18 (.11)
Per cent of females married	− 90.45 (19.41)	− 3.59 (3.89)	− .60 (.17)	− 84.44 (16.44)	− 7.52 (1.99)	− .25 (.09)
Per cent male	17.80 (32.80)	16.53 (6.57)	.37 (.28)	156.75 (33.69)	13.26 (4.08)	.54 (.18)
Per cent in urban areas	− 12.67 (3.79)	− .75 (.76)	− .04 (.03)	.31 (2.37)	.53 (.29)	.03 (.01)
Per cent over 12 years education	5.12 (12.16)	2.05 (2.44)	.14 (.10)	− 4.22 (8.01)	− .31 (.97)	− .01 (.04)
Per cent nonwhite	8.49 (4.20)	1.89 (.84)	− .03 (.04)	1.89 (3.36)	.19 (.41)	.01 (.02)
Population per dwelling unit	−1,166.33 (384.48)	−19.00 (77.05)	−8.22 (3.31)	−507.92 (321.52)	−91.89 (38.97)	1.03 (1.74)
Multiple correlation coefficient: R^2	.7971	.5473	.7358	.7708	.6885	.7900
R^2 corrected [a]	.7195	.3742	.6348	.6832	.5693	.7097

FORMULA: $\dfrac{\text{No. of observation units}}{\text{No. of observation units} - \text{No. of variables}} \times (1 - R^2) = \text{corrected } (1 - R^2); \ 1 - \text{corrected } (1 - R^2) = R^2 \text{ corrected}.$

the linear model does not entail much sacrifice in terms of "fit." [14] The 1960 multiple correlation coefficients for admissions and length of stay were higher than those for 1950; for both years the coefficient for length of stay was higher than for admissions. However, the reverse was observed for patient days per one thousand, which had a higher multiple correlation coefficient for 1950 than for 1960. These high coefficients for patient days, 0.72 for 1950 and 0.68 for 1960, suggest that the wide variations in utilization among the states are not a matter of accident, but rather reflect to a large extent the differences in the characteristics of the states.

This tends to confirm the original premise of this study, that these characteristics should be considered in the process of estimating demand, and provides some justification for the use of this model to develop estimates of bed needs. Such estimates of bed needs will be presented in Chapter 6. The remainder of this chapter will examine the association between each of the individual area characteristic variables and the various components of utilization or demand.

THE SOCIODEMOGRAPHIC VARIABLES

Age Distribution

Perhaps the most striking finding of the parameter estimation was the weak association of the age variables, particularly the proportion of the population over sixty-four years of age, with the utilization of short-term general and special hospitals.[15]

In 1950, the proportion of population under fifteen years of age showed no significant relationship to any of the utilization measures. The proportion over age sixty-four did display some relationship, but the direction of this relationship is difficult to explain. For example, with respect to patient days per one thousand population, the observed relationship was the reverse of that anticipated. When the other characteristics were held constant (see partial coefficient in

---

[14] A multiple correlation coefficient of 1.0, positive or negative, would mean "perfect" correlation, that is, *all* variation in utilization among the state units observed would have been accounted for by the area characteristic variables included in the analysis, a most improbable finding, of course.

[15] In all regression estimates, the 5 per cent level of significance was used; that is, the regression coefficient shows a significant causal relationship between the demand variable and the area characteristic variable if it is approximately two times its standard error. However, a variable is said to have some association to utilization if its coefficient is larger than its standard error.

Table 3), a greater proportion over age sixty-four was associated with a lesser utilization in terms of patient days and length of stay. However, this age variable showed a positive relationship with the admissions rate.

No significant association is noted in the 1960 relationships, but

TABLE 3

CORRELATIONS BETWEEN UTILIZATION OF HOSPITAL FACILITIES AND SOCIODEMOGRAPHIC AND ECONOMIC VARIABLES: 1950 AND 1960

Variables	1950 Correlation Coefficients		1960 Correlation Coefficients	
	Raw	Partial	Raw	Partial
Patients Days per 1000 Population				
Charges for 2-bed room	.4159	−.2669	.2282	−.6094
Per cent over $5999 income	.5589	.1022	.2466	.1588
Per cent under $2000 income	−.6514	−.4444	−.3683	−.3373
Per cent hospital coverage	.4229	−.0617	.6339	.4244
Per cent over age 64	.5258	−.1699	.4487	.1530
Per cent under age 15	−.6324	.0972	−.4133	.1890
Per cent of females married	−.2000	−.6244	−.2800	−.6609
Per cent male	.1324	.0926	.0180	.6237
Per cent urban	.3751	−.4970	.0522	−.0226
Per cent over 12 years education	.4259	.0720	−.0176	−.0900
Per cent nonwhite	−.6004	.3277	−.4686	.0963
Population per dwelling unit	−.5630	−.4615	−.3284	−.2615
Admissions per 1000 Population				
Charges for 2-bed room	.0788	.0280	−.0891	−.5019
Per cent over $5999 income	.2059	−.0588	−.0280	.0514
Per cent under $2000 income	−.3100	−.2210	−.1488	−.3878
Per cent hospital coverage	−.0194	.2038	.1573	.2178
Per cent over age 64	.1841	.2446	.2131	.0706
Per cent under age 15	−.0897	.1071	.0962	.3985
Per cent of females married	.2707	−.1563	.1443	−.5431
Per cent male	.5186	.3960	.3976	.4866
Per cent urban	−.1162	−.1660	−.3533	−.3008
Per cent over 12 years education	.4522	.1426	.1487	−.0553
Per cent nonwhite	−.3619	.3590	−.4139	.0808
Population per dwelling unit	−.3195	−.0423	−.0947	−.3749
Average Length of Stay				
Charges for 2-bed room	.4950	−.2194	.4413	−.3867
Per cent over $5999 income	.4723	.0310	.4214	.0984
Per cent under $2000 income	−.4882	−.1840	−.4234	−.1024
Per cent hospital coverage	.6010	−.2445	.7498	.4078
Per cent over age 64	.4162	−.4554	.3818	.1190
Per cent under age 15	−.7050	−.0853	−.6950	−.2651
Per cent of females married	−.5556	−.5279	−.5074	−.4296
Per cent male	−.3682	−.2214	−.4055	.4563
Per cent urban	.6442	−.1916	.4765	.3623
Per cent over 12 years education	.0111	−.2219	−.1411	−.0528
Per cent nonwhite	−.3581	−.1548	−.2487	.0988
Population per dwelling unit	−.3490	−.3923	−.3909	.1010

the direction of influence is positive, an observation more in line with expectations.

The implication of the findings is underlined by the observation, shown in Table 3, that in both years the raw correlation between population over age sixty-four and patient days per one thousand was positive, 0.53 in 1950 and 0.45 in 1960. This indicates that those states with higher proportions of population over age sixty-four also tended to be the states with the higher utilization. However, when the other variables being examined are held constant, as shown in the partial coefficients in Table 3, the correlations between patient days per one thousand and proportions of population over age sixty-four were as follows: 0.17 for 1950 and 0.15 for 1960. In both years the association manifested between these variables tends to be greatly reduced when the levels of the other variables are specifically considered.

The association between the proportion of population under fifteen years of age and patient days per one thousand is also reduced greatly when the other variables are held constant. In 1950 the raw correlation was as follows: 0.63 and the partial correlation was 0.10; in 1960 the raw and partial correlations were as follows: 0.41 and 0.19 respectively.

The findings do not necessarily mean that utilization does not increase as people age. It is possible, for example, that areas with a higher proportion of population in the older age groups may also be areas with a high number of alternative facilities such as nursing homes and long-term chronic disease hospitals, and that a lower utilization of general and special short-term hospital facilities conceals an overall higher utilization of all medical care facilities by the older age groups. It is also possible that a positive relationship, if it does indeed exist, might be found at a different level of aggregation, that is, if the Public Health Service areas, rather than the states, had been the geographic units observed.

With respect to the development of estimates of utilization that will distinguish among the states on the basis of area characteristics, the fact that the age variable showed no strong differentiating impact was in itself of importance. The lack of independent relationship between either of the age variables and utilization leads to the conclusion that, at the state level of aggregation used in this study, the factor of age does not prove as relevant to policy formation as expected, *provided all of the other area characteristics are explicitly considered.*

Sex Distribution

The sex variable, the proportion of the population over age fourteen who are male, showed little association with utilization in 1950 or 1960. The raw correlations with patient days (Table 3) were estimated as 0.13 in 1950 and 0.02 in 1960. In 1950 there was little change when the levels of the other variables were held constant, and the regression coefficient (Table 2) was about one-half its standard error. In 1960, however, there was a significant change; the partial correlation rose to 0.62, and the regression coefficient was almost five times its standard error.

Although the direction of influence of the proportion of males is as anticipated in both years, the results are particularly striking for 1960. One aspect of this variable which differs from expectation is the strong positive relationship between proportion of males and the admissions rate. Other studies, made on a less aggregated level, imply that, while males use more hospital facilities, the impact is felt in length of stay rather than in the admissions rate, which is generally higher for women. At the state level of aggregation used in this study, this does not show up; indeed, the 1950 results, while not significant, present the reverse picture, showing positive association between the proportion of males and the admissions rate and a negative association between the proportion of males and length of stay.

Marital Status

The relationship between marriage and utilization of hospital facilities was, in all cases and for all types of utilization, negative; and, with the exception of the 1950 admissions rate, it was significantly so. This conforms to the behavior of the persons-per-dwelling-unit variable. In both cases the explanation is that being married and having a family involve both unavoidable responsibilities at home and the existence of a place other than the hospital where care can be received. The fact that both of these influences show up at the state level of aggregation suggests that if other facilities were available, such as home care, convalescent homes, and so on, there might be a substitution of these other types of facilities for hospitalization. The association between each of these two variables and utilization is reflected mainly in length of stay, which supports the hypothesis stated above. In 1960, however, the relationship between length of stay and population per dwelling unit was positive, though not significant.

Degree of Urbanization

In 1950 the proportion of population living in urban areas was negatively associated to a significant degree with patient days per one thousand, but there was no significant relationship with either admissions rate or length of stay. In 1960 there was no significant relationship between the urban variable and patient days per one thousand, but a positive relationship was found with length of stay and a negative one with admissions.

Part of the explanation for this difference may lie in the changing distribution of facilities and incomes within nonurban areas. The reasons supporting the hypothesized greater utilization of hospital facilities in rural areas concern the relative shortage of doctors and the large amount of travel time involved in making house calls or getting patients to the hospital. It is possible that the difficulty of getting to the hospital encourages the use of the hospital for preventive care in that some patients may be directed to the hospital prior to examination. In addition, patients may be kept longer in the hospital to conserve the scarce time of the physician and to minimize patients' travel. If this is so, it may be that the improvement in distribution of facilities as well as improved transportation has made these factors less important over the ten-year period.

Distribution by Race

The impact of the nonwhite proportion of the population on utilization was positive in both 1950 and 1960, but was significant only in 1950. It is notable that the relationship is positive, since the characteristic of nonwhiteness is so highly correlated with other characteristics that are associated negatively with utilization (e.g. income and educational level). Other studies, which do not utilize actual examinations of individuals for morbidity information, find that nonwhites tend to use fewer services in all areas of medical care. If income levels are held constant, however, this is less evident. The relationship implied by the positive associations developed here is consistent with existing mortality and morbidity information, even though the raw correlations (Table 3) between patient days and proportion of population nonwhite were −0.60 and −0.47 for 1950 and 1960 respectively.

Educational Level

The influence of educational levels on utilization was not significant in either year. In 1950 the raw correlation between patient days and educational level was 0.43, but in 1960 even the raw correlation, −0.02, was not significant. The independent impact on utilization generated by educational levels is rather small at the state level of aggregation. The recent popularization of medical care problems and issues may have reduced the influence of the educational level on utilization of medical services.

THE ECONOMIC VARIABLES

Income Distribution

The income variable manifested much the same relationship in both years under study. The constraining impact of a higher proportion of families with low incomes was significant in both years, the partial correlations with patient days being −0.44 and −0.34 for 1950 and 1960. Although the proportion of high incomes was positively associated with utilization, it was not significant in either year. This may imply that, once beyond the constraining range of incomes, the demand for hospital facilities is not so income-elastic as has been supposed. For the most part, the behavior of the income variables conforms to the expectations discussed in Chapter 4 and is much the same in the two periods examined.

Price Variations

The price variable is consistent with the economist's expectations in that it exhibits a negative influence on utilization in the estimates of the demand relationship. The regression coefficient was not significant in 1950, even though it was 1.6 times greater than its standard error (significant at approximately the 10 per cent level, though not at the 5 per cent level). In 1960, however, the price coefficient was significant for all three utilization measures at less than the 1 per cent level. This increase in the influence of price as a factor in utilization may be the reflection of two changes during the decade: higher family incomes and increases in insurance coverage, both of which had the effect of increasing the element of choice in utilization.

Although the influence of incomes did not change, the level of incomes over all observations was higher (Table 1). This observation, together with the fact that the admissions rate was higher over all states, implies that a greater number of individual "stays" were purchased. If there were no significant changes in the incidence of morbidity, then it would seem reasonable to assume that at least part of this increase in purchases reflects a higher qualitative level of consumption, encompassing proportionately more elective services for which the price elasticity of demand is presumably greater. In other words, a decrease in the proportions of admissions that are nonelective implies that in 1960 there was a greater element of choice in the market for medical services of all kinds, and particularly for hospital services.

The second change, increase in insurance coverage both in the number of individuals covered and in the scope of benefits, had a similar effect. Insurance benefits, by paying a portion of the costs for essential hospital services, frees a larger proportion of consumer income to pay for elective services.

Proportion with Insurance

The insurance variable, which is a pseudo-price variable, shows much the same type of behavior as does the price variable, but in the opposite direction. In 1960 the independent impact of insurance coverage was significant and positive. In 1950, however, the association between utilization and the proportion of population covered by hospital insurance was negligible when the other variables were held constant, the partial correlation being -0.06. The explanation suggested for this difference in impact is that the insurance variable meant different things in 1950 and 1960. The scope of benefits was rather limited in 1950, and it is likely that the amount of benefits did not affect the real price of hospital facilities enough to influence the decision of the consumer significantly. By 1960, however, both the coverage and the scope of benefits were much broader, and in many cases insurance paid significant proportions of the total bill.

The increase in coverage would probably consist largely of benefits for nonelective hospital services, in the consumption of which there is the least element of choice. The increase in insurance coverage may feed back to the impact of price on utilization by placing an element of choice (with respect to the timing of expenditures) on nonelective admissions. The ability to prepay enables the consumer to transfer a greater proportion of out-of-pocket (noninsured) purchases into the realm of choice.

"STRUCTURAL" CHANGE OVER TIME

Once the behavior of each of the variables had been related to the two time periods for which estimations were made, it seemed desirable to estimate the significance of the difference between the two demand relationships as entities. A dummy time variable,[16] which took a value

---

[16] *Editors' note:* Refer to Appendix II for a discussion of dummy variables.

of 0 for 1950 observations and a value of 1 for 1960 observations, was added to the original twelve independent variables. The total observations for both years were pooled and a new relationship was estimated, with the three utilization factors as the dependent variables and the twelve original variables, plus the time variable, as independent variables. The results of this estimation are presented in Table 4, which shows that the multiple correlation was quite

TABLE 4

DEMAND RELATIONSHIPS FOR POOLED OBSERVATIONS,
1950 AND 1960 COMBINED

Independent Variables	Regression Coefficients and (Standard Errors)		
	Patients Days per 1000 Population	Admissions per 1000 Population	Average Length of Stay
Constant	5,090.24	−79.00	44.35
Charges for 2-bed room	− 30.70 (7.64)	− 2.09 (1.20)	−0.13 (0.06)
Per cent over $5999 income	12.26 (3.78)	.57 (.59)	.05 (.03)
Per cent under $2000 income	− 12.00 (3.53)	− 1.54 (.55)	− .00 (.03)
Per cent hospital coverage	2.12 (1.46)	.41 (.23)	.00 (.01)
Per cent over age 64	5.48 (21.78)	5.62 (3.41)	− .30 (.16)
Per cent under age 15	18.19 (14.71)	4.68 (2.30)	− .14 (.11)
Per cent females married	− 75.43 (12.05)	− 5.16 (1.89)	− .35 (.09)
Per cent male	72.28 (22.53)	12.98 (3.53)	.05 (.16)
Per cent in urban areas	− 6.30 (1.94)	− .74 (.30)	.00 (.01)
Per cent over 12 years education	3.25 (6.89)	.81 (1.08)	− .03 (.05)
Per cent nonwhite	3.74 (2.50)	.94 (.39)	− .03 (.02)
Population per dwelling unit	−726.67 (227.41)	−57.99 (35.61)	−2.36 (1.64)
Time period	−322.50 (119.86)	−39.80 (18.77)	−0.07 (0.87)
Multiple correlation coefficients:			
R^2	.7220	.5896	.6910
R corrected	.6734	.5178	.6381

high. The "time period" regression coefficients show that both the relationships for patient days and admissions per one thousand population displayed a significant difference with respect to time. It is also noteworthy that there was no significant difference in the length-of-stay relationships between the two periods.

The most interesting aspect of these relationships is the negative coefficient for the time period. This means that, for any given set of characteristics, there would have been a lesser utilization in 1960 than in 1950. It follows, therefore, that the increases in utilization noted over the ten-year period resulted from changes in overall social, demographic, and economic characteristics in the United States, rather than from an increasing propensity to consume hospital services at a given level of these variables. In economic terms, a different demand relationship may exist for every combination of tastes and preferences. For any given combination, it might be inferred that there was a downward shift in this demand relationship during the decade.

SUMMARY

It might be said that the impact of the economic variables on utilization of hospital services was such that the role of consumer choice was significantly greater in 1960 than it had been in 1950. It is suggested that this is the result of rising levels of living, as well as the greater availability of both services and methods of obtaining these services. The increased share of disposable income spent on services of all kinds as income levels rise plays a significant part in this process. As consumption of medical services of all kinds encompasses a greater proportion of elective services, one would expect greater price elasticity with respect to alternative expenditures. The decision between a summer vacation and cosmetic surgery presents the traditional elements of a problem in consumer choice, but an emergency hospital service will inevitably result in changes in the allocation of the balance of the consumer budget.

The noneconomic variables also show a marked response to alternatives, since the variables which are most significant relate to family and marital status. As previously mentioned, a household with more than one responsible adult presents an alternative to hospitalization. In the final chapter of this section some of the implications of alternative facilities, either in the home or elsewhere, are discussed.

REFERENCES

Health Information Foundation: Health insurance benefits and the American family. *Progress in Health Services,* Feb. 1957.

U.S. Public Health Service: *National Health Survey: Proportion of Hospital Bill Paid by Insurance.* Public Health Service Pub. No. 584-B30, Washington, D.C., U.S. Dept. of Health, Education, and Welfare, 1961.

Appendix C—A Curvilinear Model of Demand

The assumption of linearity which is implicit in the model presented in the text has certain theoretical drawbacks.[17] It has been

---

[17] Wold, H. and Juréen, L.: *Demand Analysis.* New York, John Wiley and Sons, Inc., 1953, p. 3.

APPENDIX TABLE 1
DEMAND RELATIONSHIPS BASED ON A CURVILINEAR MODEL: 1950 AND 1960

Independent Variables	1950 Regression Coefficients and (Standard Errors)			1960 Regression Coefficients and (Standard Errors)		
	Patient Days per 1000 Population	Admissions per 1000 Population	Average Length of Stay	Patient Days per 1000 Population	Admissions per 1000 Population	Average Length of Stay
Constant	35.6894	−17.6255	53.2982	−0.0977	1.3479	−0.9473
Charges for 2-bed room	−0.15 (0.23)	0.34 (0.31)	−0.49 (0.20)	−0.65 (0.18)	−0.46 (0.14)	−0.22 (0.12)
Per cent over $5999 income	.28 (.26)	.22 (.34)	.06 (.22)	.33 (.30)	.15 (.24)	.22 (.21)
Per cent under $2000 income	− .55 (.41)	.23 (.58)	− .78 (.36)	− .25 (.24)	− .27 (.19)	.04 (.17)
Per cent hospital coverage	.09 (.09)	.22 (.11)	− .13 (.07)	.39 (.16)	.17 (.13)	.23 (.11)
Per cent over age 64	− .12 (.44)	.81 (.58)	− .93 (.38)	.21 (.22)	.09 (.17)	.10 (.15)
Per cent under age 15	.81 (.90)	.85 (.18)	− .04 (.78)	.57 (.84)	1.54 (.66)	− .99 (.58)
Per cent of females married	−5.52 (1.74)	− .15 (2.29)	−5.36 (1.52)	−5.27 (1.23)	−3.13 (.97)	−2.25 (.85)
Per cent male	.12 (2.27)	3.94 (2.98)	−3.83 (1.97)	7.36 (1.89)	3.99 (1.49)	3.35 (1.31)
Per cent in urban areas	− .73 (.25)	− .31 (.33)	− .42 (.22)	− .05 (.18)	− .19 (.14)	.14 (.13)
Per cent over 12 years education	.18 (.24)	.34 (.31)	− .16 (.21)	− .08 (.15)	− .05 (.12)	− .01 (.11)
Per cent nonwhite	.03 (.04)	.02 (.05)	.00 (.04)	.00 (.03)	− .01 (.02)	.01 (.02)
Population per dwelling unit	−3.93 (1.80)	.56 (2.36)	−4.49 (1.56)	−1.46 (1.18)	−2.09 (0.93)	0.63 (0.82)
Multiple correlation coefficient:						
R^2	.7643	.4826	.7212	.7242	.6638	.7570
R^2 corrected	.6742	.2847	.6146	.6187	.5214	.6641

noted earlier that the theoretical relationship between demand and at least some of the variables which affect it, i.e. price and income, is primarily a nonlinear one. Although it was decided that a linear approximation was sufficient for the purposes of this paper, an alternative nonlinear model was also estimated. The particular model was a curvilinear multiple regression which was obtained by estimating a linear relationship between the logarithm of utilization and the logarithms of the independent variables used in the previous estimates. The estimating model is as follows:

$$\log Y = \log a + b_1 \log x_1 + b_2 \log x_2 + \cdots + b_{12} \log x_{12} + e$$

where the variables are identical to the original model. This yields a curvilinear relationship where

$$Y = a x_1^{b_1} x_2^{b_2} \ldots x_{12}^{b_{12}}$$

The results of this estimation are presented in Appendix Table 1.

In general, the results from the two models do not differ significantly. Most significant is the fact that the nonlinear model does not show as strong an influence with respect to the constraining effect of a greater proportion of low incomes. In addition, the influence attributed to insurance coverage in 1950 was greater in the nonlinear model than in the linear model. However, there do not seem to be any clear-cut grounds for preferring one model over the other for the purposes of this study.

Chapter Six

PRODUCTION AND COST

P RODUCTION is one of the basic and essential activities of any economic system. Without it, all economic activity, and even life itself would cease. Even water (commonly viewed as a gift of nature) is produced, in that it must be located, possibly purified, and transported from its origin to its place of ultimate use, activities that entail elements of production.

Although production theory is usually conceived of as being part of the body of managerial knowledge aimed at achieving maximum profit for any enterprise, it is equally applicable to that sector of the economy that is not profit oriented. The absence of a profit motive does not eliminate the need to economize, as all endeavors are confronted with the basic economic fact of life, the scarcity of resources. By maximizing the efficiency of any productive process, more goods or services can be provided with a given set of resources, or the same output can be achieved at lower cost. Both of these options, greater output and lower costs, are of concern to members of the health team responsible for the provision of health care.

This chapter presents an overview of the productive process, an economic schema for analyzing production including a discussion of two economic concepts associated with production, diminishing returns and economies of scale, and a brief derivation of cost curves. Differential calculus and linear programming are introduced in their simplistic form and reviewed as means of applying production theory to concrete problem areas. (In all cases the mathematical presentations follow a diagrammatic exposition of the concept; the reader who chooses to can omit these sections without jeopardizing his understanding of the material in the remainder of the chapter) .

101

THE PRODUCTION PROCESS

The production process involves the use and combination of various *inputs* to produce a desired *output*. The output can be a good or service, a final product or an intermediate product that will be used in the subsequent production of another item. Economists traditionally classify production inputs into three categories: *land, labor,* and *capital.* These three input categories are also known as the three *factors of production.* To facilitate quantitative discussions of production, the various productive inputs are often expressed in dollar terms; the dollar value used being determined by the prevailing actual or imputed "shadow" price for each input. Although a monetary measure is often an imperfect estimate of an input's true value, because it may be distorted by various institutional factors such as monopoly control leading to price fixing (for example, unionization), it is the easiest obtainable and only universally understood common denominator of economic activity.

Land represents all the natural resources used in production. Its remuneration is called *rent.* Labor represents the effort of man, and includes all categories of human input ranging from unskilled effort to that of the most highly trained individual. The labor category can be defined to encompass not only those people employed in the actual productive process but also the person or persons responsible for the development and/or adaptation of the particular productive process. Labor's share in the proceeds of production are *wages* or *salaries,* and *profit* (if the developer or innovator is included in the labor category). Capital represents the physical inputs such as machines, tools, and fixtures. Monetary assets are also referred to as capital since money represents the command over physical capital in the sense that with money one can buy machines. Consequently, the term capital as used in this chapter will represent either the physical or the monetary types.[1] Capital's remuneration is designated as *in-*

[1] A recent use of the term capital, human capital, refers to the investment embodied in individuals. It is the human component which, together with ability, differentiates skilled from unskilled labor. This concept of human capital will be further elaborated upon in Chapter Eight.

terest. It is not uncommon for any individual engaged in the productive process to contribute more than one type of input. A person may own land, contribute his labor, and also own machinery, tools, or fixtures. In such a case, his remuneration for participating in the productive process includes rent, wages or salaries, and profits.

The presentation of production theory in the following sections focuses on three basic production assignments: a) produce a desired output level (one good or service) with a minimum of input cost, b) produce a maximum level of output (one good or service) with a fixed input budget, and c) produce a maximum combination of outputs (two or more goods or services) subject to specified input limitations. The analysis of the first two assignments will be based on the concept of production functions, while analysis of the third assignment will draw upon the concept of transformation curves. Before turning to these elements of production theory a discussion of the problem of applying production theory to health care issues is warranted.

Within the health field, researchers have had relatively little difficulty in identifying and quantifying the various productive inputs. No uniformly acceptable measure has been advanced for identifying and quantifying output—the maintenance or improvement of health. Indices of morbidity or mortality are usually used to represent health, but many students of the health field are dissatisfied with these statistics as they are currently constructed or used.[2] Within the medical sector of the health field there is even less agreement on a proxy measure for the output of medical care. While measures of physician and hospital care have been employed,[3] there is almost universal agreement among health officials on the need for a more representative measure for the output of medical care. Although output measures of health and medical care are recognizably imperfect, this

[2] For a discussion of the problems involved in constructing a health index, see Sullivan, Daniel F.: *Conceptual Problems in Developing an Index of Health.* Public Health Service Publication No. 1000, Series 2, No. 17. Washington, D.C., U.S. Government Printing Office, 1966.

[3] These measures are, in actuality, inputs into the medical process rather than outputs. Their use as output proxies can be rationalized as a "second best" solution.

imperfection does not negate the value of a knowledge of production theory as a guide to conceptualizing productive behavior.

PRODUCTION FUNCTIONS

The output generated by the combination of inputs to produce output is governed by technological relationships. Engineering studies design the various alternate ways the different inputs can be combined to produce output. These engineering relationships are summarized in mathematical notation as follows:

$$Q = f(X_1, X_2, X_3) \tag{1}$$

where Q represents output, and X_1, X_2, X_3, inputs.[4] The relationship represented by equation (1) is called a *production function;* it denotes that the amount of production (output) is related in a functional manner to the various inputs.[5]

Equation (1) contains a generalized version of a production function; an example of a more specific production function is the following:

$$Q = 2X_1 + 5X_2 + 9X_3 \tag{2}$$

Whereas equation (1) reveals that output is only dependent on X_1, X_2, and X_3, it does not disclose the precise nature of the dependence. Equation (2) specifies the functional dependence; it states that the combination of 2 units of X_1, 5 units of X_2, and 9 units of X_3 results in the production of 1 unit of output, Q.

Although a number of production techniques may exist for producing any specified output, the choice among alternate production technologies is dictated by their relative cost and prevailing institutional and legal arrangements specifying the various factors that must be employed. Whatever the prevailing institutional environment, the method by which the good or serv-

---

[4] Although three inputs are specified in the above illustration to correspond to the three major input categories (land, labor, and capital) the number of inputs in any production process can range from one to a very high number, the range being determined by technological factors and the refinement used in designating any input. For example, all types of labor can be included in a broad labor category or subdivided into a number of categories by function and/or skill level.

[5] Refer to Appendix I for a discussion of functional relationships.

ice is generated can be summarized into a production function. Assume that the following production function represents a given health related activity

$$Q = 50C^{\frac{1}{2}}L^{\frac{1}{2}} \tag{3}$$

where C represents a capital input and L a labor input.[6] Table XVIII and Figure 6 illustrate the properties of this production function.

TABLE XVIII

SELECTED OUTPUT VALUES [1] FOR
PRODUCTION FUNCTION $Q = 50C^{1/2}L^{1/2}$

CAPITAL UNITS									
5	112	158	194	224	250	274	296	316
4	100	141	173	200	224	245	265	283
3	87	123	150	173	194	212	229	245
2	71	100	123	141	158	173	187	200
1	50	71	87	100	112	123	132	141
	1	2	3	4	5	6	7	8

LABOR UNITS

[1] Rounded to the nearest whole integer.

The series of curves shown in Figure 6 are known as *isoquants*. An isoquant is a line of equal quantities. In the context of production, it is a line (curve) representing various combinations of inputs each of which yield the same amount of output. Referring to Table XVIII and Figure 6 it is seen that an isoquant representing 100 units of output passes through the following points: 4 capital units and 1 labor unit; 2 capital units and 2 labor units; and 1 labor unit and 4 capital units. On a theoretical level it can be surmised that any capital-labor combination represented by a point on that isoquant would also yield 100 units of output.[7] It can be further seen that isoquants further from the origin represent greater output; isoquants closer to the origin, less output.

Efficiency in production is defined either as the achievement of a specified output at minimum cost or as producing the maximum

[6] Although actual production functions would require a much more complex formulation, a two input model is chosen to simplify the ensuing pedagogical and geometric presentation.

[7] This presentation assumes that the production inputs are fully substitutable for each other. In reality this is not usually the case. Consequently, actual isoquant curves would not be as smooth as those in Figure 6.

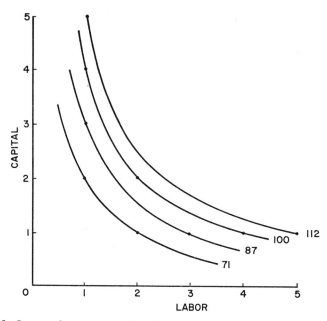

Figure 6. Geometric representation of selected values of production function
$Q = 50C^{1/2}L^{1/2}$.

output given a specified budget level. Production functions and
their diagrammatic representation, isoquants, do not provide sufficient information for the choice of the efficient method of production as they embody only technological data on possible output levels. Additional information representing the cost (prices)
of the various inputs are required. By including cost factors in
production considerations and by comparing the cost and technological aspects of input (factor) substitution, the optimal production point is determinable either geometrically through the
ascertainment of a tangency solution or mathematically through
the use of the tools of calculus. The following examples diagrammatically illustrate the attainment of productive efficiency.

From a technological viewpoint, the substitutability of inputs
in the production process is derivable from an isoquant map.
That is, the points on an isoquant map indicate the various combinations of the factors of production which will yield a designated output level. However, costs must also be considered. The
cost aspect of input substitution is determined by input prices.

If capital costs 8 dollars a unit and labor 2 dollars a unit, 4 units of labor are substitutable in terms of cost for 1 unit of capital. This cost relationship is represented geometrically by an *isocost* line, a line whose slope reflects relative input costs. Based on the hypothetical capital and labor costs of 8 dollars and 2 dollars per unit, respectively, an isocost line would have a slope

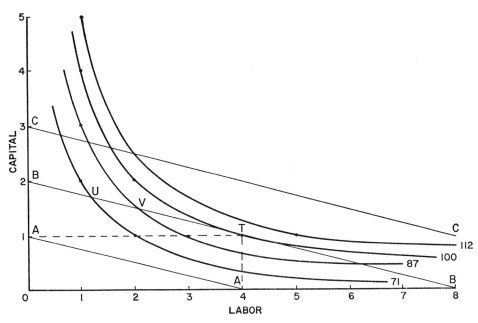

Figure 7. Geometric determination of production efficiency.

of 4 (8/2).[8] In Figure 7 several lines with a slope of 4 are super-imposed on the isoquant map representing production function $Q = 50 \ C^{1/2} L^{1/2}$; these isocost lines are labeled AA, BB, and CC, respectively. The minimum cost for any output level is indicated by the tangency[9] point between an isocost line and *an* isoquant representing the desired output level. Any other point on that isoquant represents higher costs of production. Thus in the previous example, the combination of capital and labor which minimizes the cost of producing 100 units of output is 1

[8] Refer to Appendix I for a discussion of the mathematical concept of a slope.
[9] Refer to Appendix I for a discussion of the mathematical concept of tangency.

capital unit and 4 labor units, derived from the tangency point (T) between the isoquant representing 100 units of output and isocost BB. This combination costs 16 dollars $(1 \cdot 8 + 4 \cdot 2)$; the other two input combinations yielding 100 units of output, 2 capital units and 2 labor units or 4 capital units and 1 labor unit cost 20 dollars $(2 \cdot 8 + 2 \cdot 2)$ and 34 dollars $(4 \cdot 8 + 1 \cdot 2)$ respectively.

Similarly, the maximum output obtainable with a given budget is determined by the tangency point of an isoquant with a budget line. Assuming a budget of 16 dollars and per unit capital and labor costs of 8 dollars and 2 dollars respectively, a budget line is constructed by determining the maximum quantity of capital purchasable with 16 dollars if no labor is brought—2 units of capital (16/8), and the maximum amount of labor that can be purchased with 16 dollars, if no capital is bought—8 units of labor (16/2). A straight line drawn between these two points represents all possible combinations of capital and labor obtainable at this budget level. Referring to Figure 7, isocost line BB is also the budget line for a budget of 16 dollars, as its slope represents the purchasable combinations of capital and labor. Thus the maximum output achievable with a budget constraint of 16 dollars and input prices of 8 dollars and 2 dollars for capital and labor respectively is 100 units; it is determined by finding the tangency point between the budget line and the isoquant curve. Although points U and V are also on budget line BB (refer to Fig. 7) they both represent lower output levels, 71 and 87 units, respectively, compared to the tangency point value of 100 output units. Output levels greater than 100 units cannot be achieved unless the budget is increased.

The geometric method for the attainment of production efficiency has its mathematical analogue. Given equations for the production function (isoquant), isocost line or budget line, the combination of inputs yielding the maximum output or minimizing cost for a designated output is ascertainable through the use of the mathematical tool of differentiation.[10] For example, the budget constraint in the previous example can be expressed mathematically as

---

[10] For a description of this process, refer to Appendix I.

$$B = P_1X_1 + P_2X_2 \tag{4}$$
$$16 = 8X_1 + 2X_2$$

where X_1 and X_2 are the capital and labor inputs, P_1 and P_2 the respective price of each input used, and B represents the budget. Equation (4) states that the amount of labor and capital inputs, times their respective prices (8 dollars and 2 dollars), cannot exceed 16 dollars (the budget constraint). Alternately equation (4) can be interpreted as stating that the value of the number of inputs used, times their prices, minus 16 dollars must equal zero $(0 = 8X_1 + 2X_2 - 16)$. The values of X_1 and X_2 that lead to overall cost minimization for a stated output, 100 units, given production function $Q = 50X_1^{\frac{1}{2}}X_2^{\frac{1}{2}}$ is determined by using the lagrange multiplier method [11] as expressed below:

$$Z = 8X_1 + 2X_2 - 16 + \lambda\,(100 - 50X_1^{\frac{1}{2}}X_2^{\frac{1}{2}}) \tag{5}$$

where, λ is a new variable, the lagrange multiplier and Z is the cost function to be minimized. Equation (5) is now differentiated with respect to X_1 and X_2 and λ, the resulting differentials are set equal to zero and solved for values of X_1 and X_2. The second derivatives of X_1 and X_2 are then calculated to ascertain whether the values of X_1 and X_2 are true minima. (A step by step solution to this cost minimization problem appears in an appendix to this Chapter).[12] A similar technique is employed to solve an output maximization problem. Assuming equation (6) represents a budget constraint

$$C = 4X_1 + 7X_2 - 6 \tag{6}$$

the maximum output, Z, is determinable by constructing an equation such as equation (7), using the lagrange

$$Q = 50X_1^{\frac{1}{2}}X_2^{\frac{1}{2}} + \lambda\,(4X_1 + 7X_2 - 6) \tag{7}$$

multiplier, differentiating equation (7), and solving for the values of X_1 and X_2 by the same method as described above (and detailed in the appendix to this chapter).

[11] For a definition of the lagrange multiplier concept and a description of the use of this method see, Baumol, William J.: *Economic Theory and Operations Analysis.* Englewood Cliffs, New Jersey, Prentice Hall, Inc., 1961, pp. 54–58.

[12] For additional illustrations of this procedure see, Lewis, J. Parry: *An Introduction to Mathematics for Students of Economics.* New York, St. Martin's Press, 1962, Chapter 21.

DIMINISHING RETURNS AND RETURNS TO SCALE

Two important concepts concerning production can be seen from an analysis of the function $Q = 50 \ C^{\frac{1}{2}}L^{\frac{1}{2}}$, *diminishing returns* and *returns to scale*. The concept of diminishing returns, more correctly identified as the *law of decreasing marginal (incremental) returns to a factor,* states that as more and more of one factor input is utilized in the production process, while all other inputs are held constant, less and less additional output will be produced. Referring to Table XVIII, it can be seen that there is a continuous decline in output increments derived from continually adding either capital or labor to a fixed amount of the other factor input. For example, if the production process initially utilizes 3 capital units and 1 labor unit, the addition to output achieved by adding only more labor units are as follows:

Labor Units	Additional Output Units
2	36
3	27
4	23
5	21
6	18
7	17
8	14

A similar outcome would be attained if either 1, 2, 4, or 5 capital units are taken as the fixed factor (input) or if the quantity of labor is assumed to be the fixed input and additional capital units are introduced.

The attribute of diminishing returns is not unique to the production function $Q = 50 \ C^{\frac{1}{2}}L^{\frac{1}{2}}$ but rather is a common attribute of production in general. It results from the fact that as one input is increased with all others being held constant, each additional unit of input has relatively less of the fixed factor (s) with which to interact, thereby limiting its ability to increase output by the same amount as the preceding units. An example will help to clarify this situation. Assume the existence of a hospital laboratory with a certain amount of equipment but no laboratory technicians. Without labor (technicians) there will be no output, where output is defined as the performance of laboratory tests, since one unit of labor is required to activate even the most automated equipment. As technicians are incrementally hired and employed, total output will increase but the average output per technician will decline. This is due to the amount of equipment being fixed. Each additional technician can add something to output by relieving the other technicians of some tasks. However, the marginal contribution of each new technician is bound to fall since the new tasks performed are less and less meaningful in terms of marginal output. Another way of looking at this phenomenon is that each technician has less of the fixed input (equipment) to work with, as the fixed stock of capital and materials is spread over more and more labor. Naturally, the last technician will not be able to add as much to production as the previous one.

The phenomenon of decreasing marginal returns to a factor (diminishing returns) may not exist at the initial stages of production (although it does occur in our hypothetical production model). For example, in the case of the hospital laboratory, the first technician would initially have to undertake all the labor activities involved in a laboratory. The addition of a second technician would permit specialization and hence greater production for both. However, a point must soon be reached where diminishing incremental output results from the addition of more technicians.[13]

Returns to scale refer to the effect on output as *all* productive input are increased proportionately. By referring to Table XVIII it can be seen that output increases in the same proportion as an equal increase in both inputs. Increasing the scale of production from 1 capital unit and 1 labor unit to 2 capital units and 2 labor units (an increase of 100 per cent) results in an increase of output from 50 units to 100 units (an increase of 100 per cent). Similarly, an increase in input use from 1 capital unit and 2 labor units to 3 capital units and 6 labor units (an increase

[13] Another aspect of the concept of diminishing returns is the technological possibility of negative marginal returns to a factor. An example would be the continual addition of technicians into the laboratory to the point where the technicians are so crowded that they bump into one another while attempting to work, thus causing everyones work to suffer. Presumably management never permits this situation to occur.

of 200 per cent) results in an increase of output from 71 units to 212 units (an increase of 200 per cent). Since this result is found for every set of inputs, one can conclude that production function $Q = 50C^{1/2}L^{1/2}$ exhibits <u>*constant returns to scale,*</u> i.e. output increases by the same multiple as any increase in all inputs.

Constant returns to scale is not a general economic law. Cases of *increasing* and *decreasing returns to scale* are quite common.[14] Increasing (decreasing) returns to scale is defined as a condition wherein when all inputs are increased by some multiple, output is increased by a larger (smaller) multiple. Increasing returns to scale is commonly referred to as *economies of scale* and decreasing returns to scale as *diseconomies of scale.* A small enterprise increasing its scale of operation to the point where automated machinery can be used is an example of economies of scale. Many machines are not made in all sizes, e.g. autoanalyzers or systems for multiphasic screening. A certain critical volume of use is necessary for their employment. When such capital is utilized, output goes up by an amount more than proportional to the increase in labor and capital. On the other side of the spectrum, a size may sometimes be reached where management may no longer have effective control over production.[15]

Both of these production conditions, diminishing returns and returns to scale, are independent of each other. There is no logical conflict when a certain production function displays constant returns to scale and decreasing returns to a factor. Both properties are characteristic of production function $Q = 50C^{1/2}L^{1/2}$. Constant returns to scale refers to a situation where *all* factors of production (inputs) are being increased by the *same* multiple; decreasing returns to a factor refers to a situation where *one* factor increases while *all others remain fixed.* It should be the goal

---

[14] Formally, the returns to scale relationship of any production process can be ascertained from its production function. For a general Cobb-Douglas production function,

$Q = aC^{\alpha} L^{\beta}$, (an example of which appears in equation (3))

   if $\alpha + \beta = 1$ constant returns to scale prevail;

   if $\alpha + \beta > 1$ increasing returns to scale prevail; and

   if $\alpha + \beta < 1$ decreasing returns to scale prevail.

   ($>$ and $<$ stand for greater than and less than respectively).

[15] The traditional solution for this problem is decentralization.

of management to ascertain the conditions unique to its production process and to establish the appropriate expansion policies.[16]

TRANSFORMATION CURVES

Whereas production functions focus on the production of a single output, *transformation curves* relate the use of fixed inputs to produce several outputs. The focus of transformation curves, also known as *production possibility curves*, can be expressed mathematically as follows:

$$Q_1, Q_2 = f(X_i) \tag{8}$$

where X represents each of the i factors of production employed, and Q_1 and Q_2 represent output levels of the goods or services produced.

Transformation curves can be empirically determined by tracing out the boundary of feasible combinations of outputs, delineated by the availability of inputs and the nature of their utilization in the production of Q_1, Q_2, or both. The four lines (AA, BB, CC, DD) in Figure 8 represent, through the use of linear line segments, hypothetical input restraints, i.e. how much of each output could be produced given existing input limitations. For example, AA represents an input used only in the production of Q_1. The amount of AA available limits the amount of Q_1 to OA but does not limit and has no effect on the output of Q_2 as it never hits the horizontal axis. CC represents an input used in the production of both Q_1 and Q_2. The slope of line CC indicates the number of units of Q_1 that must be sacrificed if one unit of input C is shifted from the production of Q_1 to the production of an additional unit of Q_2. Thus the amount of CC available limits the output of both Q_1 and Q_2. The boundary (transformation curve) formed by the intersection of all the input constraints, OAEFGB, indicates that the maximum feasible output ranges are either OA units of Q_1, OB units of Q_2, or any combination of Q_1 and Q_2 lying on the surface of curve OAEFGB.

---

[16] For example if both conditions described above prevail, diminishing returns to a factor could be endured in the short run, but long-term expansion should seek to capitalize on the constant returns to scale phenomenon.

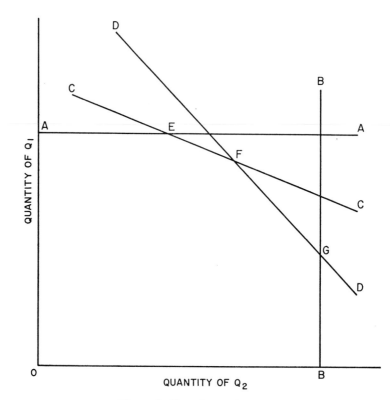

Figure 8. Transformation curve.

The determination of which of the output combinations of Q_1 and Q_2 is optimal depends on the relative valuation of Q_1 and Q_2, that is, the relative importance of Q_1 and Q_2 to a predetermined production goal. As in the previous section, where production efficiency with regard to a single output was examined, production efficiency in a situation of multiple outputs can be determined geometrically or mathematically.

Geometrically, a line (or a series of lines) whose slope indicates the relative importance of outputs Q_1 and Q_2 to the predetermined production goal, called an *isocontribution* line, is added to a diagram containing a transformation curve. For example, if Q_1 is valued ¾ as much as Q_2, the isocontribution line reflecting this valuation would have a slope of 0.75. As in the case of isocosts or budget lines, the higher (further to the right) the isocontribution lines the greater the quantities of output.

The geometric solution of production efficiency is determined by finding the tangency point between the transformation curve and the highest isocontribution line, as seen in Figure 9 where a series of isocontribution lines with a slope of 0.75 (XX, YY, and ZZ) have been imposed on the transformation curve derived in Figure 8. The tangency point solution (point F) indicates that the optimal levels of Q_1 and Q_2 are Oq_1 and Oq_2 respectively. Any other output combination on the transformation curve yields a lower valued combination of output because it falls on a lower isocontribution line.

The determination of the optimal production combination embodied in the transformation curve-isocontribution line analysis is determinable mathematically through the use of linear pro-

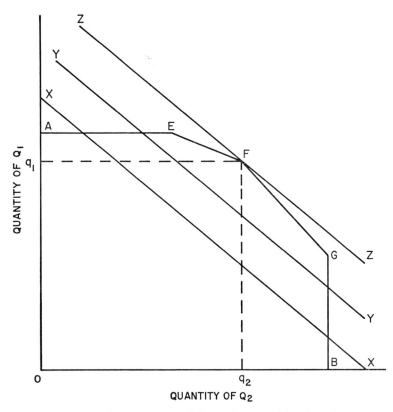

Figure 9. Geometric determination of the optimal combination of two outputs with fixed input specifications.

gramming. The mathematical statements used in linear programming represent the relative valuation of the outputs (isocontribution line), and the structural input limitations from which a
transformation curve is derived.

The basic linear programming approach can be summarized
as follows:

$$Z = a_1q_1 + a_2q_2 \tag{9}$$

$$b_1q_1 + b_1q_2 \leq c_1 \tag{10}$$

$$b_2q_1 + b_2q_2 \leq c_2 \tag{11}$$

$$b_3q_1 + b_3q_2 \leq c_3 \tag{12}$$

$$b_4q_1 + b_4q_2 \leq c_4 \tag{13}$$

where Z symbolizes the production goal (s) of the enterprise; q_1,
q_2 are the quantities of goods (or services) Q_1 and Q_2; a_1, a_2 are
weights reflecting the contributions of q_1 and q_2 to the production
goal; b_1 . . . $_4$ are the utilization rates of the inputs in the production of the respective q's; c_1 . . . $_4$ are the availabilities of each
of the inputs. Equation **(9)** is a mathematical representation of
the isocontribution curves appearing in Figure 9, and equations
(10) through **(13)** represent input constraints represented by
lines AA, BB, CC, and DD in Figure 8.[17] The goal of the linear
programming exercise is to maximize Z subject to the basic conditions that both q_1 and q_2 be greater than or equal to zero
$(q_1, q_2 \geq 0)$. In spite of its title, the structural nature of the
linear programming process is easily adaptable to include nonlinear relationships and to account for many additional aspects
of production. As the mathematical solution of a linear programming model requires a knowledge of matrix algebra, a mathematical tool rarely used in the health economics literature and
consequently not developed in the mathematical appendix (Appendix I), an example of a solution to a linear programming
model will not be presented here.[18] A linear model of hospital

[17] For those inputs used in the production of only Q_1 or Q_2, the respective b coefficient is assigned a value of zero.

[18] For a rigorous discussion of the linear programming technique including the
various methods of solving the mathematical model see either Buffa, Edward S.:
Models for Production and Operations Management. New York, John Wiley, 1966;
or Spivey, W. Allen: *Linear Programming: An Introduction.* New York, Macmillan,
1963.

operations solvable by linear programming is, however, presented in the Baligh and Laughhunn article reproduced in the next chapter.

DERIVATION OF COST CURVES

An enterprise's cost of production curve is easily derivable from its production function and budget constraint. As total production costs are determined jointly by technological factors embodied in the production function (and reflected in the isoquant

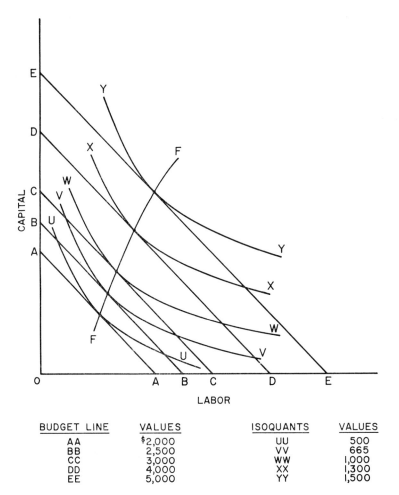

Figure 10. Production expansion path.

BUDGET LINE	VALUES	ISOQUANTS	VALUES
AA	$2,000	UU	500
BB	2,500	VV	665
CC	3,000	WW	1,000
DD	4,000	XX	1,300
EE	5,000	YY	1,500

map) and the enterprise's available budget, the series of tangency points between various isoquants and budget lines representing higher outlays traces out the enterprise's path of production expansion. Figure 10 contains a series of hypothetical isoquants and budget lines; [19] the line connecting the series of isoquant-budget line tangency points, FF, is the production expansion curve. At budget level 2,000 dollars (AA), 500 (UU) units of output can be produced, at budget level 2,500 dollars (BB), 665 (VV) units of output can be produced, at budget level 3,000 dollars (CC), 1,000 (WW) units can be produced, at budget level 4,000 dollars (DD) 1,300 (XX) units can be produced and at budget level 5,000 dollars (EE), 1,500 (YY) units of output can be produced. Plotting the various budget-output combina-

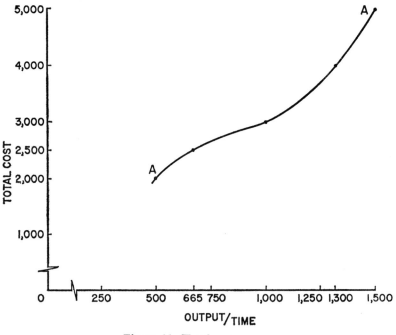

Figure 11. Total cost curve.

[19] The isoquants appearing in Figure 6 are not reproduced in this example as they display constant returns to scale throughout the production range. For pedagogical purposes, ranges of increasing, constant, and diminishing returns to scale are desirable for the current presentation.

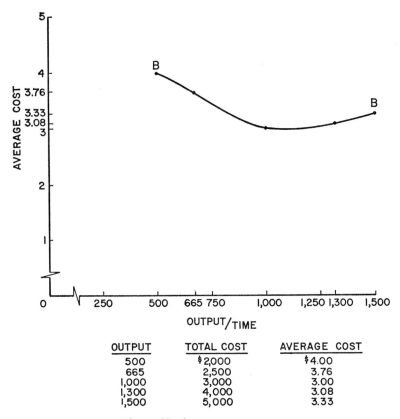

OUTPUT	TOTAL COST	AVERAGE COST
500	$2,000	$4.00
665	2,500	3.76
1,000	3,000	3.00
1,300	4,000	3.08
1,500	5,000	3.33

Figure 12. Average cost curve.

tion points and connecting these points yields a total cost of production curve; curve AA in Figure 11.

Between output levels 500 and 1,000 total costs are increasing at a decreasing rate (cost per unit of output declines from 4 dollars to 3.76 dollars to 3 dollars); between output levels 1,000 and 1,500 total costs are increasing at an increasing rate (cost per unit of output increases from 3.08 dollars to 3.33 dollars). This cost-output relationship is highlighted when average rather than total costs are reported, as can be seen in the average cost curve, BB, appearing in Figure 12. Over the output range where total cost increases at a decreasing rate, average cost (total cost divided by quantity) declines; when total cost increases at an increasing rate, average cost increases.

The concept of returns to scale is often used as a basis for explaining the approximate U-shaped form of the average cost curve. Economies of scale bring down average cost as quantity (scale) increases and diseconomies of scale lead to increasing cost with expansion. If a segment of the production process displays constant returns to scale, the average cost curve would resemble an elongated U, i.e. ⌊⎯⌋ .

Appendix: Mathematical Derivation of Minimum Cost Solution

Problem: Ascertain minimum cost solution for the following production function and budget constraint:

(1) Production Function and Budget Constraint:

$$Z = 8X_1 + 2X_2 - 16 + \lambda (100 - 50X_1^{\frac{1}{2}}X_2^{\frac{1}{2}})$$

Step 1: Differentiate (1) with respect to X_1, X_2, and λ and set the differentials equal to zero.

(2) $\dfrac{\partial Z}{\partial X_1} = 8 - 25\lambda X_1^{-\frac{1}{2}}X_2^{\frac{1}{2}} = 0$

(3) $\dfrac{\partial Z}{\partial X_2} = 2 - 25\lambda X_1^{\frac{1}{2}}X_2^{-\frac{1}{2}} = 0$

(4) $\dfrac{\partial Z}{\partial \lambda} = 100 - 50X_1^{\frac{1}{2}} X_2^{\frac{1}{2}} = 0$

Step 2: Solve equations (2), (3), and (4) for X_1, X_2, and λ.

(5) $25\lambda X_1^{-\frac{1}{2}}X_2^{\frac{1}{2}} = 8$
$3.125\lambda X_1^{-\frac{1}{2}}X_2^{\frac{1}{2}} = 1$
$9.766\lambda^2 X_2 = X_1$

(6) $25\lambda X_1^{\frac{1}{2}}X_2^{-\frac{1}{2}} = 2$
$12.5\lambda X_1^{\frac{1}{2}}X_2^{-\frac{1}{2}} = 1$
$156.25\lambda^2 X_1 = X_2$

(7) $100 = 50X_1^{\frac{1}{2}}X_2^{\frac{1}{2}}$
$2 = X_1^{\frac{1}{2}}X_2^{\frac{1}{2}}$
$4 = X_1 X_2$
$4/X_2 = X_1$

(8) [substitute the value of X_1 from (7) into (5)]
$4/X_2 = 9.766\lambda^2 X_2$
$4 = 9.766\lambda^2 X_2^2$
$X_2^2 = 4/9.766\lambda^2$
$X_2 = 2/3.125\lambda$

(9) [substitute the value of X_1 from **(7)** into **(6)**]

$156.25\lambda^2 (4/X_2) = X_2$

$156.25\lambda^2 (4) = X_2{}^2$

$625\lambda^2 = X_2{}^2$

$25\lambda = X_2$

(10) [substitute the value of X_2 from **(9)** into **(8)**]

$25\lambda = 2/3.125\lambda$

$78.125\lambda^2 = 2$

$\lambda^2 = 0.0256$

$\lambda = 0.16$

(11) [substitute value of λ from **(10)** into **(9)**]

$25(0.16) = X_2$

$X_2 = 4$

(12) [substitute value of X_2 from **(11)** into **(7)**]

$X_1 = 4/4$

$X_1 = 1$

Step 3: Test whether the solution arrived at in Step 2 indicates maximum or minimum values of X_1 and of X_2. A minimum cost solution has been attained if:

$$\frac{\partial^2 Z}{\partial X_1{}^2} > 0, \qquad \frac{\partial^2 Z}{\partial X_2{}^2} > 0,$$

and

$$\left(\frac{\partial^2 Z}{\partial X_1{}^2}\right)\left(\frac{\partial^2 Z}{\partial X_2{}^2}\right) > \left(\frac{\partial^2 Z}{\partial X_1 X_2}\right)^2$$

Calculate the required second derivates.[20]

(13) $\dfrac{\partial Z^2}{\partial X_1{}^2} = 12.5\lambda X_1{}^{-\frac{3}{2}} X_2{}^{\frac{1}{2}}$

$= 12.5 \, (0.16) \, (1)^{-\frac{3}{2}} \, (4)^{\frac{1}{2}}$

$= \dfrac{12.5 \, (0.16) \, (2)}{1}$

$= 4$

(14) $\dfrac{\partial Z^2}{\partial X_2{}^2} = 12.5\lambda \, X_1{}^{\frac{1}{2}} X_2{}^{-\frac{3}{2}}$

$= 12.5 \, (0.16) \, (1)^{\frac{1}{2}} \, (4)^{-\frac{3}{2}}$

$= \dfrac{12.5 \, (0.16) \, (1)}{(0.125)}$

$= 16$

[20] The following mathematical property of exponents, $X^{-\alpha} = \dfrac{1}{X^\alpha}$, is used in the solution of equations **(13)**, **(14)**, and **(15)**.

(15) $\dfrac{\partial Z^2}{\partial X_1 \partial X_2} = -12.5\lambda\ X_1^{-\frac{3}{2}}\ X_2^{-\frac{1}{2}}$

$\qquad\qquad = -12.5\ (0.16)\ (1)^{-\frac{3}{2}}\ (4)^{-\frac{1}{2}}$

$\qquad\qquad = \dfrac{-12.5\ (0.16)}{(1)\ (2)}$

$\qquad\qquad = -1$

(16) $\left(\dfrac{\partial Z^2}{\partial X_1^2}\right)\left(\dfrac{\partial Z^2}{\partial X_2^2}\right) = 4 \cdot 16 = 64$

(17) $\left(\dfrac{\partial Z^2}{\partial X_1 \partial X_2}\right)^2 = 1^2 = 1$

Since $64 > 1$ a minimum cost solution has been attained.

Chapter Seven

PRODUCTION STUDIES

THE APPLICATION of production theory to health administration issues is one of the newer developments in the health
literature. This feature notwithstanding, research on health institution production functions and on productivity within the
health care domain has already highlighted many crucial questions with a direct impact on administration and planning issues. Among the issues researched are, for example, the questions
of: a) how to define the output of a health care institution, b)
the existence of economics of scale in larger institutions, and
c) the development of broad production models intended both
for simulating industry behavior and establishing a reference
frame for applying management science techniques. Each of the
two articles reproduced in this chapter deals with at least one of
the three areas enumerated above. Both articles focus on the issue of deriving a measure of hospital output and, having established the criteria for estimating output, turn to other production related issues.

Harold Cohen, in his article, "Variations in Cost Among Hospitals of Different Sizes," addresses the question of whether
economies of size exist, and if they do, what is an optimal size for
a short-term general hospital. Before addressing this issue he
notes the need to adjust hospital cost data for varying wage scales
prevailing in different sectors of the country and develops a
formula for the required adjustment. He further develops a formula for deriving a measure of hospital output based on a
weighted average of in-patient admissions, out-patient visits, and
utilized ancillary service procedures. The weights used for the

averaging are the relative costs of each of the output components.

Having derived an output measure, Cohen utilizes linear multiple regression analysis to estimate hospital average cost curves. The estimated regression equation is then used to calculate the output level representing the minimum cost point on the average cost curve. This output level, measured in terms of number of beds, is found to be approximately two hundred beds for short-term general hospitals providing nonspecialized patient care.

Helmy H. Baligh and Danny J. Laughhunn, in their article, "An Economic and Linear Model of the Hospital," dispute the utilization of an output measure which is based on services rendered.[1] They propose an output measure based on the individual institution's perception of a patient's relative value to the institution. The institution is viewed as attempting to maximize an output function where output is measured as the sum of each patient's projected *value*. In addition to specifying a general form for an output equation, the authors construct representative equations to reflect the existence of resource, budget, patient,[2] and policy constraints.

Baligh and Laughhunn's economic model of a hospital also demonstrates the type of equations required for a linear programming analysis. Such a formulation is a valuable aid in establishing policy regarding the type of specialized services an institution should strive to provide, given the goals that it has set for itself. The type of services, in turn, largely determine the patient and, to a lesser degree, the research and teaching mix that an institution will attract.

Both the Cohen and Baligh and Laughhunn articles are highly technical and geared to a specialized readership group. They are, however, representative of the quantitative research that is ap-

[1] For an in-depth discussion of the relative merits of an output measure based on services rendered versus an output measure based on the *outcome* of the services rendered see, Donabedian, Avedis: Evaluating the quality of medical care, *Milbank Memorial Fund Quarterly, 44:* (3) , 166, 1966.

[2] Patient constraints result from the fact that most health institutions cannot always obtain the patient mix that they might desire on medical, research, or financial grounds.

pearing in the literature. Recognizing the complexity of health institutions and the new generation of management science techniques that are pervading the health field, one can expect to see a proliferation of research studies along these lines.

In both of the articles reproduced in this chapter, the authors indicate that their studies are initial attempts at applying elements of production theory to health administration and planning issues. Additional refinements and extensions will undoubtedly be introduced in these areas as better data sources are developed and existing theoretical production models are adopted to reflect the operation of nonprofit enterprises.[3]

* * *

VARIATIONS IN COST AMONG HOSPITALS OF DIFFERENT SIZES [4]

HAROLD A. COHEN

Much money and effort today is going into the development of the nation's medical facilities; the federal government, acting under the Hill-Burton program, is spending a great deal on the construction of general, "short-term" hospitals (i.e. for an average patient-stay of less than thirty days) ; and there is an increasing amount of planning for regional health care facilities. The most efficient size for a hospital should be carefully ascertained in order that the available funds be utilized in the best fashion. The question of optimal hospital size becomes especially important as the population becomes more concentrated in urban centers where larger and larger hospitals could be effectively utilized. The purpose of this chapter is to explore two aspects of cost variation with respect to hospital size among general, "short-term" hospitals.

---

[3] For some initial efforts in this respect see, Brown, Max: An economic analysis of hospital operations, *Hospital Administration, 15*:60, 1970; Dowling, William L.: The application of linear programming to decision making in hospitals, *Hospital Administration, 16*:66, 1971; Lee, Maw Lin: A conspicious production theory of hospital behavior, *Southern Economic Journal, 38*:48, 1971; and Newhouse, Joseph P.: Toward a theory of nonprofit institutions: An economic model of a hospital, *American Economic Review, 60*:64, 1970.

[4] Reprinted with permission from *The Southern Economic Journal, 33*, No. 3, January, 1967, pp. 355–366. Copyright © 1967 by the Southern Economic Association.

Studies comparing the costs of hospitals of different sizes have generally incorporated at least one of two biases. One is a failure to recognize salary and wage differentials due to factors other than hospital size. Such differentials are very large in this nonunionized field. These cost differentials inflate the costs of urban hospitals relative to the costs of hospitals in nonurbanized areas. The other bias stems from the use of "adult and pediatric patient days" as a measure of the output of hospitals, without adjustment for auxiliary services, the use and availability of which vary greatly among hospitals of different sizes. The use of the simple "patient days" measure in cost comparisons tends to inflate the costs of larger hospitals, which generally offer more of the specialized and expensive auxiliary services, relative to the costs of smaller hospitals. Together these two sources of bias tend to exaggerate the difference between the costs of large urban hospitals and the costs of small, nonurban hospitals.

WAGE DIFFERENTIALS

Wages and salaries paid by hospitals vary greatly among the major geographic regions of the United States, as shown in Table 1. There

TABLE 1
AVERAGE HOURLY WAGE RATES BY REGION

Occupation	United States	Northeast	South	North Central	West
General Duty Nurse	$2.16	$2.16	$1.92	$2.21	$2.34
X-ray Technician	2.09	2.09	1.91	2.09	2.29
Medical Technician	2.38	2.26	2.22	2.40	2.76
Nursing Aids (women)	1.32	1.46	.99	1.32	1.58
Nursing Aids (men)	1.46	1.55	1.14	1.52	1.66
Licensed Practical Nurses	1.61	1.72	1.35	1.66	1.82
Clerks	1.90	1.92	1.76	1.89	2.06
Kitchen Helpers	1.26	1.37	.89	1.30	1.50
Finishers, Flatwork Machine	1.21	1.27	.88	1.29	1.48
Maids and Porters	1.30	1.39	.90	1.36	1.61
Engineers, Maintenance	2.54	2.47	2.34	2.75	3.29

Source: United States Bureau of Labor Statistics: *Industry Wage Survey: Hospitals-Mid-1963*, Bulletin No. 1409, U.S. Government Printing Office, Washington, D.C., June 1964.

are also significant differentials between rural and urban wages for similar occupational classes. These differences appear to be primarily attributable to two factors: the relative number of alternative employment opportunities open to trained hospital personnel and the relative salary levels currently prevailing for untrained personnel in the community.[5] In many small communities the hospitals are understaffed monopsonists or oligopsonists [6] that would have to offer considerably higher wages to attract trained personnel into the area but can pay fairly low wages to people, largely immobile wives, already in the area. These hospitals often choose to alter the ratio of skilled personnel to auxiliary and less skilled personnel rather than bid up wage levels significantly. Thus in comparing costs for hospitals of different size, differences among hospitals in starting salaries should be eliminated because such differences are induced exogenously by factors other than size.

A questionnaire was sent to virtually all accredited short-term general hospitals in a six-state northeastern region asking for starting salaries in representative employee classifications in 1962. Of the 339 questionnaires sent only 82 were returned.[7] The urban-rural wage differential in this region is shown in Tables 2 and 3. The range of starting salaries is substantial. Of the "low" starting salary figures, all occurred in small towns, eight of which were in Delaware or Vermont. Four of the nine "highs" reported from New York City, the other five from urban areas in Connecticut, New Jersey, and

TABLE 2

STARTING HOURLY WAGE RANGES IN NORTHEAST

Occupation	High	Low	High/low
General Duty Nurse	$2.38	$1.50	1.59
X-ray Technician	2.40	1.46	1.65
Medical Technician	2.67	1.73	1.54
Nursing Aid	1.52	.86	1.76
Orderlies	1.52	.86	1.76
Licensed Practical Nurses	1.85	1.20	1.54
Clerks	1.72	1.00	1.72
Laundry Workers	1.44	.96	1.50
General Maintenance	2.00	1.11	1.80

Source: Table 1.

[5] A study by the American Nurses' Association shows median salaries for registered nurses working in doctor's and dentist's offices to vary nationally in the same way as hospital salaries. Highest-Pacific States (415 dollars per month), next in order Great Lakes Region, New England States, Southeastern States. *American Journal of Nursing,* September 15, 1965.

[6] *Editors' Note:* Monopsony and oligopsony refer to market situations where one buyer or a few buyers confront a large number of sellers.

[7] Evaluating the quality of the product is not discussed here but only hospitals accredited by the American Hospital Association were used in the various samples of this study. Of the 82 questionnaires returned, 35 were from New York State, 12 of which were from metropolitan New York City, 25 from Massachusetts, 9 from New Jersey, 7 from Connecticut, 5 from Vermont and 1 from Delaware.

TABLE 3

AVERAGE STARTING HOURLY WAGE RATES IN
NEW YORK STATE

Occupation	"Down-state" [a]	"Upstate"	D/U
General Duty Nurse	$2.22	$1.93	1.15
X-ray Technician	2.15	1.78	1.21
Medical Technician	2.22	1.95	1.14
Nursing Aid	1.36	1.22	1.11
Orderlies	1.44	1.33	1.08
Licensed Practical Nurses	1.66	1.45	1.14
Clerks	1.56	1.33	1.17
Laundry Workers	1.34	1.21	1.11
General Maintenance	1.70	1.54	1.10

[a] "Downstate" refers to New York City plus Nassau and West-chester Counties.

Source: See source note to Table 1.

Massachusetts. While this questionnaire does not prove conclusively that urban starting salaries are always higher than rural, the pattern is very clear. Especially interesting is the difference in starting salary levels between New York City (including Nassau and Westchester Counties) and the remainder of New York State, as shown in Table 3.

The analysis of relative hospital cost for this sample or for almost any sample of geographically scattered hospitals should take into account these differences in starting wages, if these differences do in fact reflect exogenous factors in the labor market rather than differences in labor quality. Otherwise, the exclusively urban location of larger hospitals distorts the cost picture. Such an adjustment would be necessary even if all hospitals in a sample were from one state, but there were significant concentrations of population and job alternatives within the state.

Within the above sample of 35 New York State hospitals, a factor contributing to the city-upstate differentials in starting salaries is the possible bargaining power of New York City hospital employees due to union organization. Many hospital employees in the city are unionized although they do not have the right to strike. In 1962 the New York State legislature refused a bill sponsored by the New York City delegates that would have extended the right to collective bargaining to hospital employees on a statewide basis. In Nassau and Westchester County hospitals employees are not unionized but receive substantially the same wages as employees in New York City hospitals, since hospitals in these counties are competing directly with city hospitals for the same pool of workers.[8]

[8] *Editors' Note:* This was repealed in 1965 in favor of statewide collective bargaining.

The procedure that will be used here to make adjusted cost comparisons is described by the formula below. In effect, this procedure assumes that cost differences attributable to differences in starting salary should be eliminated. To the extent that large hospitals can attract a sufficient staff only by paying higher starting salaries than small hospitals pay, such an assumption reverses rather than corrects the bias in the cost figures. It is hoped that by adjusting wage differentials but not fringe benefit differentials, the possibility of overcompensation is minimized. It is also assumed that starting salary differentials are locked into the system but wage raises are largely determined by employee productivity.[9]

Similarly, differences in starting wages of the various classes of nurses within individual hospitals (Directors of Nursing, Supervisors, Head Nurses and General Duty Nurses) are assumed to be based on relative productivity. For this reason, only starting salaries, and not salary levels, need to be known.

Data from only 53 of the 82 answering hospitals are used in comparing hospital costs adjusted for wage differentials. Of the remaining 29, 16 were excluded because they had contract laundry services which, as will be shown later, invalidates the analytic procedure used. Other hospitals were excluded due to partial completion of questionnaires, information deficiencies in the Guide Issue of *Hospitals,* or for possessing only one of two types of laboratories.[10] (The last factor will be explained later.)

The formula for adjusting total cost is as follows:

$$A^K = C^K + \Sigma[(S_i - S_i{}^k)(P_iE^k52H_i)]$$

where

A^k = Total adjusted cost for Hospital k
C^k = Total costs reported by hospital k
S_i = Median starting salary for ith occupation among hospitals in the sample
$S_i{}^k$ = Starting salary for ith occupation reported by hospital k
P_i = Proportion of employees in ith occupation
E^k = Total employment in hospital k
$52H_i$ = Yearly hours per employee in ith occupation

The mid-1963 Hospital Wage Survey presented a set of occupational classifications covering 70 per cent of all employees in North-

---

[9] This might be approximately true even though 45% of metropolitan hospitals report raises based solely on length of service and 2% have a single rate system.
[10] American Hospital Association: *Hospitals,* August 1, 1962. (Referred to as *Guide Issue.*)

eastern hospitals. From the occupational distribution it was possible to establish the average percentage of hospital employees in each covered occupational category. Total employment for each of the fifty-three hospitals in the sample was then found from the August *1962 Guide Issue* of *Hospitals*. The total personnel figure is multiplied by each of the occupational percentages. The resulting estimate of the number of employees in each category is multiplied by the average annual hours for that category. This result is then multiplied by the difference between a starting salary chosen to represent that occupation and that hospital's starting salary. The product is then added to total cost as reported in the 1962 Guide Issue. In this way, all hospital wage levels are made to conform to an identical wage rate schedule for the 70 per cent of employees covered. The assumed starting salaries, per cent of employees covered, and average weekly hours for each occupation are shown in Table 4.

TABLE 4

Occupation	Assumed starting salary (S_i)	% Employees Covered (P_i)	Weekly hours per employee (H_i)
General Duty Nurse	$1.85	.14	39.5
X-ray Technician	1.85	.02	39.0
Medical Technician	2.05	.03	39.0
Nursing Aid	1.20	.14	39.5
Orderlies	1.25	.02	40.0
Licensed Practical Nurse	1.45	.07	39.5
Clerk	1.30	.09	39.0
Laundry Worker	1.20	.18	39.5
General Maintenance	1.70	.01	39.5

Admittedly, this is a very rough procedure, especially in relying upon published cost figures to be mutually comparable. Such figures were used primarily because they were readily available. Total adjusted cost, when derived, was plotted against the standard output measure which is adult and pediatric patient days.

Due to the surprisingly high correlation between adult and pediatric patient days, on the one hand and unadjusted costs on the other (.979), there was little room for improvement. The simple correlation, however, between adjusted cost versus adult and pediatric patient days was .983. The linear correlations were in both cases higher than the quadratic and cubic correlations. The linear regression lines, however, included sizeable negative constants, the interpretation of which is economically absurd.[11] The other regression curves were also dismissed as being economically improbable since they were characterized by negative constants or by total cost curves which eventually slope downward. We shall return to this sample after discussing the bias in the measure of output.

MEASURE OF OUTPUT

Almost all studies comparing hospital costs use adult and pediatric patient days as the measure of output. However, hospitals differ in the number and nature of the services which they offer; in general the larger a hospital is the greater is the variety of services which it provides. Many small hospitals, rather than offer a particular service at low volume and consequent high unit cost, will have an agreement with large hospitals in nearby cities to provide the service in question. Such arrangements may reflect insufficient demand in the vicinity of the smaller hospital for either specialized equipment such as Cobalt units or specialist physicians such as neurosurgeons; but these arrangements foster an appearance of relative efficiency in the smaller hospital. That is, merely using patient days as a measure of output involves a systematic bias against larger hospitals which offer many more kinds of services.

Saathoff and Kurtz have faced this problem by devising a measure

[11] *Editors' Note:* A negative constant term in a regression analysis of cost implies that a plot of cost on the vertical axis on a two quadrant diagram and output on the horizontal axis would result in a negative cost observation at zero output, as seen here. Such a finding cannot be explained based on any real world observations, because in the short run even at zero output, positive costs are incurred due to contractual commitments (salaries, leasing agreements, etc.) .

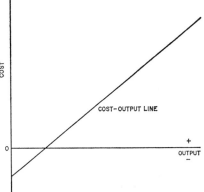

of service output that is something more than simple adult and pediatric days.[12] Their unit of service is as follows:

$$S = D + 2A + .3X + .1L + .20$$

where

S = Adjusted measure of output
A = Surgical and obstetrical admissions
X = X-ray diagnostic procedures
L = Laboratory tests and tissue exams
O = Out-patient department visits.

The weight coefficients used by Saathoff and Kurtz for items D, A, X, L, and O were based on time and motion study; here an effort will be made to develop a more inclusive measure of service output which weights each included service by its estimated average cost in dollars rather than time. To accomplish this, twenty-three member hospitals of the United Hospital Fund of New York were visited in 1963 and 1965. The Hospital Fund is a philanthropic organization which subsidizes a group of New York City area hospitals including short-term general hospitals. In order to receive its donation a hospital must submit detailed cost schedules. A worksheet is also provided which calls for a stepdown allocation of overhead to various "service cost centers" such as laboratory, x-ray department, operating room, etc. On the worksheet the hospital lists the number of units of each service such as laboratory exams, x-ray films, and operations (divided into major and minor). The methods of allocating overhead among these "service cost centers" are quite standard and acceptable to cost accountants.

The data reported to the United Hospital Fund can be attacked on several grounds. First, hospital comptrollers are subjected to an extremely long list of questions which they must answer if any of their figures are unusual. Several comptrollers report that figures were juggled to minimize tiresome questions.

Second, the U.H.F. has established certain arbitrary rulings on the reporting, such as requiring the allocation of all costs for interns and resident physicians to in-patients, even though these employees may work in other service areas. Thus in-patient costs are raised relative to the costs of the out-patient department, emergency room, and perhaps the ambulance service. Third, hospital comptrollers may use their own judgment in allocating certain other costs and in

---

[12] Donald E. Saathoff and Richard A. Kurtz, "Cost Per Day Comparisons Don't Do the Job," *The Modern Hospital,* October, 1962, pp. 14, 16, 162.

so doing their reports are rendered not strictly comparable. Services not separately specified on the form may be included under the categories of "routine patient services" and "auxiliary service cost centers."

Some comptrollers list services such as "occupational therapy," "mental health," and "neurological examinations" as routine; to the extent that these services are not in fact generally considered routine, or are not offered by other hospitals, such a practice causes "routine" patient expenses to appear high for those hospitals which do consider such services to be routine. Fourth, in many areas the medical staff may make differing judgments. For example, hospitals are told to weigh minor operations as one-third of a major operation, but the individual medical staff decides when an operation is major and when it is minor. Hospitals which would be expected to have fairly similar groups of patients have vastly different ratios of major to minor operations. Similarly, hospitals do not use the same criteria to arrive at the total number of laboratory exams. A fifth problem is that hospitals may choose, without the complete blessing of the United Hospital Fund, *not* to allocate costs to some service centers. The *Guide Issue* reports several hospitals in the UHF sample as offering services to which they do not allocate any costs. Of the services in the measure of output, those which are most neglected in this manner are electroencephalograms and therapeutic x-rays.

The failure of such hospitals to allocate costs to such services, even though they are provided, makes it impossible in this study to estimate accurately the average cost of all services; on the one hand, the number of observations on such services is reduced to the number of hospitals reporting them rather than the number of hospitals rendering them; on the other hand, since the costs of these services have been lumped in under some other headings, the cost estimates for these other headings will be distorted. So few hospitals allocate any cost to the metabolism service that it was impossible to include it in this study. Oxygen and metabolism are not routinely administered but they are routinely offered, and so their costs were included in total costs whether reported separately or not. A major problem in the measurement of output is the insufficiency of observations upon which to base acceptable estimates for the cost of rare services offered by only a few hospitals. Examples of these services are psychiatric ambulatory day care, radioisotope facilities, cardiopulmonary facilities, cobalt treatment, and ambulance service. Despite these shortcomings and omissions, the formula derived below for the measure of output is at least a further step in the right direction, or so it is hoped.

The approach to the measure of service output is similar to that of Saathoff and Kurtz inasmuch as an adult and pediatric patient day is weighted as one and the unit cost (in dollars rather than time) of other included services is divided by that of an in-patient day. To derive the weight for that service the average costs and ratios for those services for which sufficient observations were available are given in Table 5.

TABLE 5

Service Units	Average Cost [c]	Relative Cost (W_i)	Observations
Operations, weighted [a]	$114.35	4.75	22
Deliveries	56.92	2.36	15
X-rays, diagnostic [b]	3.83	.16	23
Laboratory examinations	1.66	.07	23
Physical therapy treatments	3.71	.15	19
Electrocardiograms	4.92	.20	20
X-ray, therapy treatments	9.44	.39	13
Blood transfusions (inc. Plasma)	21.74	.90	17
Newborn days	12.72	.53	14
Out-patient visits	6.72	.28	21
Electroencephalograms	17.59	.73	8
Emergency room treatments	3.97	.16	19
Adult and pediatric days	24.09	1.00	22

[a] Major operations plus $\frac{1}{3}$ minor operations.
[b] $\frac{1}{20}$ dental films plus other films.
[c] Because of the discrepancies in individual cost figures which are discussed in the text, the extremely high and low figures have been eliminated by using the mid-mean. That is, the average cost figure is the mean of the middle half of the observations for each service; other modified measures of central tendency give very similar results.

This then gives a measure of output

where

$$S^k = W_i Q_i^k$$
S^k = service output in kth hospital
W_i = weight of ith service
Q_i^k = quantity of ith service in kth hospital

Since different numbers of observations (i.e. hospitals) are used in the calculation of costs for different services, the reader might suppose that some adjustment for wage differentials might be required. If, for example, wage rates in the eight hospitals reporting electroencephalograms is higher than the average for the entire sample, then the average cost for the EEG service would be inflated. In developing these weights, however, wage and salary differences among hospitals in the sample were not adjusted. These hospitals are all competing for a common pool of employees so it is reasonable to consider wage differences to be internally caused. In addition, for development of the unit of output measure, we are interested in relative costs of the services within the hospitals. For these reasons, adjustment of costs for wage differences is not necessary.

TESTING THE MEASURE OF OUTPUT

Having established an adjusted measure of output (S^k) to be used in place of "adult and pediatric patient days," we may now proceed to consider the relationship between output and costs. We shall develop several regressions between S^k and total costs, and the qualifications which the reader should bear in mind may be summarized as follows:

1. S^k is in effect necessarily based upon data from less than half the UHF New York City sample, since the costs used in calculating the weights for S^k are mid-means.
2. The first regression, between S^k and total costs for New York City hospitals, may be made without any adjustment of total costs for inter-hospital wage differentials.
3. The later regressions between S^k and total costs for hospitals throughout six northeastern states does require an adjustment of total costs for inter-hospital wage differentials.
4. Total hospital costs in the New York City sample have been put on a more comparable basis by deducting costs for extraordinary services, such as those mentioned before (psychiatric ambulatory day care, etc.), and other costs not relating specifically to patient care. Examples of the latter are gift shops and fund raising expenses. Depreciation was not included because it was not available. Other costs were also eliminated such as extraordinary repairs, expenses associated with interns and residents, and costs associated with nursing school. The first was eliminated because such repair costs are not attributable to current patients. The second and third were eliminated for involving primarily teaching operations. While the availability of a nursing school may reduce the hospital's payments for a nursing staff, that reduction is believed to be but a small proportion of nursing school expenses borne by the sponsoring hospital.

These adjustments were not made for total hospital costs for the six-state sample because detailed information was unavailable.

5. It may be objected that the correlation between S^k and total costs will necessarily be quite high, since S^k is based on weights which are determined by costs. Hopefully the possibility of introducing biases which will inevitably lead to high correlations has been avoided in the calculations of weights (W_i); however, biases must also be avoided in those cases where Q_i^k is not reported by the individual hospitals and had to be estimated. Some hospitals reported the total cost of a certain type of service but not the output (Q_i) of that service; others did not report either cost or output, although the *Guide Issue* made it clear that the hospital in question did in fact offer the said service. Estimates of the output of service (Q_i) might have been derived in the former case by dividing reported total cost of the service by the corresponding sample wide average cost figures from Table 5; to have done this would have been to assure a high positive linear correlation between cost and the measure of output thus making the analysis "self-fulfilling" and fruitless. In the latter case, estimates of Q_i might have been omitted thus leading to the same pointless end. It was considered necessary, therefore, to estimate Q_i for those hospitals which reported no service output units. The method of estimation was as follows: It was assumed, (contrary to the general hypothesis of this analysis) that in-patient services are solely a function of patient days and that the missing service outputs should consequently be estimated on some basis of patient days. In particular, for those hospitals reporting units of the service in question the average number of units of the service per patient days was calculated and this ratio was then applied to the number of patient days reported by the hospitals which had given no service output units. For example, suppose that out of twenty-three reporting hospitals fifteen are known to offer electroencephalograms either because they list the units of this service (and the cost), as in the case of say 9, or because they reported total electroencephelogram costs but not the number of units, as in the case of say 2, or because they are listed in the *Guide Issue* as offering this service even though they reported neither costs nor units, as in the case of say 4. From the nine hospitals reporting numbers of electroencephalograms a ratio of encephalograms to patient days was computed. This ratio was then applied against the number of patient days reported by the other six hospitals.

After developing the measure of output and adjusting costs for nonpatient and other expenses, two regressions, one for 1962 data and the other for 1963–1964 observations, were made on New York City data. Second and third powers of the measure of output were included to see if a curvilinear relation was better. The results were somewhat surprising. For 1962 data the correlation between adjusted output (S^k) and costs (.973) was higher than that between unadjusted output (adult and pediatric patient days) and costs (.961) but both were much higher than expected. The first power correlations were in every case higher than the second and third power correlations but the constant term of the straight line was negative. The results for the 1963–1964 observations were similar except that the correlations were higher. The simple correlation between patient days and cost was .978 while between adjusted output and cost was a surprising .992.

For the 1963–1964 data there was a significant increase in the multiple correlation in the quadratic total cost curve (.9923 to .9962) and F levels remained above 10.0. The regression equation was as follows: [13]

$$C = \begin{array}{l} 499446.3 \ (264107.0) \end{array} + \begin{array}{l} 17.16104(S^k) \ (2.33257) \end{array}$$
$$+ \begin{array}{l} .00002395(S^k)^2 \ (.000005512) \end{array}$$
$$R^2 = .9925$$

F level to remove

$$S^k = 54.1$$
$$(S^k)^2 = 18.9$$

F level to enter

$$(S^k)^3 = .0059$$

This gives a slowly rising straight line marginal cost curve,[14] and an approximately "U" shaped average cost curve which has a low

[13] *Editors' Note:* Numbers in parentheses are standard error coefficients. The critical F values specify the range within which an F statistic (a statistic signifying statistical significance) must fall for the variable to be included in the regression analysis.

[14] *Editors' Note:* A marginal cost curve represents the incremental change in total cost for a change in quantity. Mathematically it is derived by calculating the first derivative of total cost with respect to quantity. (Refer to Appendix I for a discussion of derivatives.)

point of $24.08 at approximately $S^k = 144000$.[15] For those used to thinking of hospital sizes in other units, this represents about 85–90,000 patient days, or about 290–295 beds. Average cost is below $24.20 for a fairly wide range (120,000–175,000). This range of hospital sizes might be described as the "large but not largest" class. Of the 2,493 accredited voluntary nonprofit short-term general and other special hospitals registered with the American Hospital Association in 1964, 851 were under 100 beds, 761 from 100–199 beds, 436 from 200–299 beds, 251 from 300–399 beds and 194–400 beds and over.[16]

While the evidence based on New York City costs may be weak, it suggests building fairly large (250–350 bed) hospitals where the population is large and dense enough to be expected to support them. Larger hospitals may be necessary as centers for certain types of therapy. Smaller hospitals (under 100 beds at least) are preferable only when the increased travel cost to the patient is greater than the increased operating cost to the hospital, i.e. in sparsely populated areas.

APPLYING THE MEASURE OF OUTPUT OUTSIDE NEW YORK CITY

There are several further questions which might be asked concerning the applicability of the measure of output formula to hospitals outside the New York City area. First, weighted operations and deliveries have been used in S^k rather than "admissions," used by Saathoff and Kurtz. Probably most hospitals have operation and delivery information available. Certainly they know the number of births, which is a good estimator of deliveries. Second, the high weight given to transfusions in Table 5 is caused simply by blood being extremely expensive in New York (approximately $40.00 a pint). In many other places, blood is provided free by the Red Cross and other area blood bank organizations. I would estimate that less than half the charges allocated to the average hospital's "blood bank service center" are nonblood costs. Thirdly, differences in labor intensities of various hospital services determine the impact of geographical differences in wage levels upon the weights used in calculating S^k. If all hospital services were equally labor intensive

[15] *Editors' Note:* Refer to Chapter Six for a step by step illustration of how a minimum cost point is derived.

[16] American Hospital Association: *Hospitals,* August 1, 1965.

then geographical variations of the wage level would not generate differences in the ratio of costs of different services; this equal labor intensity would have to extend to both direct and indirect labor costs. Since, however, hospital services are not equally labor intensive geographical wage variations will affect the ratio of their costs. It was not feasible to trace all allocations to obtain the percentage of final allocated costs attributable to labor rather than other factors in all the various service categories. Work Schedule No. 1 of the United Hospital Fund's Annual Worksheet gives direct labor costs for the "auxiliary service cost centers." Direct labor costs for adult and pediatric patient days and for nursery days were not readily available because nursing labor costs were allocated at a later time between these services. The percentages of direct labor costs to total cost for most auxiliary service cost centers were taken from the work schedule for the hospitals visited in 1965. The unweighted average of the individual observations are shown in Table 6.

TABLE 6
DIRECT LABOR AS A PER CENT OF TOTAL COST

	Year		
Service	1964	1963	1962
Operating room	44.6%	42.5%	42.8%
Delivery room	45.7	40.2	43.7
X-ray, diagnostic	51.6	46.0	49.1
Laboratory	60.4	58.0	60.9
Physical therapy	46.4	48.4	49.0
Electrocardiograph	62.6	58.3	57.9
X-ray, therapeutic	33.0	34.0	33.3
Blood and blood bank [a]	7.3	7.6	8.0
Out-patient department	49.3	47.1	46.1
Emergency room	53.3	54.6	47.7

[a] Five hospitals reported no direct labor costs for blood and blood bank.

As can be seen, for most services, direct labor costs amount to 40–55 per cent of total cost; the laboratory and electrocardiograph services are more labor intensive while the therapeutic x-ray and blood bank services are less. (Even if we exclude the five hospitals which charged no direct labor to the blood bank, this service still maintains the lowest proportion of direct labor costs: 25.5% to 28%.)

Since the weights assigned in the measure of output (S^k) formula depend upon the ratio of the average cost of a particular hospital service to cost per patient day; and since variations in the wage level

have a greater or lesser effect on this ratio according to the greater
or lesser labor intensity of the hospital service (relative to the average
labor intensity of all services), the weights in the formula will be
sensibly affected by wage variations only for the services at the
extremes of the distribution of Table 6. For example, assume the
following data which have been designed to show the greater relative
cost of labor intensive services in high wage areas. The rural area is
assumed to render $\frac{1}{10}$ the service of the urban area; its wage index is
$\frac{1}{2}$ that of the urban area and the index for "other" costs is the
same in both areas. For simplicity a linear production function is
assumed for both services. It will be noticed that "operations" are
relatively more costly (and "exams" relatively less costly) in the
rural area than in the urban area reflecting the greater labor intensity of exams. This is, of course, the sort of "Heckscher-Ohlin" result
that international trade theory would have suggested before the
"Leontieff paradox." [17]

	Urban	Rural
Wage index	100	50
Annual cost of laboratory services	$100,000	$7000
Wage cost	$60,000	$3000
Other	$40,000	$4000
Number of exams	50,000	5000
Average cost of exams	$2.00	$1.40
Annual cost of operating rooms	$100,000	$8000
Wage cost	$40,000	$2000
Other	$60,000	$6000
Number of operations	500	50
Average cost of operations	$200.00	$160.00
Ratio of average costs	100:1	114:1

A fourth, and perhaps the main, problem in applying the formula
for S^k is that the services omitted in the calculation of S^k are the

[17] *Editors' Note:* The "Hecksher-Ohlin" result and the "Leontieff paradox" refer
to aspects of international trade theory reflecting on what goods or services geographic areas are expected to specialize in and export. Hecksher and Ohlin predicted, on theoretical grounds, that areas would specialize in the production and
export of goods and services whose production required the use of inputs in which
the areas had a relative surplus. Empirical studies found that the United States
exported labor intensive goods and imported capital intensive goods, which appeared to refute this hypothesis. Leontieff provided an explanation for this apparent paradox—the greater efficiency of United States labor makes its *effective* labor
supply comparatively greater than its capital supply. (Refer to Chapter Ten, for a
definition of effective labor.)

ones found in the fewest, and typically the biggest, hospitals, thereby discriminating in favor of the smaller hospitals; it is a peculiarity of the UHF sample of New York City hospitals that it was possible to subtract total allocated costs of these rare services so as to make costs more comparable. Such costs could not be taken into account for the six-state sample, however, as the *Guide Issue* did not report on the availability of rare services (other than home care or a radioactive isotope facility) in 1962. The 1965 *Guide Issue* reports on psychiatric in-patient care, cobalt and radium therapy, rehabilitation unit, and a family planning service. Further research should be directed toward the incorporation of these rare services in any formula for the quantification of hospital outputs.

Despite these drawbacks, the weights in the formula for S^k, which were derived from the UHF data, were applied to the data from the six-state sample.

On the other hand, the lack of detailed information as to the number of units of individual services which was provided by each of the hospitals in the six-state sample required some modification of the original formula for S^k. That formula was as follows:

$$S^k = \sum_i W_i Q_i^k$$

Since Q_i^k is unknown, for services other than adult and pediatric patient days, newborn days, and deliveries, it is replaced by

$$\frac{\sum_k Q_i^k}{\sum_k P_i^k} d_i^k P^k$$

where

$$\sum_k Q_i^k = \text{the total number of units of the } i\text{th service}$$

reported by UHF hospitals reporting units of the ith service

$$\sum_k P_i^k = \text{the total number of patient days reported}$$

in the hospitals reporting units of the ith service

d_i^k = dummy variable[18] signifying whether the ith service is offered in the kth hospital in the 6-state sample (1 if offered; 0 if not).[19]

P^k = number of adult and pediatric patient days in the kth hospital in 6-state sample.

This procedure assumes that all services, where available, are offered in the same ratio to in-patient days as they are offered by the hospitals reporting them in the UHF sample. However, better estimates of Q_i^k for adult and pediatric patient days, newborn days, and deliveries are available in the *Guide Issue*. For these services Q_i^k was estimated as 365 times average daily adult and pediatric census, 365 times average daily newborn census, and number of births respectively.

The measure of output, then, is derived by the formula:

$$S^k = \sum Wi \frac{\sum_k Q_i^k}{\sum_k P_i^k} d_i^k P^k$$

or from Table 7

$$S^k = \sum_i R_i d_i^k P^k$$

The correlation between adjusted costs (A^k from part 1) and adjusted output (S^k) was virtually the same as that between the unadjusted figures (C^k from part 1 and P^k): 0.980 versus 0.979. The highest correlation, 0.983, was between adjusted costs (A^k) and unadjusted output (P^k), but the only economically meaningful regression was for the adjusted figures in the quadratic form. This regression is as follows:

$$A^k = 88802.6 + 19.09026S^k$$
$$(44725.4) \quad (1.76727)$$
$$+ \quad .000013066(S^k)^2$$
$$(.000003908)$$
$$R^2 = .9679$$

[18] *Editors' Note:* The effect of this dummy variable specification is to set S^k (output) equal to zero in those instances where the particular service is not offered.

[19] All hospitals in the 6-state sample offered operating room (s), diagnostic x-rays, electrocardiograms, and both a clinical and pathological laboratory. As was mentioned above, hospitals with only one of the laboratories were not used as it was not known how to allocate the appropriate weights.

F level to remove

$$S^k = 116.7$$
$$(S^k)^2 = 11.2$$

F level to enter

$$(S^k)^3 = .0405$$

This again gives a slowly rising straight line marginal cost curve and a "U" shaped average cost curve. The average cost curve has a low point between 80–85,000 units of service or about 160–170 beds. The low point of this average cost curve is approximately $21.25. Average cost is below $21.35 for the range from 60,000–115,000 or from about 125–235 beds. This is a smaller hospital than previously appeared to be least cost but most of the range is well above the

TABLE 7

Service Units	Relative cost (Wi)	Units per patient day	Relative cost per patient days (Ri)
Operations, weighted	4.75	.033	.1568
Deliveries	2.36	a	2.36
X-rays, diagnostic	.16	.65	.1040
Laboratory examinations	.07	2.01	.1407
Physical therapy treatments	.15	.153	.023
Electrocardiograms	.20	.06	.012
X-ray, therapy treatments	.39	.03	.012
Blood transfusions (inc. Plasma)	.90	.02	.018
Newborn days	.53	b	.53
Outpatient visits	.28	.40	.112
Electroencephalograms	.73	.0055	.004
Emergency room treatments	.16	.16	.026
Adult and pediatric days	1.00	1.00	1.00

[a] Births used as units.
[b] 365 newborn census used as units.

national median size of hospitals. It must be remembered that the cost figures used include costs for other services and for nonpatient expenses. They also include costs for nursing schools and for interns and residents. Programs for the latter and often for the former are only approved in larger hospitals.

CONCLUSIONS

While this study has been somewhat introductory and many simplifying assumptions have been used, the achievement of putting hospital data, both cost inputs and outputs of services, on a more comparable basis may facilitate wise planning and meaningful cost comparisons. The main advantage found in using the adjusted figures was in the resultant economically reasonable cost curves rather than in the slightly higher correlations generally found.

While the evidence is insufficient to make any further narrowing down possible, it appears that hospitals between 150 and 350 beds are most efficient for ordinary patient care. Larger hospitals might be needed for special services but do not appear to be most efficient for the more or less routine services included in the measure of output. It also appears that on an annual basis many patient costs are variable, with marginal costs between $21.50 and $22.00 for a hospital of about 200 beds. This is the marginal cost per unit of output, as output has been measured in this paper. The composition of this unit may vary greatly. It is clear that more work must be done to broaden the measure of output and to further facilitate the planning of urban health care complexes.

AN ECONOMIC AND LINEAR MODEL
OF THE HOSPITAL [20]

HELMY H. BALIGH AND DANNY J. LAUGHHUNN

One of the most difficult problems encountered in deriving decision models to aid in hospital planning is the development of a meaningful definition of hospital output suitable to economic analysis. An excellent discussion of this problem is given by Feldstein. A definition of output often suggested is patient days during the time period of concern, but this measures only a *property* of hospital output: it is inadequate for economic analysis, since it implies that all patient days are homogeneous with respect to resource absorption. Further, this measure fails to distinguish between types of patients served with respect to the objectives of the hospital in terms of "value" of patients: in most hospitals certain types of cases are considered more important than others, on the basis, for example, of the possibility of widespread epidemics or of certain death if the patient is not treated.

Another measure of output often used is a weighted average of the number of individual services to all patients during the time period, with the individual weights determined by the average cost of providing the services. However, this provides only a measure

[20] Reprinted with permission from *Health Services Research, 4,* No. 4, Winter 1969, pp. 293–303. Copyright © 1969, by Hospital Research and Educational Trust.

of *intermediate* hospital output: the services are performed with the ultimate purpose of treating patients. Further, given the extent of aggregation involved in computing the weighted average of hospital services, this measure of intermediate output provides no information concerning *terminal* output that would be useful in economic analysis.

An alternative measure of terminal output that meets the objections to the definitions mentioned is developed here on the basis of the concept of equivalence classes of patients and on the following general assumptions, some of which are discussed in more detail in later sections:

1. Each potential patient to arrive at the hospital can be unambiguously assigned to one of m equivalence classes E_i on the basis of his "value" to the hospital and his requirements for hospital-supplied goods and services.
2. The objective of the hospital is to maximize a weighted sum of the number of patients admitted from the equivalence classes.
3. The technology of the hospital is adequately described by a linear relationship between outputs of services and inputs of resources.
4. The quantities of at least some of the resources necessary to provide treatment for patients are fixed and unalterable during the time period under analysis.
5. The time period for the analysis is fixed but arbitrary, e.g. one month or one year.
6. Patient admissions can be completely controlled by the hospital; that is, the number of patients to be admitted from each equivalence class during the time period is a variable controlled by the hospital administration.[21]

Additional assumptions are introduced and discussed in the subsequent analysis to emphasize their importance in the model development.

OUTPUT

Assume that there are n different intermediate outputs of the hospital, each a distinct good or service limited by availability of

[21] *Editors' Note:* While this assumption may at first glance appear to contradict reality, it is nevertheless true that strong administrative directives (from the administrator or chiefs of service) to attending physicians, and house staff can have a significant impact on a hospital's patient mix.

resources and by decisions on technology, budget, and policy. Given the set of all potential patients, for each patient x_i a function is assumed, specifiable for any time period, such that $f(x_i) = r^i$, where $r^i = (r_1^i, r_2^i, \ldots, r_n^i)$ is the requirement vector [22] of potential patient x_i. Any component r_k^i is the amount of the kth good or service needed by the patient if admitted to the hospital.

The function f will permit distinction between types of potential patients on the basis of their demands on the hospital's intermediate outputs and, ultimately, on its resources. But the relative value attached by the hospital to meeting potential patients' requirements is another important distinction. In order to include this in the model, a function g is assumed such that $g(x_i) = w^i$, where w^i represents the value the hospital places upon supplying the total requirements of potential patient x_i during the given period. The value of each patient to the hospital plays a major role in the definition of the hospital's objective function, and the requirements of each patient play a major role in determining the output capacity of the hospital.

The hospital's terminal output is defined as a weighted sum of the number of patients treated within each equivalence class during the period. The set of weights specified by the hospital administration reflects the basic importance of the different equivalence classes. This measure of hospital output is, in contrast to patient days, related to resource absorption, since the equivalence classes in the weighted sum are defined in terms of the value of patients within them *and* in terms of requirements for hospital resources. Also, this definition of output, unlike a weighted average of services performed, measures a patient-oriented terminal output rather than an intermediate output.

Equivalence Classes

To facilitate expressing the model in useful terms, it is necessary to simplify the specification of patients to a statement of the number of patients to be admitted from patient classes. The functions *f* and *g* serve as the bases for creating patient classes such that no potential patient belongs to more than one class and no potential patient fails to belong to a class; that is, classes that are collectively exhaustive and mutually exclusive.

The equivalence relation states that any two patients x_i and x_j

[22] *Editors' Note:* A vector, in the sense used here, represents a series of numbers detailing the amount of goods or services required per potential patient.

belong to the same equivalence class if, and only if, they fulfill the following conditions: if either has zero requirements for a given service, both have; if either requires a given service in an amount different from zero within a defined range, the other also requires that service in an amount within the same defined range; and the hospital-assigned weights on the two are equal. If desired, the latter condition could be relaxed by defining a range into which both weights must fall.

The relation thus defined may be stated mathematically and proved to be one of equivalence. It describes some total number m of equivalence classes; the number of such classes will depend on the number of distinct values of the weights w_i for all potential patients and on the nature of the individual patient requirement vectors.

Average Requirement Vectors

Let E_i denote any one of the m equivalence classes and $H(E_i)$ denote the total number of potential patients in that class. For any patient x_i in the ith equivalence class, the function $f(x_i) = r^j$ gives the hospital intermediate outputs required by that potential patient. For simplicity, an average requirement vector for the patients in an equivalence class is defined as R_i, the vector of average total requirements of the patients in E_i. The component average requirements for individual services which make up $R_i = (R_{i1}, R_{i2}, \ldots, R_{in})$ are given by the following equation: [23]

$$R_{ij} = \frac{\sum_{g=1}^{H(E_i)} r_j{}^g}{H(E_i)} \qquad (j = 1, 2, \ldots, n) \qquad (1)$$

The components of the average vector are therefore the averages of similar requirements r^j over all patients in the equivalence class.

Assume now that for any given subset of potential patients in equivalence class E_i, the total requirement for all n hospital outputs is $X_i R_i = (X_i R_{i1}, X_i R_{i2}, \ldots, X_i R_{in})$, where X_i is the number of patients in the subset. The implications of this assumption are not minor ones and deserve special emphasis. In effect, the requirements of all patients in an equivalence class have been completely homogenized, which, of course, implies the assumption that $r^i = r^j$ if x_i and x_j are in the same class E_i, when in fact the equivalence

[23] *Editors' Note:* In the equation, *g* is the index of summation and it ranges over all patients in the ith equivalence class, E_i. (Recall that $H(E_i)$ denotes the number of patients in equivalence class E_i.)

relation that defines the conditions under which x_i and x_j are in the same class implies nothing of the sort.

To illustrate this difference, consider a simple example. Let

$$E_i = (x_1, x_3, x_7)$$
$$f(x_1) = r^1 = (0, 1, 4)$$
$$f(x_3) = r^3 = (0, 2, 5)$$
$$f(x_7) = r^7 = (0, 1, 6)$$

According to the definition of the average requirement vector, $R_i = (0, 4/3, 5)$, and for any subset of two patients in E_i, the total requirement vector is assumed to be $2R_i$, or $2(0, 4/3, 5) = (0, 8/3, 10)$. But the real requirement vector for the pair of potential patients x_1 and x_3 is $r^1 + r^3 = (0, 3, 9)$; for the pair x_1 and x_7 it is $r^1 + r^7 = (0, 2, 10)$; and for the pair x_3 and x_7 it is $r^3 + r^7 = (0, 3, 11)$. Note that not one of the vectors of *real* requirements for any pair of patients is equal to the *assumed* value of the requirement vector. Except for special cases this assumption will be correct only if $X_i = 0$ or $X_i = H(E_i)$, that is, if the subset is simply the whole class. The inability to describe exactly the actual requirements of subsets of patients within an equivalence class is the "cost" associated with this problem simplification. In return for this cost, however, the planning problem has been made analytically tractable.

THE OBJECTIVE FUNCTION

It is assumed that the objective of the hospital in its planning process is to optimize the total output during the time period. To be more specific: let w_i denote the weight given to the ith equivalence class of patients, with $w_i > 0$, where $w_i = g(x_j) = w^i$ for any member x_j of the class; by the equivalence relation, all the patients in a class are assigned the same weight. The total weighted output Z of the hospital is therefore given by the expression

$$Z = \sum_{i=1}^{m} w_i(X_i + Y_i) \qquad (2)$$

where X_i is the number of paying patients treated in the ith equivalence class during the time period and Y_i is the number of indigent patients treated in the ith equivalence class during the time period.

This weighting scheme assumes that the hospital administration places equal emphasis on the treatment of regular and indigent patients within equivalence classes. However, a weighting scheme that places different weights on regular and indigent patients is possible without added complexity. Specification of the complete set of weights, i.e. the function g, is the role of a policy-making group in the hospital and reflects the hospital's objective in terms of treating and/or curing the patients in the equivalence classes. Examples of factors possibly influencing the relative values of assigned weights are moral and ethical considerations, the probability of epidemics or of the patient's death, and the existence of alternative hospitals to provide the services required.

No constraints are placed on the values of the weights assigned to equivalence classes, except that if a patient in the ith equivalence class is considered "more important" than a patient in the jth equivalence class, then $w_i > w_j$, and if $w_i > w_j$ and $w_j > w_k$, then $w_i > w_k$. There is, of course, no inherent requirement that equivalence classes must be weighted differently. If patients in all m equivalence classes are considered equally important, this is translated into the requirement $w_1 = w_2 = \cdots = w_m$, with the specific value of the common weight arbitrary for purposes of determining optimal output for the hospital.

Given any specific set of weights and an arbitrary number of patients treated for each equivalence class, Z provides a measure of total hospital output. The maximum value of Z determined by the optimal numbers of patients treated in each equivalence class, consistent with the technology of the hospital, available resources, budgetary restrictions, and hospital policies, will be defined as the output capacity of the hospital during the time period in question.

CONSTRAINTS

Resources and Technology

The optimal values of X_1 and Y_1 for each equivalence class and the optimal value of Z for a specific hospital will obviously be influenced by the fixed amounts of some of the resources at the disposal of the hospital. Relationships must therefore be established between levels of requirements for the equivalence classes and resource utilization that will describe the *feasible combinations* for optimal output in order to narrow the search.

To establish the relevant relationships, assume that all resources needed in operating the hospital and at the disposal of the hospital are divided into two broad categories: fixed and variable. The fixed category consists of all resources that cannot be altered during the time period in question, either in form or in quantity, while the variable category includes all resources that can be obtained in any desired form or quantity during the period. Examples of fixed resources are beds and various types of surgical equipment; variable resources are food and such supplies as drugs and surgical dressings. Resources are regarded as different within each category if they are not interchangeable in use: a bed designated for pediatric care only is different, by policy, from an identical one designated for post-surgical care only. Alternatively, two nurses with identical job specifications belong to the same resource group. Assume further, then, that the fixed resources are divided into K different classes, that the variable resources are divided into L different classes, and that these classes within each category are mutually exclusive and collectively exhaustive.

Now let T_k denote the total number of units of a given fixed resource in class k that are available to the hospital in treating patients during the time period in question. T_k will have a time dimension based on this period: for example, bed days, the unit of bed resource, will be found by multiplying the number of beds by the number of days in question; nurse days is the total of the number of nurses multiplied by the number of working days in the period. These represent the maximum amounts of the respective resources available to the hospital during the period. There is no upper limit on the availability of variable resources, since by definition these can be obtained in any amount required.

The relationship between service requirements R_{ij}, defined earlier as an estimate of the average requirements of a patient in the ith equivalence class for the jth service, and inputs of resources (both fixed and variable) is determined by the technology of the hospital, in the sense of the process by which a set of inputs is transformed into one or more goods or services. These goods and services, denoted arbitrarily by the set of indexes $j = 1, 2, \ldots, n$, are intermediate outputs created by the hospital in the process of treating the patients admitted, for example, meals, x-rays, blood tests, and surgery. There may be alternative technologies (or production functions) for the jth good or service that combine inputs in a manner consistent with accepted standards of medical practice. With more than one function available, the problem of choosing among them is an economic one: the hospital should adopt that technology for service j which minimizes its cost. Here, since the object is to construct a short-run planning model for an existing hospital with a given technology, it is assumed that the choice of technology has been previously made, perhaps when the hospital was designed, and the planning model is developed within the constraints imposed by this existing technology.

Given the technology, the quantity of service j provided to a patient in the ith equivalence class, denoted R_{ij}, is uniquely determined by the amounts of inputs supplied to the transformation process.[24] If $d_{1j}, d_{2j}, \ldots, d_{Kj}$ denotes the amount of each of the fixed resources, and $q_{1j}, q_{2j}, \ldots, q_{Lj}$ the variable resources used in the transformation process resulting in service j, the technology can be summarized parametrically as

$$R_{ij} = f(d_{1j}, d_{2j}, \ldots, d_{Kj}; q_{1j}, \ldots, q_{Lj}) \qquad (3)$$

The function f, a production function defining a given technology, relates the inputs used to the unique value of output that results. The technology used for each good or service, and therefore the nature of its production function, is assumed to be independent of the particular equivalence class receiving that good or service.

The total technology previously chosen by the hospital is assumed to be adequately represented by a set of individual technologies, one for each service, that exhibit proportionality between inputs and outputs and are additive in terms of resource usage. This distinguishes the assumed technologies as linear, in that resource inputs are absorbed in direct proportion to the level of intermediate output R_{ij}, that is, $d_{kj} = a_{kj} R_{ij}$, $q_{1j} = b_{1j} R_{ij}$, where a_{kj} is the number of units of a given fixed resource and b_{1j} is the number of units of a variable resource required in the production of one unit of the jth service. Inputs must expand in direct proportion to outputs; this technology is a special case of constant returns to scale.

The second distinguishing characteristic of a linear technology is that the total absorption of each resource is found by adding the individual resource usages of all services requiring the resource. This implies that there is no interference created by using a resource for the production of more than one service during the period. The usage of fixed resource k for all services produced in fulfilling the requirement R_{ij} is therefore written as

$$\sum_{j=1}^{n} a_{kj} R_{ij}$$

[24] *Editors' Note:* Refer to Chapter Six for a discussion of this process.

The resource absorption by R_{ij} for all equivalence classes is based on Equations (1) and (2); since the total resource availability T_k cannot be exceeded, the constraint on feasible values of X_i and Y_i may be expressed as

$$\sum_{i=1}^{m} \sum_{j=1}^{n} (X_i + Y_i)\, a_{kj}\, R_{ij} \leq T_k \qquad (4)$$

for each fixed resource, and only those combinations of output which satisfy Equation (4) need be considered as values of X_i and Y_i to maximize Z. There is, of course, no counterpart to Equation (4) for variable inputs, since there is no upper limit on the availability of these.

Numbers of Patients

Even though it is assumed that admissions of patients from the equivalence classes represent variables controllable by the hospital, there is an upper limit on the number available within each equivalence class. Earlier, $H(E_i)$ was defined as the total number of potential patients in equivalence class E_i, assumed to be the sum of paying and indigent patients. Availability of patients therefore generates constraints of the form

$$X_i + Y_i \leq H(E_i) \qquad (5)$$

Inclusion of these constraints in the planning model will guarantee an optimal solution consistent with availabilities of patients.

Budget

The hospital cannot operate independently of the resultant monetary flows during the time period considered. While budgetary restrictions might take a variety of forms in different hospitals, the model's structure may be illustrated by a single budgetary restriction for the entire hospital, ignoring budgetary restrictions at departmental levels. The purpose of this aggregate budgetary constraint is to relate the total revenue generated by all equivalence classes, the total cost of variable inputs used in providing service to the equivalence classes, the target level of profit G, cost per period of fixed resources F, and the external subsidy S.

Let c_l denote the cost per unit of variable input l, recalling that b_{lj} is the absorption of variable resource l in the process of producing one unit of the jth service. The total cost incurred by the hospital for variable resources is given by [25]

$$C = \sum_{i=1}^{m} \sum_{j=1}^{n} \sum_{l=1}^{L} c_l b_{lj} (X_i + Y_i) \, R_{ij} \tag{6}$$

If p_j denotes the price charged for one unit of the jth service, and price charged is independent of the equivalence class, then the total revenue I generated by all patients during the time period is

$$I = \sum_{i=1}^{m} \sum_{j=1}^{n} X_i \, R_{ij} \, p_j \tag{7}$$

Note that the provision of services to indigent patients does not generate revenue but does result in a cost to the hospital.

The budgetary restriction simply states that the total revenue I minus the total variable cost incurred must be at least equal to the target level of profit G plus the total cost of fixed resources F less the external subsidy S. This budgetary restriction is written

$$I - C \geq G + F - S \tag{8}$$

where I and C are as expressed in Equations (6) and (7).

The right-hand side of Equation (8) is general and includes as special cases hospitals with no external subsidy $(S = 0)$ and non-profit hospitals $(G = 0)$.

Policy

The policy decisions that establish the legitimate concerns of the hospital are sometimes implicit rather than explicit and may involve use of resources, accepted medical practices, or the proper output mix. These can change as experience indicates benefit, but they represent constraints on acceptable combinations of intermediate outputs just as effective as those rising from resource restrictions. Obviously the range of different possible policy constraints is too large to permit discussion of all types, but specific examples can be formulated and incorporated into the model.

Suppose, for example, that the hospital under study is a teaching hospital and, in order to guarantee a sufficient number of patients

[25] *Editors' Note:* Equation (6) involves a triple summation over all m equivalence classes, n intermediate outputs, and L variable inputs.

within each equivalence class for teaching purposes, identifies a minimum acceptable number of patients D_i from each equivalence class during the period. Assuming that regular and indigent patients in each equivalence class are completely interchangeable for teaching purposes, the constraint for each class is given by

$$X_i + Y_i \geq D_i \qquad (9)$$

This constraint is general and allows, as special cases, a nonteaching hospital ($D_i = 0$ for all i) and a teaching hospital without minimum requirements for some classes ($D_i = 0$ for some i).

Another policy constraint might arise in a hospital that has a policy objective that requires it to treat indigent patients even though they generate no revenue in return. Assume the policy states that a prespecified fraction of patients treated in each equivalence class must be indigent. Let V_i denote the minimum acceptable fraction greater than zero of indigent patients in equivalence class i. The constraint takes the form

$$Y_i(1 - V_i) - X_i V_i \geq 0 \qquad (10)$$

THE COMPLETE MODEL

The complete linear model developed for the hospital is:
Maximize

$$Z = \sum_{j=1}^{n} w_i(X_i + Y_i)$$

subject to resource constraint:

$$\sum_{i=1}^{m} \sum_{j=1}^{n} (X_i + Y_i)\, a_{kj}\, R_{ij} \leq T_k \qquad (k = 1, 2, \ldots, K)$$

patient constraint:

$$X_i + Y_i \leq H(E_i) \qquad (i = 1, 2, \ldots, m)$$

budgetary constraint:

$$\sum_{i=1}^{m} \sum_{j=1}^{n} X_i\, R_{ij}\, p_j - \sum_{i=1}^{m} \sum_{j=1}^{n} \sum_{l=1}^{L} c_l\, b_{lj}(X_i + Y_i)\, R_{ij} \geq G + F - S$$

policy constraints:

$$X_i + Y_i \geq D_i$$
$$Y_i(1 - V_i) - V_i X_i \geq 0 \qquad (i = 1, 2, \ldots, m)$$

The model also requires that all decision variables be nonnegative, i.e. $X_i \geq 0$ and $Y_i \geq 0$ for all i.

A cursory examination shows that the task of data collection and parameter estimation necessary to make the model operational as a planning tool is likely to be difficult. The parameters needed—the patient weights w_i, prices p_j, target profit level G, and patient restrictions D_i, V_i, and H (E_i)—can be determined from policy statements and records of previous decisions; the parameters of resource limits T_k, input costs c_i, fixed costs F, and external subsidy S can be found in accounting records; but the estimation of requirements vectors R_i and technological coefficients is more complicated. Once the goods and services produced by the hospital and all inputs have been identified and the equivalence classes specified, a sample of observations on T patients served by the hospital is required, consisting of these data for each of the patients:

$q_{j,t}$ = requirement of each good or service j by patient t.

$s_{ij,t}$ = usage of each fixed input i in producing requirement j for patient t.

$u_{ij,t}$ = usage of each variable input i in producing requirement j for patient t.

If the data collected are divided into subsets corresponding to patient equivalence classes, then unbiased estimates of the components of the requirements vector for each equivalence class (assuming at least one observation in each class) can be obtained:

$$R_{ij} = \frac{1}{T_i} \sum_{t=1}^{T_i} q_{j,t}$$

where T_i is the number of patient observations in equivalence class E_i. Similar estimates of the technological coefficients can be calculated from

$$a_{ij} = \frac{1}{T} \sum_{t=1}^{T} \frac{s_{ij,t}}{q_{j,t}}$$

and

$$b_{ij} = \frac{1}{T} \sum_{t=1}^{T} \frac{u_{ij,t}}{q_{j,t}}$$

This set of estimates is unbiased, of course, only if the technology of the hospital is linear as assumed, though the model could be extended to handle nonlinear objective functions also. (Feldstein discusses the problem of linearity and provides a test for the assumption.)

It should be noted that in linear models the optimal decision is often relatively insensitive to variations in data input; but given the cost of data collection, decisions based on fairly crude estimates are adequate. The only way to measure the sensitivity of such a decision model to data inaccuracies is to use it in conjunction with a set of preliminary data estimates. The technique of sensitivity analysis is available to evaluate the range of data values over which the same optimal decision will be indicated. This range, once determined, identifies those data inputs which require more thorough investigation prior to final use of the model for decision making.

CONCLUSION

It is not certain that the manner in which hospitals classify patients today meets the defined conditions for equivalence classes. Present practice may not distinguish properly between patients on the basis of total demands on the hospital's fixed resources. "In-patient" and "out-patient" are classes based on requirements of patients for only one of many relevant resources, bed hours. Furthermore, present classes are not always mutually exclusive, since the bases for their creation are not always the same incomplete set of requirements. To illustrate a patient classification method compatible with the model: suppose that patients had only four types of requirements—physician hours, nursing hours, bed hours, and food; that only three nonoverlapping and exhaustive levels of each of the four requirements—zero, high, and low—are distinguished; and that all patients are of equal value. There would be 4×3 equivalence classes; one might be defined as "low, high, zero, zero," where the first component is that for physician hours, the second for nursing hours, and so on. This class, with low physician–high nursing requirements, could also be called "out-patient." The name chosen is irrelevant so long as the conditions on equivalence, which in a real hospital involve many more types of requirements, are met.

The model represents a system in which a decision is to be made on the number of patients to be admitted from each equivalence class. The optimal values of these numbers of patients are those that maximize the hospital's terminal output consistent with its resources and goals, expressed as economically defined determinants of capacity: hospital objectives, available quantities of fixed resources, technology, cost of variable inputs, requirements vectors of equivalence classes, external subsidies, target level of profit, cost of fixed resources, and hospital policies. The output capacity so determined is thus not a physical but rather an economic concept. Its optimized value may be useful in economic analysis of many areas of hospital function in addition to providing a goal for admissions planning.

REFERENCES

Feldstein, M. S.: *Economic Analysis for Health Service Efficiency.* Amsterdam: North-Holland Publishing Company, 1967; Chicago, Markham Publishing Company, 1968.

Peters, W. S. and Summers, G. W.: *Statistical Analysis for Business Decisions.* Englewood Cliffs, N.J.: Prentice-Hall, 1968.

Dantzig, G. B.: *Linear Programming and Extensions.* Princeton, Princeton University Press, 1963.

Chapter Eight

INVESTMENT

THE PRECEDING chapter emphasized the attainment of economic efficiency in production. Production decisions were implicitly assumed to entail decisions of a relatively short-run nature, such as how to produce a given product or product range more efficiently given a specified technological production function and varying amounts of factor inputs. The decision of whether to produce at all, or to invest in the production of the labor skills and capital equipment to be used in the production process was not addressed as such decisions are, by their very nature, usually considered to be of a long-run nature.[1] Investment theory, the area of economic theory presented in this chapter, addresses itself to the attainment of long-run efficiency.

Investment theory is applicable not only in internal institutional management, be it of an administrative or planning nature, but also in analyzing whether certain goods or services which display the characteristics of an investment should be provided either privately or by government acting as an agent of society. Economists generally think of goods or services as having either consumption or investment characteristics. Consumer goods or services are those which yield immediate satisfaction. Consumer goods can be dichotomized into two groups: nondurable and durable. The former yield immediate satisfaction while the latter yield satisfaction in both the present and the future.

---

[1] There are no clear-cut guidelines to distinguish between the short and long run as their duration is a function of the particular activity under investigation. In most cases the distinction must be intuitive. However, a one year period has often been used as the divider between short and long-run periods.

Automobiles and phonographs are examples of durable consumer goods; food and newspapers are nondurable consumer goods. Investment goods or services are ones which are intended primarily for use in the production of future goods. The difference between durable consumer goods and investment goods is that the latter yield satisfaction only through their ability to influence consumption in the future while the former also yield direct satisfaction.

Investment is an extremely important aspect of a modern economy. It is through investment that indirect methods of production can be undertaken, thereby leading to greater output for each labor input. It is an established technological fact that more total output can be generated and greater productive efficiency attained if some labor effort is first applied to the production of physical capital and this capital is then utilized together with the remaining labor effort, than if all the labor is applied directly to the task at hand.

Health care has many attributes which qualify its inclusion primarily in the investment category. Few would assert that the process of acquiring health care is inherently pleasant although, once acquired, health care may enable one to achieve greater appreciation and enjoyment of all of one's activities. On the other side of the ledger, there are definite financial payoffs to acquiring health care. Acquiring health care in the present increases the probability of one's earning more and hence consuming more in the future.

As investment theory draws heavily upon the use of an interest rate, the causes and functions of interest are discussed in the first section of this chapter. Second, the concept of present value is introduced. Next, two techniques based on the use of present value calculations and used in investment decision-making—benefit-cost ratio, and internal rate of return, are presented and evaluated. The fifth section notes the similarity between the planning-programming-budgeting technique and general investment theory. A discussion of how cost-benefit concepts are applied to investments in human beings is presented in the concluding section.

INTEREST: CAUSES AND FUNCTIONS

The *interest rate* is the rental cost of capital.[2] It is primarily a function of three factors: the size of capital's contribution to production, the time period under consideration, and the market supply and demand for loanable funds. The first two factors determine the *existence* of an interest rate, the third explains the prevailing *level* of interest rates.

The basic determinant of interest stems from a generally accepted trait of human behavior. Given the choice between current consumption and future consumption, people generally tend to favor current consumption since present needs are perceived more accurately and acutely than future needs. If one gives up immediate satisfaction such as that derivable from the current use of a resource, greater satisfaction in the future than that foregone in the present is expected as a compensation for waiting. Furthermore, the postponement of current consumption and the allocation of the *saved* resource or resources to current production leads to greater production and consumption in the future.[3] Part of the increased production is used as a payment for the use of the saved resource. Both of these factors, time preference and capital's contribution to production, account for the *pure* interest rate.

Four other factors, in addition to the pure rate of interest, determine the existence of interest. They are the following: inflation, risk, transaction costs, and liquidity. Inflation leads to an erosion in the purchasing power of money; if an inflationary period is anticipated, a payment is required as compensation for this erosion. The greater the expected inflation, the greater the required compensation.

The investment process by its very nature usually embodies a certain amount of risk. There is the risk that the proceeds of the investment will not equal original expectations. At the extreme, there is a risk of total loss. A component of the interest

[2] The term capital, when applied to production refers to physical capital (equipment), and when applied to loans (monetary investment) refers to money capital.
[3] This is the rationale for investment.

rate is thus a payment for the endurance of such risk. The greater the risk, the greater the required payment.

The exchange of resources surrounding an investment (the transfer of funds) gives rise to transaction costs. A borrower's credit rating must be established, a contract specifying the nature of the agreement between borrower and lender must be drawn up, and resources may have to be physically transferred from one location to another. All of these steps entail a cost, whether they are done formally by lawyers or by the individuals involved themselves, and these costs are reflected in the interest rate. The greater the transaction costs the greater the positive increment in the interest rate.

Finally, the lending of any resource means that it is no longer available to its owner for immediate use if it should be needed. The foregoing of this option, described in monetary terms as a liquidity option, requires compensation. Part of the interest rate is thus a premium for illiquidity. The smaller the possibility of converting the debt certificate (I.O.U., bond, etc.) into a liquid asset (money) the greater the required liquidity premium.[4]

It is the summation of the factors embodied in the pure interest rate, inflation and risk premiums, transaction cost, and liquidity adjustment that establish the interest rate. As investment options differ with respect to risk, liquidity, transaction costs and duration (and hence the threat of inflation), a series of interest rates, rather than a uniform rate, exist at any one point in time, as can be seen in Figure 13. However, these factors (inflation, risk, etc.) do not explain the fluctuation in the interest rate for any one type of investment or security. A casual perusal of Figure 13 indicates the magnitude of such fluctuations over the last several years. The *level* of any given type of interest rate is determined by demand and supply factors operating in the financial market (the market for loanable funds).

The supply of loanable funds is primarily determined by income and tastes. When individuals real income increase, more funds are left over after taking care of absolute essentials. One

---

[4] Government and corporate bonds are considered to be quite liquid as established markets exist for their exchange. No established markets exist for the sale of personal I.O.U.'s.

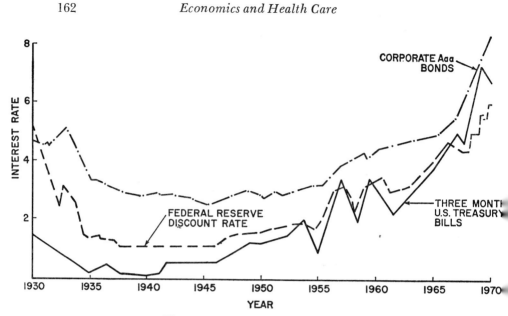

Figure 13. Coexisting interest rates.

Key: Corporate Aaa bonds—an average for the highest grade of corporate bonds.

Federal Reserve discount rate—the rate charged on loans to member banks by the Federal Reserve Board.

Three month U.S. Treasury bills—the most liquid interest bearing debt of the federal government.

of the uses to which these funds can be put is the acquisition of bonds and other commercial or bank debt certificates such as saving accounts.[5] Indeed, savings which lead to the acquisition of bonds and commercial debt certificates has an income elasticity greater than 1; as income increases, savings increase by an even greater proportion.

A second determinant of the supply of loanable funds is tastes or preferences. Attitudinal changes stemming from changes in family status, the state of the economy, or a person's confidence in the safety of an investment, affect an individual's choice be-

[5] A saving account is a bank debt certificate as the bank assumes the obligation to repay the amount deposited in a saving account, plus accrued interest, upon the receipt of the required notification. Saving account deposits, in turn, are one important factor determining a bank's ability to lend money or buy commercial debt certificates.

tween current consumption and saving or investing (future consumption). Tastes and income, respectively, determine the shape (curvature) and position of the supply of loanable funds curve. At any income and preference level, the higher the price paid for the use of loanable funds (the interest rate), the greater the attractiveness of using income for making loans among all the possible uses of income, and the greater the resulting quantity of loanable funds supplied.

The demand for loanable funds is largely determined by investment opportunities. The existence of investment opportunities such as the need for slum clearance and environmental control, color television production, and bread baking create the demand for loans. The more numerous the opportunities, the greater the demand. Investment opportunities, however, are perceived through human eyes; the human interpretation of the investment opportunity rather than its mere existence determines shifts in demand. At any perceived level of investment opportunities, the lower the cost of loanable funds (the interest rate) the greater the quantity of loanable funds demanded.

Just as with other goods and services in the economy, the market allocates the scarce resource, loanable funds, among competing uses. The interaction of supply and demand forces, as expressed in the market, determines the *level* of the interest rate—the price of loanable funds. If demand exceeds supply, the interest rate will rise until the market is cleared (an equilibrium point is reached); if supply exceeds demand, the interest rate will decline.[6]

PRESENT VALUE

The basic question surrounding any investment activity is whether an anticipated or guaranteed future outcome is worth foregoing the present consumption required to allow the investment. The answer to this question lies in the use of an interest rate to calculate the investment's *present value*, a concept al-

[6] This discussion assumes that the market is allowed to function unimpeded. Actually, rationing is often the mechanism utilized, as anyone knows who has tried to borrow money from a financial institution during a period of tight money.

ternately referred to as present discounted value.[7] The present value of any option is defined as *the current value* (the value today) *of the expected future outcome* (return or cost). As most investment options differ with respect to duration and the time flow of the anticipated returns, or costs, a common denominator is required in order to allow a systematic comparison of the various options. The common denominator is the option's current value, its present value.

Present value (PV) is calculated through the use of the following discounting formula.

$$PV = \frac{F_t}{(1 + r)^t} \tag{1}$$

where F is the value of anticipated outcome, r is an interest rate, and t represents the time period under consideration. The procedure embodied in equation (1) entails the discounting (calculating the present value) of F_t by an interest rate r. For example, at an interest (discount) rate of 10 per cent the present value of 5,000 dollars receivable in one year is $4,545.45.[8] If the same return were receivable in year two, its present value would be $4,132.23;[9] while a similar return receivable in year five would have a present value of $3,105.59.[10] If an interest (discount) rate of 5 per cent rather than 10 per cent had been used, the resulting present value of a 5,000 dollar return in one, two, and five years would be $4,761.90, $4,545.45, and $3,906.25 respectively.[11]

[7] Knowledge of an investment's present value also provides the answer for the question, how much should one be willing to pay for a promise of a specified return in some future time period.

[8] $PV = \dfrac{5000}{(1 + 10)^1} = \dfrac{5000}{1.10} = 4{,}545.45$

[9] $PV = \dfrac{5000}{(1 + .10)^2} = \dfrac{5000}{1.21} = 4132.23$

[10] $PV = \dfrac{5000}{(1 + .10)^5} = \dfrac{5000}{1.61} = 3105.59$

[11] $PV = \dfrac{5000}{(1 + .05)^1} = \dfrac{5000}{1.05} = 4761.90$

$PV = \dfrac{5000}{(1 + .05)^2} = \dfrac{5000}{1.10} = 4545.45$

$PV = \dfrac{5000}{(1 + .05)^5} = \dfrac{5000}{1.28} = 3906.25$

The results of these examples illustrate two fundamental characteristics of any present value calculation: the longer (the further in the future) the payoff period the lower the present value, and the lower the interest rate used the higher the present value. The reverse of these two properties also hold: the shorter the payoff period the higher the present value, and the higher the interest rate used the lower the present value.

The present value/time span relationship stems from the fact that interest is compounded periodically; in each time period capital earns a return. In the first period capital, C, earns an interest payment X; in the second period interest is paid on amount $C + X$; in the third period interest is paid on $C + X + X$ and so forth. As the value of the original capital used continually increases due to its factor payment (interest) accrued in the previous periods, a greater compensation must be forthcoming the longer the time period. The present value/interest rate relationship is explainable by noting that the interest rate reflects the return on loanable funds prevailing in the entire financial market at any point in time. The higher the prevailing return for the *general* use of capital, the higher the necessary return required for any *specific* use of capital to insure that the specific investment materializes.

The discussion up to this point explicitly or implicitly assumed that the return from an investment was payable in only one time period, that the interest rate remains constant throughout the period under consideration, and that the outcome was assured. The present value formula can easily be extended to include investment options with multiple period payoffs, fluctuations in the interest rate, and uncertain outcomes.

The present value of a series of future payments is simply the summation of the discounted value of each payment:

$$PV = \sum_{t=1}^{n} \frac{F_t}{(1+r)^t} = \frac{F_1}{(1+r)^1} + \frac{F_2}{(1+r)^2} + \frac{F_3}{(1+r)^3}$$

$$+ \cdots + \frac{F_n}{(1+r)^n} \quad (2)$$

where n is the last time period (t) under consideration and sigma, Σ, is a notation representing the sum of several terms which differ only in the value of t. Referring to the previous example, if an investment option had a 1,000 dollar return in the first year, a 2,000 dollar return in the second year, and a 2,000 dollar return in the fifth year, its present value at a 10 per cent interest rate would be:

$$PV = \frac{1000}{(1+.10)^1} + \frac{2000}{(1+.10)^2} + \frac{0}{(1+.10)^3} + \frac{0}{(1+.10)^4}$$
$$+ \frac{2000}{(1+.10)^5}$$
$$= 909.09 + 1652.89 + 0 + 0 + 1242.23 = 3804.21$$

Although this investment option yields a total payment of 5,000 dollars, its present value is greater than a similar option where the entire yield is receivable in year five (PV = $3105.59) because under the multiple period payoff option three-fifths of the return (3,000 dollars) is received after only two years and can be reinvested (with interest) in other areas. Under the single payoff period option all the capital is tied up until the payoff period (year five) is reached. As capital is productive and can be constantly reinvested, investments which return all or part of the capital in earlier periods at any given interest rate have a higher present value.

Equation (3) contains the appropriate present value formula for a multiple payoff period investment where the interest rate differs by period. In calculating the present value of an option under such conditions the distinctive interest (discount) rate pre-

$$PV = \frac{F_1}{(1+r_1)} + \frac{F_2}{(1+r_1)(1+r_2)} + \frac{F_3}{(1+r_1)(1+r_2)(1+r_3)}$$
$$+ \cdots + \frac{F_n}{(1+r_1)(1+r_2)(1+r_3)\ldots(1+r_n)} \qquad (3)$$

vailing in each period is used.

Similarly, uncertainty of payoff can be included in the present value formula by attaching a probability value, p, to each expected outcome, with the value of the probability coefficient reflecting the degree of uncertainty. Total certainty would result in a probability coefficient of 1, which is what has been implicitly used in previous calculations. The degree of uncertainty would be reflected in probability values ranging from 0 to 1 with higher values reflecting greater certainty. Equation (4) is a modification of equation (3), the modification being the addition of uncertainty to the option whose present value is to be calculated.

$$PV = \frac{p_1F_{1a} + p_2F_{1b} + p_mF_{1o}}{(1 + r_1)} + \frac{p_1F_{2a} + p_2F_{2b} + \cdots + p_mF_{2o}}{(1 + r_1)(1 + r_2)}$$
$$+ \cdots + \frac{p_1F_{na} + p_2F_{nb} + \cdots + p_mF_{no}}{(1 + r_1)(1 + r_2) \ldots (1 + r_n)} \quad (4)$$

$F_a \ldots F_o$ represent all the possible outcomes considered for any given year and $p_1 \ldots p_m$ are the probability coefficients attached to each outcome.[12] The reader should easily be able to modify equations (3) and (4) for use in calculating the present value of an option that has only one payoff period in the future under conditions of both a constant and variable interest rate.

The choice of an interest rate to be used in any present value calculation is crucial. A different interest rate can affect both the absolute present value of any investment, as seen in a previous example, and the relative ranking of two or more investment options. The following example illustrates these points.

	Returns		*Present Value at*	
Investment	*Today*	*In 10 Years*	*20%*	*10%*
A	$100	$ 500	$180	$293
B	0	$1,000	$162	$386

The present values of both investment A and B are higher at 10 per cent than at 20 per cent. However, at an interest rate of 20 per cent investment A has a higher present value; at an interest rate of 10 per cent the reverse is true.

In the absence of an interest rate there would be no systematic way to calculate and compare the value of alternate investment options. The substitution of purely political or personal criteria can result in an overall social loss if these criteria fail to reflect society's desires as expressed by the market supply and demand for loanable funds (investments), or the fact that capital is productive and its productivity may differ in alternate endeavors.

[12] For any given year $p_1 \ldots p_m$ must equal 1.

BENEFIT-COST RATIO

The *benefit-cost ratio* is the crucial indicator used in *cost-benefit studies*. As an investment decision making rule the cost-benefit approach decrees that an investment should be undertaken only if the anticipated benefit derivable from it equals or exceeds the cost that must be borne to make it. The benefit-cost ratio is calculated from the following formula.

$$B/C = \frac{\sum_{t=1}^{n} \dfrac{F_t}{(1+r)^t}}{\sum_{t=1}^{n} \dfrac{C_t}{(1+r)^t}} \qquad (5)$$

B/C refers to the benefit-cost ratio, and F and C refer to the absolute benefits and costs, respectively.

A B/C value of 1 indicates that the present value of the benefits exactly equals the present value of costs; a B/C value greater than 1 indicates that in terms of their present values, benefits exceed costs, while a B/C value less than 1 indicates the reverse. The discounting process involved in present value calculations is applied to costs as well as benefits because costs may also occur over a protracted period of time.

The benefit-cost ratio can be used as an investment guide in evaluating a single investment or a series of investment options. In the latter case, a B/C ratio is calculated for all the options and the one with the highest B/C value is chosen, as that option appears to have the greatest positive benefit-cost ratio. Similarly if the same benefits can be expected from an investment with two alternate designs (cost profiles), a B/C ratio can be calculated for each design option.

One must remember that the interest rate used in any present value calculation, and thus in the B/C ratio calculation, influences the numerical outcome. The choice of an interest rate rather than the anticipated benefits and costs can easily determine whether or not an investment appears justified.[13] Choosing an interest rate which does not reflect the prevailing cost of capital has often led to an erroneous investment choice. In an attempt to overcome this limitation inherent in a cost-benefit analysis, researchers usually postulate two or more interest rates covering a wide range and imply that an investment is proven viable only if its B/C ratio is above 1 for the interest rate deemed most reasonable.

INTERNAL RATE OF RETURN

A commonly encountered investment decision making alternative to the benefit-cost ratio, which is not affected by the choice of an interest rate to be used in the discounting process, is the *internal rate of return* criteria. The use of the internal rate of return criteria implies the following investment decision making rule: invest if the internal rate of return exceeds some predetermined cut-off rate; and when a choice among alternate investments must be made, choose the investment with the highest internal rate of return.

The internal rate of return is calculated by assuming a B/C ratio value of 1 in equation **(5)** and solving for r, which is then

---

[13] Consider the following potential investment: benefits (guaranteed) of 15,000 dollars, payable at a rate of 5,000 dollars for three years; costs of 14,500 dollars, payable at a rate of 7,250 dollars for two years. At an interest rate of 5 per cent this potential investment has a B/C of 1.01; at an interest rate of 10 per cent the B/C ratio is 0.99.

$$\text{B/C} = \frac{\dfrac{5000}{(1+.05)^1} + \dfrac{5000}{(1+.05)^2} + \dfrac{5000}{(1+.05)^3}}{\dfrac{7250}{(1+.05)^1} + \dfrac{7250}{(1+.05)^2}} = \frac{4761.90 + 4545.45 + 4329.02}{6904.76 + 6590.91}$$

$$= \frac{13636.37}{13495.67} = 1.01$$

$$\text{B/C} = \frac{\dfrac{5000}{(1+.10)^1} + \dfrac{5000}{(1+.10)^2} + \dfrac{5000}{(1+.10)^3}}{\dfrac{7250}{(1+.10)^1} + \dfrac{7250}{(1+.10)^2}} = \frac{4545.45 + 4132.23 + 3759.40}{6490.91 + 5991.73}$$

$$= \frac{12437.08}{12582.64}$$

$$= 0.99$$

called the internal rate of return, as it is the discount rate that is internal to the particular investment under consideration. By setting B/C equal to 1 and rearranging terms, equation (5) can be written as

$$\sum_{t=1}^{n} \frac{F_t}{(1+r)^t} = \sum_{t=1}^{n} \frac{C_t}{(1+r)^t} \qquad (6)$$

or

$$\sum_{t=1}^{n} \frac{F_t - C_t}{(1+r)^t} = 0 \qquad (7)$$

Either of these formulations, equations (6) or (7), can be used in determining the internal rate of return.

Computers can easily be programmed to solve either of these equations by means of an iterative process.[14] Alternately, the present value of the net benefits, defined as $\sum_{t=1}^{n} \dfrac{F_t - C_t}{(1+r)^t}$, can be plotted diagramatically at various discount (interest) rates as seen in Figure 14; the interest rate at which this curve intersects the horizontal axis (x-axis) is the internal rate of return, as the present value is equal to zero at that interest rate.

The internal rate of return rule for investment decision making can break down in cases where benefits *and* costs are incurred over more than one time interval. In such cases a unique solution may not exist as a polynomial equation (an equation with values to a power greater than one, or stated differently a nonlinear equation) can have more than one solution satisfying the mathematical properties of the equation.[15] Instances where this would occur in the medical field are the use of surgical techniques in period two after the failure of a chemotherapy treatment administered in period one for some illness fails, or cases where due to

[14] The iterative process involves choosing an interest rate and seeing whether its use satisfies the equality specified in equation (6) or (7). If not, a higher (or lower) rate is substituted and this process is continued until an interest rate is found which satisfies the equality.

[15] For example, quadratic equations of the type $Y = a + bX + cX^2$ have two unique solutions for X.

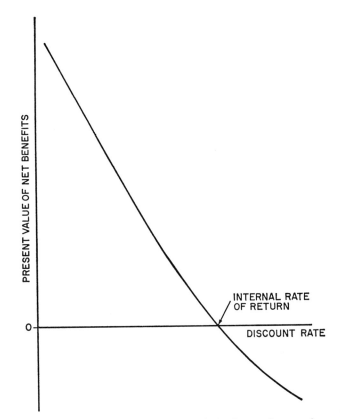

Figure 14. Geographic determination of the internal rate of return.

a limited annual budget and a large population requiring treatment, a treatment is provided to X per cent of the population annually until all those requiring the treatment have obtained it. Examples of the former would include coronary care, while the latter situation would include a limited methadone maintenance program for drug addiction. In such cases a cost-benefit approach involving the calculation of a benefit-cost ratio may be preferable.

PLANNING-PROGRAMMING-BUDGETING

Planning-programming-budgeting studies, commonly referred to as PPB studies, have recently become quite fashionable in various governmental and institutional circles. The analytical thrust of these studies, as opposed to the conceptual or structural thrust, is based completely on the tools of investment theory outlined above. The uniqueness of these studies lie in the conceptual or structural approach that is adopted.

The first step in any planning-programming-budgeting study involves a reorientation away from a departmentalized or micro approach to an end-objective or macro approach. For example, within a hospital, a departmentalized approach would focus on, for example, pharmaceutical, laundry, dietary, housekeeping, x-ray, nursing, surgery, obstetrics-gynecology, pediatric, and medical departments. The ultimate goal for which the services of these departments are used may never be considered explicitly. By adopting an end-objective approach the goal or goals of any enterprise are explicitly stated and clearly visualized. A hospital may state its goals as in-patient care, ambulatory care, teaching, and research, in that order of priority. The activity of each department is then considered in light of the department's contribution to the stated goal or goals rather than in a vacuum, and resource allocation is then based on a department's contribution to the stated goals (end-objectives).

The second step in the planning-programming-budgeting process is analytical. It involves gathering or generating the necessary data to determine the merits of alternative courses of action that can achieve the stated objectives, and evaluating these actions once they have been undertaken. The techniques used in this process are those associated with cost-benefit and rate of return studies. The final stage of planning-programming-budgeting involves the actual budgeting, the allocation of resources, to all the participating departments in any venture.

INVESTMENT IN HUMAN CAPITAL

All of the concepts presented in this chapter, interest rates, present value, and the techniques of investment decision making, can be brought together in the consideration of investments in human beings. Two primary areas where these techniques have been applied are manpower training and the acquiring of education. In general, each person can profitably acquire more education or training as long as the present value of the benefits anticipated from this investment are equal to or exceed the present value of anticipated costs.

The primary economic benefit stemming from an investment in education or training is the increased productivity of the person receiving the education or training. A common assumption made by researchers applying investment theory to manpower issues is that the wage or salary a person is paid is equal to or closely reflects his contribution to production. Based on this assumption, one can state that the increased productivity derived from the educational or training investment will have a positive effect on the person's earnings. The costs of such an investment are the resources utilized in acquiring it, including the person's time (opportunity costs). The expenditure of these resources can therefore be treated as an investment which entails a stream of costs and yields a stream of future benefits, increased earnings.

Internal rate of return and benefit-cost ratios have been calculated for various health occupations. Recently researchers have addressed the question: is it economically profitable to enter, for example, a career in nursing or medicine. In both cases internal rates of return have been calculated under a series of different assumptions reflecting alternate paths to acquiring the educational credentials and subsequent alternate career patterns.[16] The results of these studies are then used as evidence of whether the profession is economically attractive. The relative economic attractiveness of a profession is in turn used as evidence in analyses of the causes of manpower shortages (rate of return is too low to lure people in) or effects of barriers to entry (rate of return is kept at a high level by deliberately restricting entry) in advocating public policy change.

A similar technique can be applied in evaluating the outcome of any manpower retraining project from the point of view of the

---

[16] See for example, Hansen, W. Lee: Shortages and investment in health manpower, in Axelrod, S.: (Ed.). *Economics of Health and Medical Care.* Ann Arbor, Bureau of Public Health Economics, University of Michigan, 1964; Yett, Donald: Lifetime earnings of nurses in comparison with college trained women, *Inquiry,* 5 (4) :35, 1968; and Fein, Rashi: *Financing Medical Education.* New York, McGraw-Hill, 1971, Appendix C.

trainee and the funding organization. In both cases the central question is do the anticipated benefits equal or exceed the costs? Unless the return anticipated by the institution providing the training equals or exceeds the costs of the training, the resources expended on this endeavor could be better utilized elsewhere. Similarly unless the rewards accruing to the trainee equal or exceed his costs, he will not be willing to undertake any retraining. Insuring that an equitable allocation of both costs and benefits between the funding institution and the trainee prevail is an important prerequisite for the success of any training program.

Chapter Nine

INVESTMENT STUDIES

WHILE THE TOOLS of investment theory, such as cost-benefit calculations, have undoubtedly been extensively employed on an *ad hoc* basis at both the administrative and planning levels, rigorous cost-benefit studies have only recently begun to appear in the health literature. The two articles reproduced in this chapter are representative of the latter group.

Burton A. Weisbrod's study, "Costs and Benefits of Medical Research: A Case Study of Poliomyelitis" develops a methodological framework for assessing both the costs and benefits associated with applied medical research in specific disease areas. Having delineated the various cost and benefit components, internal rates of return are calculated for an assumed series of demographic, medical, and economic conditions.[1] In the aggregate, Weisbrod concludes that the economic return to the practically total eradication of poliomyelitis approximates 12 per cent. Had non-economic considerations been added to the benefit component of the calculation, the calculated return would have been much higher.

Two primary economic benefits are attributable to the eradication of poliomyelitis: increased production due to decreased morbidity and mortality, and a decline in the resources required to treat and rehabilitate polio victims. The economic gains from each of these benefit categories are then estimated over a designated time spectrum. Similarly, two major cost areas are highlighted:

---

[1] As noted by Weisbrod in his article, the internal rate of return statistics are biased in that *discounted* rather than *absolute* benefit estimates were utilized in the study. While this aspect of the study should be recognized, it by no means detracts from the accuracy of the theoretical technique developed.

175

pure research costs and application costs (which in the case of poliomyelitis take the form of vaccination costs). As in the case of
the benefit estimates, various cost projections are made for the
estimated duration of the disease eradication period.

Two conceptual issues incorporated in Weisbrod's study merit
further attention. Estimates of the economic loss attributable to
mortality are made on a net rather than gross basis. Net losses
are defined as the total loss of production, represented by the
earnings that a person could have accumulated in the absence of
mortality [2] minus a deduction for the person's future consumption. The rationale for this procedure is that the termination of
life also leads to the termination of consumption and society will
be required to produce fewer goods and services due to the sub-
traction of one consuming unit from the overall consuming
population.

Many researchers have disputed this procedure, claiming that
production alone is not the only goal of an economy. Enjoyment
(consumption) is also a goal of economic activity. Consequently,
the loss due to mortality consists of both a production component and a loss of enjoyment (consumption) component.[3] If this
interpretation of the goals of an economy are accepted, an adjustment for decreased consumption underestimates the true economic loss.

The cost of vaccination is viewed as consisting of both a direct
pharmaceutical cost of the vaccine and the labor cost of the individual administering the vaccine, and an indirect cost in the
form of the time required to receive the vaccine. The latter cost,
called an opportunity cost,[4] while relatively minor in the case of
poliomyelitis, could be quite substantial in the treatment of other
diseases. Its omissions from a cost-benefit calculation would
seriously bias the results by grossly underrepresenting the total
cost of attaining health care.

The second article reproduced in this chapter, "Cost Effective-

---

[2] A common assumption in economic research is that a person's earnings reflect
the value to society of his production.

[3] For an elaboration of this argument see, Fein, Rashi: *The Economics of Mental
Illness.* New York, Basic Books, 1958, Chapter 2.

[4] Refer to Chapter Four for a detailed discussion of this concept.

ness Analysis Applied to the Treatment of Chronic Renal Disease," by Herbert E. Klarman, John O'S. Francis and Gerald D. Rosenthal, adopts a variant of a cost-benefit study—cost-effectiveness—and analyzes the optimal combination of hospital dialysis, and kidney transplantation for chronic renal disease, given existing medical and economic conditions. As noted by the authors, cost-effectiveness analysis represents a special type of cost-benefit study; a study where it is assumed that the resources are available to meet the given costs and alternate ways are assessed for obtaining specific benefits.[5]

Based on the current state of medical knowledge for treating chronic renal failure, Klarman, *et al.*, conclude that economic considerations favor a maximum utilization of transplants rather than dialysis, if appropriate kidney donors are available in sufficient quantity. Barring maximum utilization of surgical techniques, home dialysis is deemed preferable to hospital dialysis because of the significantly lower costs associated with the home environment.

Klarman, *et al.* adopt two unorthodox, but nevertheless interesting, procedures in deriving their cost-effectiveness estimates. They attempt to attribute a monetary value to mental anguish associated with disease. In their particular study, they recognize the negative psychological attributes of dialysis stemming from the fact that a person realizes that his life is literally in the hands of a dialysis machine, and arbitrarily assert that the *quality* of life of a patient with a transplanted kidney is greater than that of a patient on dialysis care by a factor of one-quarter of each life-year gained. Recognizing the controversial nature of this adjustment, the economic benefits of transplantation are reported both with and without this quality adjustment.

The authors utilization of a *net* discount rate is a further diversion from conventional cost-benefit methodology. An initial discount rate of 6 per cent is chosen, as it is assumed to reflect an appropriate discounting factor from a societal (social) perspective. This rate is then adjusted for the anticipated increase in

---

[5] For a detailed comparison of cost-effectiveness and cost-benefit studies see, Smith, Warren F.: Cost-effectiveness and cost-benefit analyses for public health programs, *Public Health Reports, 83*:899, 1968.

the cost of providing home or hospital based dialysis above and beyond general increases in price levels. The adjustment takes the form of reducing the discount rate by 1 and 2 percentage points, respectively, for home and hospital dialysis. The rationale for this procedure is that a gross discount rate reduces the dollar value of the factor being discounted, to reflect the fact that future dollars are worth less than present dollars. However, costs of medical care are rising faster than costs in general.[6] To adjust for this phenomenon the gross discount rate is deflated by a differential cost factor (1 and 2 percentage points in this case) ; the net effect of the adjustment is to lower the effectiveness of the procedure under analysis, in cost terms, by recognizing and allowing for increased cost. As noted in Chapter Eight, a lower discount rate yields a higher present value. Since costs of care are being discounted, the *net* discount rate increases the cost values commensurate with the authors estimate of the differential for providing a specific medical care service.

Although the data utilized in the two studies reproduced here are estimates, and in a few instances preliminary estimates, the insights derived from such studies can be of extreme importance in guiding the allocation of scarce resources among a host of competing projects.

* * *

COSTS AND BENEFITS OF MEDICAL RESEARCH: A CASE STUDY OF POLIOMYELITIS [7]

BURTON A. WEISBROD

Medical research has come to attract large and growing expenditures; the United States government alone spent more than 1.6 billion dollars in 1969–1970, up from 450 million dollars in 1959–

[6] The *Medical Care Price Index* has been rising faster than the general *Consumer Price Index*. For a confimation of this differential trend, see Chapter Three.

[7] Reprinted with permission from *The Journal of Political Economy, 79*, No. 3, May–June 1971, pp. 527–542. Copyright © by the University of Chicago, 1971.

1960 and from only 69 million dollars a decade earlier (Skolnik and Dales, 1970). Yet little is known about the economic efficiency of medical research—an activity which, having a substantial collective-consumption or public-good component,[8] is financed in large part either by the federal government or by "nonprofit" organizations.

This paper examines costs and benefits of a particular medical research program that would generally be regarded as a medical "success"—the research which led to the development of vaccines (Salk and Sabin) against poliomyelitis. No attempt is made to generalize our findings to other medical research programs, either ongoing or prospective, although the paper does conclude with some brief comments on the possible wide applicability of the approach used here.[9]

Why undertake a case study? What can be learned from it? First, if other case studies of medical research are undertaken, we may someday be able to develop generalizations as to the nature of the probability distribution of rates of return from various "types" of medical research and application programs. That is, theories may grow out of observations. Second, this case study will help to point up the relationship between research and its application and the relevance of both to assessment of the social "profitability" of discovering new knowledge.

Third, the form in which the rate-of-return calculation is presented here can be thought of as constituting a checklist of items about which the informed public decision maker might seek information prior to making allocations of research funds among competing research programs.

The approach involves estimating the following: the time stream of research expenditures directed toward the disease (poliomyelitis); the time streams of a number of forms of benefits resulting from (or predicted to result from) the application of the knowledge generated by the research; and the cost of applying that knowledge. Finally, internal rates of return on the research expenditures are computed using several alternative sets of assumptions regarding costs and

[8] *Editors' Note:* Goods from whose consumption people cannot be easily excluded (e.g. water fluoridation) and/or goods whose consumption yield benefits to a larger group than the one consuming it (e.g. smallpox vaccination) are called public goods.

[9] *Editors' Note:* This concluding discussion, appearing on pages 542–3 of the original article is omitted here as it presents a theoretical treatment of an economic issue not developed in this text.

benefits.[10] In effect, we consider the rate of return that would have been obtained on polio research depending on which of a number of alternative states of events transpired and which alternative policy choices were (are) made subsequent to the technical success of the polio research program in 1957.

Evaluating benefits from medical research poses a problem not often encountered in other research. How should one evaluate a life saved or a lifetime of paralysis avoided? The complexity of the philosophical and empirical issues is clear. In this paper only a subset of the varied but elusive benefits from medical research is considered; these include: a) the increased production and b) the reduced costs of treatment for persons who would have become ill or died from polio were it not for the successful research. Since total benefits are thus understated, our estimates of rates of return on costs will also be understated.

The internal rate of return on medical (polio) research, the rate which equates the time stream of research costs with the stream of benefits, is r in the denominator of the following expression:

$$\sum_{t=0}^{T} \frac{R_t - [B_t(N_t - W_t) - V_t]}{(1 + r)^t} = 0,$$

where R is research costs, B is the benefit per case of the disease prevented (or the loss per case occurring), N is the number of cases occurring in the absence of a successful program of research and application, W is the number of cases occurring after a successful program of research and applications; so that $N - W$ is the number of cases prevented—V is the cost of applying the research findings, t is a particular year, and T is the terminal horizon year, the year beyond which the values of variables are asserted to be irrelevant (T could take on any value, including infinity).

The bracketed terms in the equation express the research benefits in year t, net of the cost, V, of applying the research knowledge. In the following sections, the operational form of each variable is discussed in the order in which it appears in the equation, with attention focused on the disease, poliomyelitis.

---

[10] Internal rates of return have been estimated for various public expenditure programs, for example, education (Hansen, 1963) and water resources (Haveman, 1965, pp. 111–12), but to only one governmental or nonprofit research effort, on hybrid corn (Griliches, 1958), and, as far as I know, to not a single medical research program.

RESEARCH COSTS

The nature of medical research is such that identifying an expenditure with a particular disease is frequently not easy. Expenditures on "basic" research (not directed at any disease) may contribute nonetheless to the development of an operational method for preventing some specific disease. Research aimed at a particular disease may produce results that are useful in dealing with some other disease. As a result, it is often not clear precisely what should be included in an estimate of the cost of research "on" a particular disease, for example, the research leading to the polio vaccines.

The conceptual problem is matched by the empirical problem of obtaining data. In Table 1, column (2) shows the time series of

TABLE 1

ESTIMATED AWARDS FOR POLIOMYELITIS
RESEARCH, 1930–56 (thousands
of dollars)

Year (1)	Current Dollars (2)	Price Adjusted (1957 = 100) (3)
1930	...	100
1931	...	200
1932	...	300
1933	...	300
1934	...	300
1935	...	300
1936	...	300
1937	...	300
1938	...	300
1939	...	300
1940	...	300
1941	...	100
1942	...	100
1943	...	100
1944	...	100
1945	...	100
1946	242	356
1947	492	631
1948	746	891
1949	1,513	1,823
1950	1,729	2,064
1951	2,609	2,883
1952	2,744	2,967
1953	2,022	2,170
1954	1,920	2,051
1955	2,176	2,332
1956	1,962	2,072

Source: Col. (2), Science Information Exchange; col. (3), for 1946–56, adjustments of data in col. (2) by CPI (1957 = 100); for 1930–45, author's estimates.

amounts awarded for polio research, on the basis of information obtained by the Science Information Exchange (SIE). The data represent awards, not actual expenditures, and then only those research awards (grants and contracts) registered with the SIE by national granting agencies. The SIE series begins with 1946, and I have arbitrarily extended it back to 1930 in the interest of tolerable completeness. Because of the incompleteness of the SIE expenditure data and because of the necessarily arbitrary nature of the extrapolation, two alternative assumptions about the accuracy of the data are utilized in the calculations described below.

The research data in column (2) are in current dollars. In order to take account of price level changes, and in the absence of a truly satisfactory basis for doing so, the author used the *Consumer Price Index* to adjust the expenditure estimates to the 1957 level of prices. The results appear in column (3).

BENEFITS PER CASE PREVENTED

In principle, "benefits" include *all* favorable effects in whatever forms are deemed relevant. As measured here, however, benefits from prevention of polio are only the sum of: a) the market value of production lost because of premature *mortality* due to polio; b) the market value of production lost as a result of *morbidity*—illness and disability—caused by polio; and c) the cost of resources devoted to *treatment* and *rehabilitation* of polio victims. The basic methodology by which each of these three components was estimated is described in detail in *Economics of Public Health* (Weisbrod, 1961; Chaps. 7 and 8; hereinafter cited as EPH) and will only be summarized briefly here. The present paper extends this earlier work, which dealt only with the benefit side, to an analysis in which the costs incurred to discover the effective vaccines and the costs of vaccinating people, applying the new knowledge, also are considered.

Mortality losses for people of specified ages had been estimated previously (in EPH) as the present value of expected future earnings,[11] utilizing 1951 earnings data and United States life tables for

---

[11] Alternative discount rates of 10 and 5 per cent were used, but the 10 per cent calculations are utilized in the present paper. Except for the fact that the present-value estimates were already available from my earlier work (EPH), the undiscounted data would have been entered into the internal-rate-of-return formula (Equation 1) above. In addition, were it not for the fact that these estimates were already available, more recent data, for example, on earnings and life expectancies, would have been used.

1949–51.[12] For women, the market earnings data were supplemented by estimates of the value of household services (EPH, Appendix 2). From these gross-loss figures were subtracted my estimates of the marginal consumption expenditures attributable to an incremental person in a household—the point being that mortality involves the loss of a consumer as well as a producer.[13] The resulting values of net future earnings were weighted by the actual reported number of deaths attributable to polio among males and females, by age, to obtain the estimated "premature mortality" loss per death from polio (EPH, table 6).

Morbidity losses, those resulting from the temporary loss of a producer, were derived from the same age-specific and sex-specific earnings-productivity data used for the mortality-loss estimates, it being assumed that an average of one-fourth of a year of work time was lost per case because of temporary or permanent disability (EPH, Table 9 and accompanying discussion). For the permanently and totally disabled, the entire remaining working lifetime was lost, but the overwhelming majority of cases produced little or no loss of work time—in part because the effects were very short-term and occurred among children.

Treatment losses are the third form of social cost of polio that had previously been estimated. Prevention of a disease makes treatment costs unnecessary, thereby liberating resources for alternative uses.[14] The range of treatment costs for polio victims has been great, running into many thousands of dollars when respiratory equipment was utilized, but for the large proportion of cases, which have been non-paralytic, these costs have been far smaller. Earlier, the author estimated the mean at around 550 dollars per case as of 1950 (EPH, p. 80).

These three forms of losses were summed to give an estimated

[12] EPH, Tables 2 and 3. The assumption was made that age-specific and sex-specific incidence rates for other diseases are independent of those for polio. Thus, a reduction in the incidence of polio, as would result from a successful prevention program, was assumed to leave unchanged the incidence rates, morbidity, and morality rates from other diseases.

[13] For details of the estimation procedure see EPH, esp. 33–34, Tables 2, 6, and 12, and appendix 1.

[14] It might be noted that a freeing of resources from treatment activities would produce no direct effect on the GNP, since treating the sick is not regarded as a final output. Notwithstanding the absence of a change in measured GNP, it would seem clear that such a reallocation of resources, made possible by a successful disease-prevention program, would increase economic welfare.

mean loss per case of 1,150 dollars—the estimate of the expected benefit per case prevented (EPH, p. 90). It is possible that a successful prevention program could bring about a significant change in the labor supply (and, hence, in the marginal productivity of labor) or in the demand for treatment; and in this case the 1,150 dollar figure would be invalid. In the case of polio, however, the disease was not so widespread that substantial effects on factor supply or demand were likely to result from a successful prevention program.

Thus, it was assumed that for each case of polio prevented, a benefit of at least 1,150 dollars resulted—"at least," because, as noted above, benefits in such important forms as reduced pain and suffering have not been considered. This estimated benefit per case prevented is derived from data for various years between 1949 and 1954, but because the data were largely from around 1950, the 1,150 dollar figure was assumed to apply to that year. This figure has been adjusted to prices in 1957—the year of research "success," when the Sabin oral vaccine first became widely available—by the arbitrary use of the CPI, thereby producing a figure of 1,350 dollars in 1957 prices. In some of the calculations described below, a productivity-growth adjustment was also made; more about this later.

NUMBER OF CASES PREVENTED

We turn next to determination of the number of polio cases prevented. This requires estimation of the number of cases expected for each year following 1957, with and without the research success.

Expected Cases—No Research Success

During the period 1920–1956 the trend in reported cases of polio was upward, although there was substantial year-to-year variation (Department of Health, Education, and Welfare 1962, p. 17). Some of the "increase" was the result, simply, of improved reporting, and so the incidence rates for the later years should be given heavier weight in a forecast. The procedure actually used, therefore, was to calculate the mean rate for the ten years ending with 1956. This gave an average of some twenty-one new cases annually per 100,000 persons in the population. For the United States population in 1957, 168 million, this produced an estimate of 36,000 new cases for each year after 1957, holding constant the size and age distribution of the population in that year.[15] Since the U.S. population is actually grow-

---

[15] The age distribution is relevant because the incidence of polio is markedly age-specific. The incidence among persons over fifty has been virtually zero.

ing, and for reasons quite independent of the incidence of polio, the absolute number of polio cases would be expected to rise in the absence of a successful research program. The assumption of population constancy is relaxed, later, to assess the sensitivity of the rate of return to this assumption.

Expected Cases—Successful Research Program

Granted that in the absence of the research, 36,000 new cases of polio could be expected each year, it is necessary next to estimate the degree of success of the research. Here an important, if simple, point must be reiterated: knowledge without application is valueless. Since application of new knowledge is rarely costless, we can expect application of new knowledge to be less than complete and immediate. Polio vaccine illustrates this generalization. There are costs of producing and delivering vaccine, and there are implicit costs, in the form of time, for the individual taking it. Thus, we cannot except the vaccine to be utilized by less than the entire vulnerable population under fifty, and, consequently, the number of new cases of polio may well not fall to zero.[16] In any event, we must take these application costs into account when we turn to the net benefits of the polio research effort, and this will be done below.

The number of new cases expected in a given year after the successful research is a function of the amount of resources devoted to vaccinating people over the previous forty to fifty years or so. The larger the expenditures on application of knowledge, that is, the more people vaccinated, the smaller the number of expected new cases.

In the procedure utilized in this paper, the number of cases expected after 1957 was assumed to equal zero, but alternative assumptions were employed regarding the number of persons who had to be vaccinated and, hence, the total cost of vaccination—in order to produce this result. Alternative assumptions also were made regarding the cost per person vaccinated. Thus, in the equation above, $N_t - W_t$, the number of cases prevented was assumed to equal 36,000, the number of cases expected in the absence of a successful research-vaccination program.

---

[16] Since the number of cases prevented as well as the costs of prevention vary directly with the expenditures on applying knowledge, there is an economic optimum level of application; this may well involve less than complete vaccination of the population. In fact, as of 1970, 4.6 per cent of all U.S. persons under age twenty are estimated to have had no polio vaccinations and an additional 15.2 per cent had less than full protection, that is, less than three doses of either the oral or the injected vaccines (Department of Health, Education, and Welfare 1970, p. 13).

APPLICATION (VACCINATION) COSTS

Turning to the vaccination costs, V, it was assumed that to eliminate polio would have required a) vaccinating the entire 1957 population under fifty,[17] b) vaccinating all or, alternatively, none of the subsequent newborn children, assumed constant at the 1957 level of 4.25 million, and c) incurring a vaccination cost per person of either $0.66 or $3.00 of direct cost plus an opportunity cost of time. The $0.66 figure assumes three "shots" (actually impregnated sugar cubes) at a cost of $0.22 each. This is an estimate of how low the cost might be if mass vaccination techniques were used.[18] It includes the purchase price of the drug, advertising costs, and my estimate of the implicit cost of the time donated by physicians, dentists, pharmacists, and others (utilizing 1959 income data for these occupations, from the 1960 census). The total cost, so computed, was simply divided by the number of persons vaccinated to obtain the average cost estimate of $0.22 per shot, or $0.66 per person receiving the series of three. The $1.00 per shot alternative cost is a rough estimate of the charge made by private physicians (in 1957 prices).

Obtaining a vaccination also requires some of the time of the persons being vaccinated. In my calculations, the average opportunity cost of time per shot received was judged to be around $1.00 for adults and $0.50 for children. These figures are "guesstimates." I assumed that about a half hour, including travel time, was required for each of the three shots at an opprotunity cost of $2.00 per hour per adult. The lower figure for children (under eighteen) was based on the assumptions that, typically, a mother would take more than one child at a time, so that even if the mother herself were not also obtaining a vaccination, the opportunity cost to her of the time required would be well under the $1.00 per hour figure; in addition, in many instances, the vaccination would coincide with a physician visit for some other purpose, thus making the marginal time required rather modest.

RATES OF RETURN

We can now relate the data on benefits and costs in order to obtain estimates of internal rates of return on polio research. Table 2

---

[17] The Sabin vaccine provides lifetime protection.

[18] The figure is derived from information provided by the Dane County (Madison), Wisconsin, "Sabin Oral Sunday" program. I have simply assumed that the costs of this program are representative of such programs generally.

represents the rates of return under various assumptions about the variables, and with alternative time horizons.[19] Column (2) indicates

TABLE 2

INTERNAL RATE OF RETURN ON POLIO RESEARCH UNDER
A VARIETY OF ALTERNATIVE ASSUMPTIONS

Ex-ample (1)	Savings per Case Prevented (2)	Vaccination Costs (Millions of Dollars)		Research Costs: Ratio of Actual to Reported (5)	Rate of Return (%)	
		In 1957 (3)	After 1957 (per Year) (4)		1930–80 (6)	1930–2200 * (7)
I......	Constant (at $1,350)	350	9	1	8.4	9.7
				5	5.1	7.0
		625	19	1	0.4	4.5
				5	− 0.7	3.7
II......	Growing	350	0	1	13.4	14.2
				5	9.0	10.4
		625	0	1	7.9	10.0
				5	5.8	8.4
III......	Growing	350	9	1	11.7	12.9
				5	7.8	9.6
		625	19	1	4.5	8.1
				5	3.0	7.1

Source: Cols. (2)–(4), see discussion in text; col. (5), for "reported" data, see Table 1 above; cols. (6)–(7), author's calculations.
* The rates in this column are also the asymptotic limits as the time horizon is extended.

the saving per case prevented (equivalent to the loss per case occurring, B in the rate-of-return equation above). In Example I the assumption is made that the saving per case will remain constant over time, at the 1957 level of 1,350 dollars. By contrast, Examples II and III assume that the saving per case will increase through time. The reasoning is this: nearly half (actually 625 dollars) of the 1,350 dollar figure consists of productivity (earnings) lost because of illness and premature mortality of polio victims. Since labor productivity may be expected to increase through time, a productivity-growth

[19] The rate-of-return estimates are not, strictly, internal rates of return. The reason is that I utilized previously estimated data on benefits per case prevented, and these data included estimates of mortality loss which were, in turn, present values of expected future earnings, discounted at 10 per cent (see EPH, tables 2 and 3).

factor of 3 per cent per year was applied in Examples II and III to the labor-productivity portion of the 1,350 dollar loss per case.[20]

As discussed in a previous section, the author estimated that an average of some 36,000 new cases of polio could be expected annually in the absence of a successful vaccine, assuming a constant population with constant age distribution. In making the estimates of the rate of return on polio research, the author assumed, further, that the number of cases subsequent to 1957 would be negligible (strictly, zero) if everyone under age fifty were inoculated in 1957 and if, alternatively, a) pessimistically, all newborn babies after 1957 would have to be inoculated in order to sustain the complete polio control (Example III), or b) optimistically, no further inoculations of newborns would be required after 1957, the disease having been completely and permanently eliminated by the vaccination program in 1957 (Example II). The truth, no doubt, is between these extremes; the object, however, is to assess the sensitivity of the rate-of-return estimate to a wider range of values of the variables.[21]

Columns (3) and (4) of Table 2 reflect these and other alternative assumptions as to the cost of a completely successful vaccination program (V in the equation). The total vaccination costs in 1957 and, if necessary, thereafter are a function, of course, of the number of persons vaccinated and the cost per person. In each of the three examples in Table 2 the assumption was made that the number of newborn children remained constant at the 1957 level of some 4.25 million. Later, this assumption is dropped.

Vaccination costs, as noted above, include the direct cost of producing and distributing the vaccine and also the opportunity cost

[20] By adjusting the treatment-cost portion for price-level changes only, I have assumed implicitly that real costs of treatment would remain constant in the absence of a successful program.

[21] W. Lee Hansen has speculated that this procedure understates the expected rate of return because the poor are less likely to be vaccinated and their marginal productivity (as measured by earnings) is below average.

Some recently available data confirm his prediction about vaccination. As of 1969, the proportions of the United States population age one to twenty that were fully protected against polio by virtue of having at least three doses of either the oral or the injected vaccine were as follows: central cities poverty groups, 68.6 per cent; central cities nonpoverty groups, 78.2 per cent; other poverty groups, 78 per cent; other nonpoverty groups, 83.3 per cent. The differences in percentages between "poverty" and "nonpoverty" (unfortunately not defined in the report) are significant at far better than the .01 level (Department of Health, Education, and Welfare 1970, p. 13 and p. 52, table B).

of the time required to obtain the vaccination. In column (3) the cost of vaccinating the 1957 population under age fifty is shown for each of the three examples: first, under the low-cost assumption, $0.22 per shot plus opportunity cost, and second, under the high-cost assumption, $1.00 per shot plus opportunity cost. The respective total costs are $350 million and $625 million.

Column (4) is similar to column (3). It shows the estimated costs of vaccinating all newborn children in the years after 1957 under the low-cost and high-cost assumptions, which produce total costs of, respectively, $9 million and $19 million per year for the case of a constant number of newborns. (In Example II, it is assumed that no post-1957 vaccinations are required.)

Column (5) reflects two alternative assumptions as to the accuracy of the data on polio research expenditures (awards) which appear in Table 1.

The rate-of-return estimates thus may be examined to see their sensitivity to substantial underestimates of the research-expenditure series. It is quite likely that the research series in Table 1 understates the volume of resources entering polio research, in particular because it excludes expenditures by the pharmaceutical industry as well as expenditures on vaccine testing and on basic research that contributed to the eventual success of polio research efforts, but the degree of understatement remains a question. The rate-of-return estimates in Table 2 have been made under the alternative assumptions that a) the research-expenditure series in Table 1 is essentially correct or b) the true expenditures were five times as great as the figures in Table 1.[22]

There is some possibility, however, that the polio research series in Table 1 actually overstates expenditures devoted directly to polio research. For example, Watson (1968, p. 132) comments that he had a Polio Foundation fellowship while doing research on the tobacco mosaic virus and on the DNA molecular structure—research that ultimately led to the Nobel Prize for physiology and medicine in 1962 (shared with Francis H. D. Crick and Maurice H. F. Wilkens). It seems either that such expenditures should not be included fully in polio research costs or that the total benefits of polio research should be recognized as including external benefits—those extending

---

[22] A report by the American Medical Association states that the National Foundation spent "for research related to vaccine development and for field trial studies" some 41.3 million dollars. This is approximately twice as large as the total indicated in Table 1 above (American Medical Association 1964, p. 45).

beyond that specific disease. Either way, the result would be to raise the rates of return estimated in this paper.

Similarly, John F. Enders, Frederick C. Robbins, and Thomas H. Weller, who shared the Nobel Prize for physiology and medicine eight years earlier, in 1954, won it for discovering a simple method of growing polio virus in test tubes (*World Book Encyclopedia*, 1965, *14*:347); yet their polio-related research had far more general value, for it "showed that viruses could be grown outside the body in tissues that they do not usually attack within the body" (*World Book Encyclopedia*, 1965, *6*:223). Here again, we see that research produced a finding whose applicability was considerably wider than to polio alone.

Finally, a decision was required as to the time horizon relevant for the analysis. How far into the future should the savings from polio research be assumed to occur? Again, the procedure employed was intended to assess the implications of various choices of horizons. Five horizons were considered (1980, 1990, 2000, 2100, 2200), but the results for only two of them, 1980 and 2200, have been presented in Table 2 (cols. [6] and [7]). There may be little justification for selecting a horizon as near as 1980; yet it may well be true that current vaccines will eventually (as soon as 1980?) yield to new strains of polio, and when that occurs the economic life of present vaccines will have ended.

The more distant the horizon, the larger the rate of return on polio research, although it is clear from Table 2 that the rate-of-return estimates are not highly sensitive to the horizon choice. Among the dozens of cases considered (only some of which are reported in Table 2) the extension of the horizon from the year 2100 for an additional 100 years never made a difference of more that one-tenth of 1 per cent, and the extension from the year 2000 to 2100 seldom increased the rate of return by more than 1 percentage point. Considering the variety of alternative assumptions, the range of rates of return seems modest. Even extending the time horizon by 100 years or more beyond 1980 does not make a substantial difference in most of the cases examined. Generally speaking, the internal rates of return are within the range of 4–14 per cent.

The "most likely" rate of return would seem to be about 11–12 per cent. This conclusion was reached in the following way: a) Since labor productivity (earnings) can be expected to continue to grow, Examples II and III (Table 2) seem to be more relevant than Example I. b) The most likely assumption regarding the need for post-1957 vaccinations is somewhere between the opposite extremes assumed in Examples II and III, column (4), and so my choice of a rate of return will be bounded by these two examples. c) Research expenditures reasonably ascribable to polio were probably less than three times as great as those reported in Table 1 (although one certainly cannot be confident about this). d) With respect to the social cost of applying the polio research knowledge, the low-cost-vaccination assumption seems to be preferable (for the high-cost assumption rests on an estimate of physician charges for individual vaccinations—charges which are likely to exceed the level of the marginal social cost that is possible when more efficient, mass inoculation techniques are used). A time horizon extending to the year 2100 or 2200, it makes virtually no difference which is selected, is reasonable.

These five judgments lead to the conclusion that the most likely rate of return on polio research is between an upper bound of around 12 per cent—the mean of the figures in column (7), fifth and sixth rows (Example II), and a lower bound of 11 per cent, the mean of the figures in column (7) ninth and tenth rows (Example III) [23]

Polio is a contagious disease, and as a result, vaccinations produce external as well as internal benefits; because of this public-good nature of the commodity vaccination, our rate-of-return estimates would be even greater if the assumption were made that only a portion of the vulnerable population were vaccinated. The point is that, because of the external economies resulting from a vaccination, an increase in the proportion of population vaccinated will, up to some point, bring about a greater relative drop in disease incidence.[24] Beyond

[23] Although these estimates apply to the case of a medically successful research effort, not all expenditures on polio research contributed to the ultimate success of the Salk and Sabin vaccines. Thus, the estimated rates of return are, implicitly, weighted averages of the much larger rates of return on the "useful" lines of polio research and much smaller—perhaps even negative—rates of return on the less fruitful lines of polio research. (Griliches [1958, pp. 426–27] notes the same circumstances with respect to the research on hybrid corn.)

[24] To illustrate: 1969 incidence data (obviously unavailable in 1957) show that 95.4 per cent of the United States population under age 20 had received some polio vaccination protection, and 80.2 per cent had full protection (3 doses of either the oral or the injected vaccine); but the number of reported new cases of polio has fallen by 99.9 per cent and the number of deaths from polio has fallen by 100 per cent! Cases decreased from between 15,000 and 57,000 per year during the 1950–56 period to only 17 in 1969, and deaths dropped from 556 in 1956 to zero in 1969. Source: U.S. Department of Health, Education, and Welfare, *Morbidity and Mortality Weekly Report*, "Surveillance Summary: Poliomyelitis," various issues.

that point, diminishing external and internal benefits result from vaccination of additional persons.[25]

All of the rate-of-return estimates in Table 2, however, may well be biased toward the low side—even with respect to the so-called economic consideration they are intended to reflect. For one thing, the benefits accruing outside the United States have been disregarded. (It is true, on the other hand, that research costs incurred outside the United States have also been ignored, but the sums involved are probably quite small.) For another, the risk aversion which doubtless characterizes most people's preferences has not been considered,[26] benefits from reduced incidence of polio being estimated at their actuarial level.

Moreover, in order to be conservative, the productivity loss attributable to mortality from polio was taken to be net of the victim's expected individual consumption. Since death takes a consumer as well as a producer, this approach has some merit. Such a *net-*productivity view examines the losses from polio as they are seen by nonvictims, for whom the excess of a victim's productivity over his own consumption may be most relevant.

Alternatively, however, the point of view could be the entire society, including the victims who, of course, cannot be identified *ex ante*.[27] This would imply estimating mortality losses by *gross* productivity. Were this done, the mortality losses per case of polio would be increased by some 15 per cent, but the total loss per case (including also treatment and morbidity losses) would rise by only some 5 per cent.[28] Such an increased loss per case would raise the Table 2

[25] It does not follow, however, that a restricted vaccination program would necessarily be efficient, for the internal rate of return is not the appropriate maximand. For discussion of the latter point see, for example, Baumol (1965, pp. 439–45).

[26] *Editors' Note:* Risk aversion is characterized by a willingness to pay for a benefit more than its expected value. The expected value of a set of possible occurrences is equal to the sum of the probability of each possible occurrence times the value imputed to that occurrence. Thus including a premium for risk aversion would lead to higher benefits from the vaccine because cost savings equal to the amount of money people would have been willing to spend on any device or service which they believed would reduce the risk of poliomyelitis is realized.

[27] Alternative points of view regarding definitions of "society" are discussed in EPH, pp. 35–36.

[28] Measuring mortality losses by gross productivity adds only some 15 per cent because of the manner in which consumption was estimated. Specifically, the concept was used of the *marginal* family consumption with respect to a change in family size; the marginal consumption, as expected, is considerably less than average consumption, the portion of aggregate income devoted to consumption. For additional

estimates of internal rates of return by only about one-half of 1 per cent.

Another conservative assumption was that the number of newborn children would be constant at the level in 1957. If this number were assumed to increase at the rate of 2 per cent per year—a figure somewhat larger than that which actually occurred in the United States during the decade 1950–60 [29]—the rate of return would rise by about 2 percentage points above the levels shown in Table 2. Although the assumption of increase in the number of newborns raises vaccination costs, it also raises the number of cases of polio subsequently prevented.

Finally, but very significantly, some analysis of the importance of application costs is in order. The economic efficiency of research cannot properly be isolated from the costs of applying any new knowledge it generates. Expansion of knowledge and application of that knowledge are joint inputs, both of which are essential if benefits are to be obtained from any research. One implication of this point is that an efficient choice among alternative research strategies should take into account the costs of applying the research once it has become successful. A higher-cost research approach may be more efficient than a less costly one if the latter would entail greater application costs.[30]

To underscore the significance of application costs in the case of polio research, the rates of return summarized in Table 2 have been reestimated under the assumption that successful research could be applied without cost, thus eliminating all vaccination costs. The results appear in Table 3. The rates of return shown therein differ from those in Table 2 for only one reason—the different assumptions regarding vaccination costs. (In the interest of expository simplicity, Table 3 compares only some of the examples from Table 2, specifically those involving the higher cost [1 dollar per shot] vaccination cost assumption. These appear in Table 2, third, fourth, seventh, eighth, eleventh, and twelfth rows.)

---

discussion and computational details, see EPH, pp. 49–51 and appendix I, pp. 100–113.

[29] See *Statistical Abstracts of the U.S.,* 1964 (1964, p. 48). Since 1961, the absolute number of births has actually been decreasing.

[30] Medically successful research that entails very great costs of application, for example, kidney dialysis machines, presents a most difficult social choice; either enormous costs must be incurred to provide sufficient machines or decisions must be made as to which ill people will have access to the limited supply of machines and which ill people will die.

TABLE 3

INTERNAL RATES OF RETURN ON POLIO RESEARCH,
WITH AND WITHOUT VACCINATION COSTS

		Rate of Return (%)			
	Research Costs:	1930–80		1930–2200 *	
Ex-ample (1)	Ratio of Actual to Reported (2)	With Vaccination Costs (3)	Without Vaccination Costs (4)	With Vaccination Costs (5)	Without Vaccination Costs (6)
I............. 1	1	0.4	20.0	4.5	20.1
	5	−0.7	11.9	3.7	12.3
II.............	1	7.9	21.0	10.0	21.1
	5	5.8	13.2	8.4	13.6
III.............	1	4.5	21.0	8.1	21.1
	5	3.0	13.2	7.1	13.6

Source: Cols. (3) and (5), table 2 above; cols. (4) and (6), author's calculations.
Note: The results in cols. (4) and (6) for Examples II and III are identical. The reason is that these two examples differed in table 2 only with respect to their assumptions about post-1957 vaccination costs.
* The rates in cols. (5) and (6) are also the asymptotic limits as the time horizon is extended.

Comparisons in Table 3 between the rates of return in columns (3) and (4) and in columns (5) and (6) are striking. Whereas the assumptions of Example I produced a rate of return of only 0.4 per cent for the period 1930–80, this would soar to 20 per cent if there were no application (vaccination) costs. If there were no vaccination costs, it appears that, *ceteris paribus*, the internal rate of return on polio research surely would have been satisfactory even by ordinary market standards—for the lowest rate of return shown in Table 3 is 11.9 per cent. If we disregard the costs of application, an erroneously high rate of return might have been assigned to the research effort alone. This would ignore the fundamental fact that research and its application are joint inputs to any disease control program.

This discussion of application costs grew out of the concern with returns from research, together with recognition of the relationship between research and application. The approach and the data presented here can also be used, however, to estimate the rate of return on programs to *apply* existing knowledge, taking as given the existence of the required knowledge and ignoring the sunk costs of research. In the case of polio, the research costs were small relative to estimated application costs, and so the expected rates of return, as of 1957, on a mass vaccination program are generally only 1–2 percentage points greater than the estimates in Table 2, which reflect costs of research as well as vaccination.

CONCLUSION

The resources devoted to polio research in the United States have produced vaccines that are both safe and effective in preventing polio. The analysis in this paper shows that, except under the most extreme assumptions, this research is raising output and reducing treatment expenditures in amounts producing a rate of return on the research and application costs of at least 5 per cent, or more probably 11–12 per cent.

Because of the narrowness of the operational measure of benefits used in this paper, including its abstraction from the pain and anguish accompanying disease,[31] there is little doubt that the real value of the medically successful polio research, and the price that buyers would pay for the vaccinations, is greater than what is estimated in this paper. The "value" of reduced illness and increased longevity is, one might guess, greater than simply the effects on earnings. In addition, even the more strictly financial benefits are probably understated, in part because of the disregard for the benefits occurring outside the United States.

Empirical findings as to the rate of return on polio research cannot be generalized to other medical research. The approach presented here, however, may have wider applicability.

In the case of some medical research programs, it may be possible to identify the disease or diseases that will be affected if and when the research is fruitful; the closer the research is to the "applied" end of the applied-basic spectrum, the greater the likelihood that such an identification can be made. When it can—when the output of medical research is expected to take the form of a reduction in the incidence, prevalence, or severity of one or more particular diseases—the variables in the internal-rate-of-return equation above constitute a checklist of items about which information should be sought by persons responsible for resource allocation decisions: What is the expected cost of the research program in each period? If the research is "successful," what "benefits" will result in each future period (and with what probabilities) per case of the disease (s) prevented or made less severe? How many cases will be affected in each future period?

[31] *Editors' Note:* For an interesting discussion of the monetary value of anguish see, Klarman, Herbert E.: Measuring the benefits of a health program—The control of syphilis, in, Dorfman, Robert (Ed.) : *Measuring Benefits of Government Investments.* Washington, D.C., The Brookings Institution, 1965, pp. 367–410.

What application costs, in each future period, will be required in order to realize these benefits from the medical research?

These questions will probably never be easily answered, and any answers will be uncertain. Uncertainty has not been considered explicitly in this paper; implicitly, however, variables have been evaluated in terms of expected values—a procedure that is not entirely satisfactory. Since it seems reasonable to assume that people are generally risk averters when disease is involved, the expected value of medical research will exceed the value of the expected benefits discussed above.

REFERENCES

American Medical Association: *Report of the Commission on the Cost of Medical Care.* Vol. 3. Chicago, American Medical Assoc., 1964.

Baumol, W. J.: *Economic Theory and Operations Analysis.* 2d ed. Englewood Cliffs, N.J., Prentice-Hall, 1965.

Department of Health, Education, and Welfare: *Trends.* Washington, Government Printing Office, 1962.

———: *U.S. Immunization Survey—1969.* Washington, Government Printing Office, 1970.

Griliches, Zvi: "Research Cost and Social Returns: Hybrid Corn and Related Innovations." *J.P.E., 56* (October 1958) : 419–31.

Hansen, W. Lee: "Total and Private Rates of Return to Investment in Schooling." *J.P.E.* 71 (April 1963) : 128–40.

Haveman, Robert. *Water Resource Investment and the Public Interest.* Nashville, Tenn.: Vanderbilt Univ. Press, 1965.

Skolnik, Alfred, M., and Dales, Sophie, R.: "Social Welfare Expenditures, 1969–70." *Soc. Sec. Bull., 33* (December 1970) : 4.

Statistical Abstracts of the U.S.; 1964. Washington: Bureau of the Census, 1964.

Watson, J. D.: *The Double Helix.* New York, Atheneum, 1968.

Weisbrod, Burton A.: *Economics of Public Health.* Philadelphia, Univ. Pa. Press, 1961; referred to as EPH.

World Book Encyclopedia. 1965 ed.

COST EFFECTIVENESS ANALYSIS APPLIED TO THE TREATMENT OF CHRONIC RENAL DISEASE [32]

HERBERT E. KLARMAN, JOHN O'S. FRANCIS
AND GERALD D. ROSENTHAL

This paper attempts to answer one question: <u>Under existing conditions of knowledge regarding the cost and end-results of treating</u>

[32] Reprinted with permission from *Medical Care,* Volume VI, No. 1, (January–February 1968) , pp. 48–54. Copyright © by J. B. Lippincott Company, 1968.

patients with chronic renal disease, what is the best mix of center dialysis, home dialysis, and kidney transplantation? The question is explored through the application of cost-effectiveness analysis.

DIMENSIONS OF THE PROBLEM

It is estimated that in the United States perhaps 6,000 persons whose life spans could be appreciably prolonged through treatments already known die every year from chronic renal disease. A large majority of these persons are 15–54 years old. Currently, it is estimated, approximately 1,000–1,100 receive available treatments—850 are on dialysis and 150–200 receive kidney transplants annually.

Treatment is expensive. On the average, a kidney transplantation costs 13,000 dollars, and the annual cost of dialysis is 14,000 dollars at a hospital center and 5,000 dollars in the patient's home.

Costliness of treatment, coupled with lack of adequate health insurance coverage, is a major factor in the Federal government's support of a substantial proportion of total expenditures, through its accepted role as sponsor of medical research, demonstrations of new methods of treatment and new ways of delivering health services. The Federal government also faces decisions regarding the size and scope of such programs in its own hospitals.

Other Western nations, including Great Britain and Sweden, have assumed a commitment to provide treatment for all persons with chronic renal disease who are eligible to receive it from a medical standpoint.

WHY COST-EFFECTIVENESS ANALYSIS?

Cost-effectiveness analysis is a special, narrower form of the cost-benefit approach that economists have evolved in the past generation. Much of the original work was done in the field of water resources.

The cost-benefit approach represents an attempt to apply systematic measurement to projects or programs in the public sector, where market prices are lacking and external effects in production or consumption loom important (so that individual decisions do not reflect true economic values). The cost-benefit approach is characterized by: a) the objective of enumerating as completely as possible all costs and all benefits expected and b) the recognition that costs and benefits tend to accrue over time.

In principle, cost-effectiveness analysis partakes of both of these characteristics: a complete listing of inputs and outputs and recognition of time. The time dimension is treated by means of the discount rate, which serves to convert a future dollar into its present value. Under cost-effectiveness analysis the enumeration of benefits need not be so complete as under the cost-benefit approach. Rather, certain results are specified and all other results are regarded as held constant or perhaps of secondary importance.

Cost-effectiveness, rather than cost-benefit, is employed when various benefits are difficult to measure or when the several benefits that are measured cannot be rendered commensurate. Under cost-effectiveness analysis costs are calculated and compared for alternative ways of achieving a specific set of results.

In performing a cost-effectiveness analysis it is taken for granted that the results sought can be "afforded."

AVAILABLE TREATMENTS

Chronic renal disease, resulting in irreversible kidney failure, stems from a variety of disease processes. No measures known today can be applied to a population with the resonable expectation that the number of persons who develop chronic renal disease will be reduced.

In some patients kidney function deteriorates to the point of cessation. The patient dies of poisoning within a short time, unless certain relatively new and radical treatments are applied. Two specific modalities are available: hemodialysis (the patient's blood is cleansed of impurities by an artificial kidney) and kidney transplantation. As previously implied, dialysis can take place at a hospital center or in the patient's home. The center may be a teaching hospital or a community hospital related to it. Dialysis at home usually is performed under close supervision of hospital center personnel. In transplantation the kidney may be taken from a live donor, usually a blood relative, or from a cadaver just deceased with kidneys intact.

An obvious difference between dialysis and transplantation is that dialysis continues over the patient's lifetime, whereas transplantation is a one-time procedure, with due allowance for the careful and prolonged follow-up that it requires. When a transplanted kidney fails, the patient may survive and can submit to another operation or shift to dialysis permanently.

TABLE 1

LIFE YEARS—COHORT OF 1,000 INDIVIDUALS
STARTING ON A CHRONIC HEMODIALYSIS
PROGRAM

| End of year | No. of individuals | | Average dialysis life years |
	Dead	On dialysis	
1	150	850	925
2	85	765	808
3	77	688	727
4	69	619	654
5	62	557	588
6	56	501	529
7	50	451	476
8	45	406	428
9	41	365	385
10	37	328	346
11	33	295	311
12	30	265	280
13	27	238	251
14	24	214	226
15	21	193	203
16	19	174	183
17	17	157	168
18	16	141	149
19	14	127	134
20	13	114	120
21	11	103	108
22	10	93	98
23	9	84	89
24	8	76	80
25	8	68	72
26	7	60	64
27	6	54	57
28	6	49	52
29	5	44	47
30	4	40	42
31	4	36	38
32	4	32	34
33	3	29	30
34	3	26	28
35	3	23	25
36	2	21	22
37	2	19	20
38	2	17	18
39	2	15	16
40	2	13	14
41+	13		160
TOTAL	1,000		9,005 *

* 9,005 ÷ 1,000 = 9.005 years of life expectancy for
each individual.

TABLE 2

EXPECTED ANNUAL MORTALITY RATES FOR
KIDNEY FAILURES BY FIVE-YEAR INTERVALS,
AGES 45–69

Age (years)	Range of annual mortality rates per 1,000 population	Assumed annual mortality rates per 1,000 pop. (normal × 2)	Adjusted rate per 100 pop. (per cent)
45–49	4.75– 6.89	11.64	1.2
50–54	7.58–10.72	18.30	1.8
55–59	11.63–16.03	27.66	2.8
60–64	17.31–24.17	41.48	4.1
65–69	26.42–35.93	62.35	6.2

Source: *Statistical Abstract of the United States*, 1966.

MEASURES OF END RESULTS

What is uniquely significant in both dialysis and kidney transplantaton is their capability for prolonging lives that otherwise would be cut short. It is no oversimplification to express their contributions in terms of the number of life-years gained by beneficiaries.

It is possible to make some allowance for certain differences in life style between patients on dialysis and those with an effective transplanted kidney. The latter have greater vitality, escape restrictive regimens, can continue to live in the same community, yet are free to travel without encumbrance or special arrangements. They enjoy a differential in the quality of life, which may be quantified as a fraction of each life-year gained. In this paper the differential is set at one-quarter of a life year. Other values may be posited; the implications of the findings are not affected.

Consideration was given to drawing a similar distinction between life-years on dialysis at the center and at home. It appears that although treatment at home is preferable for some patients, treatment at the center is preferable for others. There is yet no clear-cut evidence in either direction; accordingly, it seems best at this time to give equal value to a life-year gained at either location.

MEASURES OF COST

Cost is measured in terms of the present value of life-time expenditures for two cohorts of equal size, say 1,000 persons, each embarking on treatment with dialysis or kidney transplantation. Expenditures depend on unit cost, previously presented, and on the volume and timing of services used.

It should be noted that total expenditures are calculated, regardless of who pays for them. It is desirable—and has been found feasible— to separate the question of sources and mechanisms of financing from that of economic efficiency.

Since dialysis is a continuing treatment over the patient's life-time, the number of life-years gained is a necessary element of its cost while the same gain also serves as the measure of end results. To estimate the present value of the cost of transplantation, it is necessary to develop rates of retransplantation and of life years spent on dialysis by members of this cohort whose transplanted kidneys fail, who survive, and do not receive second kidney transplants. The cost of maintenance drugs is also taken into account.

For both cohorts it is important to tag the time when expenditures are incurred, so that they may be discounted to the present. It is realized that the choice of an appropriate rate of social discount is problematical, for there do not yet exist objective criteria for choosing one that commands general assent. In this paper a rate of 6 per cent is employed, because for diverse reasons it appears frequently in this type of analysis. Selection of alternative rates would affect the dollar amounts calculated in this paper but not the rank order of costs.

In order to facilitate calculations, projected future percentage increases in relative unit cost are combined with the initial discount rate of 6 per cent to yield a net discount rate. For transplantation and for center dialysis an extra annual rate of increase of 2 per cent (above any rise in the general price level) is posited and for home dialysis, which has a much lower labor component, an extra annual rate of increase of 1 per cent. The net rates of discount are, therefore, approximately 4 and 5 per cent, respectively.

allows for greater rt of medical cost inflation

Since transplantation occurs in the present, its estimated cost for a cohort can be estimated with greater certainty than that of dialysis, which takes place over a long time period. Reductions in the future cost of dialysis, if any, may be offset by the tendency to accept for treatment more patients with complications from other diseases.

The indispensable requirement for calculating the present value of expenditures expected to be incurred by each cohort, as well as for calculating the end results of treatment, are survivorship tables, with separate specification of years spent on dialysis and years with a functioning, transplanted kidney.

It will be noted that the total number of patients cared for has no

TABLE 3

ASSUMED DISTRIBUTION OF ANNUAL
KIDNEY FAILURES OF FIVE PER CENT
BETWEEN DIALYSIS AND MORTALITY
IN EACH FIVE-YEAR SURVIVORSHIP
PERIOD

Five-year survivorship period *	Proportion dying	Proportion to dialysis
1	$\frac{1}{4}$	$\frac{3}{4}$
2	$\frac{2}{5}$	$\frac{3}{5}$
3	$\frac{1}{2}$	$\frac{1}{2}$
4	$\frac{4}{5}$	$\frac{1}{5}$
5	All	—

* Period starts at the end of year two in Table 4.

bearing on the results of the cost-effectiveness analysis. The total cost of treatment is, of course, in part a function of the number of patients, and total cost does influence the determination of what can be afforded.

BASIC DATA

Table 1 presents life years gained by a cohort of 1,000 individuals embarking on a chronic hemodialysis program.[33] This table is based on two assumptions: (1) the death rate in the first year is 15 per cent; (2) the death rate in every subsequent year is 10 per cent. For the first six years the survival estimates are based on data accumulated from various operating dialysis centers in hospitals in the United States. Life expectancy in the longer run must be predicated on speculation, for actual experience with chronic dialysis has not yet reached 10 years, much less the 30–40 years shown in the table.

Table 4 shows the disposition of a cohort of 1,000 persons who embark on transplantation. In evaluating the experience of individuals on transplantation, it became evident that several alternatives must be considered. Patients starting on transplantation may have a successful first transplantation, may require a second transplantation, may die, or may move on to a program of long-term hemodialysis.

[33] The authors had access to the data developed for and by an expert Committee on Chronic Kidney Disease, convened by the Bureau of the Budget. Since this paper draws heavily on the Committee's data, it is not necessary to present here as detailed a documentation of sources and bases for assumptions as would be required otherwise. See Report by this Committee, Carl W. Gottschalk, Chairman, Washington, Sept. 1967.

TABLE 4

DISPOSITION AND AVERAGE LIFE YEARS OF TRANSPLANTATION
COHORT OF 1,000 BY TREATMENT MODALITY

	On trans-planted kidney	Lose kidney during interval				Average life years	
		Total	Aggregates in interval			Trans-plantation	Dialysis *
End of year			Total	Move to dialysis	Die		
1	—	—	—	—	—	875	55
2	600 **	400	400	200	200	675	200
3	570	30 ⎫					
4	552	28 ⎪					
5	524	28 ⎬ †	137	105	32	2,617	105
6	498	26 ⎪					
7	473	25 ⎭					
8	449	24 ⎫					
9	427	22 ⎪					
10	406	21 ⎬ †	106	65	41	2,035	65
11	386	20 ⎪					
12	367	19 ⎭					
13	349	18 ⎫					
14	332	17 ⎪					
15	315	17 ⎬ †	83	42	41	1,579	42
16	299	16 ⎪					
17	284	15 ⎭					
18	270	14 ⎫					
19	256	14 ⎪					
20	243	13 ⎬ †	65	13	52	1,219	13
21	231	12 ⎪					
22	219	12 ⎭					
23	208	11 ⎫					
24	198	10 ⎪					
25	188	10 ⎬ †	49	—	49	943	—
26	179	9 ⎪					
27	170	9 ⎭					
28+	Less 5% annually					3,407	
Total 34						13,350 + (480 × 8)/ 1,000 = 17.2	

* Represents persons moving to dialysis, surviving eight years.
** Assumes no information until end of year two.
† Five-year survivorship groups (see Tables 2 and 3).

Here, too, experience has been too short to enable one to generate
an expected life table with great accuracy or confidence. The assumptions taken from the Committee are that at the end of two years
approximately 50 per cent of the cohort will have a surviving first

34 *Editors' Note:* The values in the "Total" row were derived as follows: 13,350 is
the total of the geometric progression of 3,407 average life years for those with transplants at the end of year 28 adjusted for a 5 per cent annual loss; 480 is the sum
of the last column in Table 4; and 8 is the assumed survival rate in years for
patients whose transplant failed and consequently were shifted to dialysis.

transplanted kidney, 10 per cent will have a surviving second kidney transplant, 20 per cent will have died, and 20 per cent will be on long-term dialysis.

It must be emphasized that kidney failure following transplantation signifies loss of the donated kidney, not death of the patient. In case of such failure, some patients die whereas others move into a dialysis pool.

Owing to the additional alternative, given failure of a transplanted kidney, it was essential to develop criteria for dividing the failures occurring after year 2 into two categories—those dying and those moving into dialysis programs. An annual failure rate of 5 per cent was posited. The procedure adopted in this analysis follows from the evidence that the median age of people who have chronic uremia is approximately 45 years. To facilitate calculations it was assumed that the mortality rate for each age class would be approximately twice the rate for that age class in the U.S. population as a whole. Table 2 presents the expected mortality by five-year intervals from age 45 to 69, translated into annual rates. Table 3, derived from Table 2, distributes the annual kidney failure rate of 5 per cent between death and dialysis for each age class.

From the life tables for the dialysis cohort in Table 1 and the transplantation cohort in Table 4 it was possible to calculate the average life expectancy of an individual in each cohort. This was done by summing the total number of life years gained (or, where possible, taking the limit of the sum of a geometric progression) and dividing by 1,000, the number of individuals in the initial cohort. This exercise yields a life expectancy gain of 9.0 years for an individual in the dialysis cohort. The life expectancy gain for an individual entering the transplantation cohort is approximately 17.2 years—13.3 additional years on a successfully transplanted kidney and almost four years on dialysis, after the failure of a transplanted kidney. The added life years for a cohort embarking on transplantation are almost twice those of a cohort on dialysis alone, given the above assumptions.

When the adjustment is introduced for the qualitative differences between life after transplantation and life on dialysis, the differences between the results of transplantation and dialysis increases. Table 5 summarizes the calculations of cost and life years gained for each cohort.

The average increase in life expectancy with chronic hemodialysis alone is estimated to be nine years and that for transplantation, com-

TABLE 5

PRESENT VALUE OF EXPENDITURES AND LIFE
YEARS GAINED PER MEMBER OF COHORT
EMBARKING ON TRANSPLANTATION AND
ON CENTER AND HOME DIALYSIS

Modality	Present value of expenditures	Life years gained	Cost per life year
Dialysis			
Center	$104,000	9	$11,600 ←
Home	38,000	9	4,200 ←
Mean	71,000	9	7,900
Transplantation			
Unadjusted	44,500	17	2,600
Adjusted for quality	44,500	20.5	2,200 ←

Note: The cost of transplantation incorporates $24,500 for dialysis, based on a 50–50 per cent distribution of patients between the center and home.

bined with dialysis when appropriate, is 17 years. The present value of the per capita cost of the several treatment modalities is approximately $44,500 for transplantation, $38,000 for home dialysis, and $104,000 for center dialysis. If the conservative assumption of a 50–50 mix between home and center dialysis is made, the present value of the per capita cost of caring for the dialysis cohort is $71,000.

By almost every measure the maximum transplantation route appears to be the more effective way to increase life expectancy at a given cost. Further, the cost incurred is not appreciably greater than that of the least expensive dialysis program, that is, a program of home dialysis exclusively—which is not practicable.

Notwithstanding, it is noteworthy that the present value of the cost of a transplantation program does not differ a great deal from the present value of the cost of a home dialysis program. This emphasizes the degree to which it is possible to underestimate the true cost of transplantation by omitting additional hemodialysis as part of the expected experience of the transplantation cohort. It will be recalled that the additional 17 life years accruing to the transplantation cohort consist of approximately 13 years as the result of a successful transplantation plus four years on long-term dialysis, following kidney failure.

IMPLICATIONS

On the basis of the above findings it is concluded that transplantation is economically the most effective way to increase the life expectancy of persons with chronic kidney disease.

Certain factors constrain the expansion of transplantation capability. Removal of these constraints has the priority for action in the foreseeable future. More kidneys will be needed; it will be necessary to change certain state laws concerning autopsy and donation of organs and to improve the storage and preservation of kidneys. The last will depend on the outcome of research.

Successful research in tissue typing will serve to increase further the difference in cost per life year gained between transplantation and dialysis. Any improvement in the technology of dialysis might reduce the difference.

It should be noted that the amount to be spent on research in an area cannot be expressed simply as a percentage of expenditures for services. Rather, research expenditures are properly a function of the size of the problem (measured by the sum of costs due to expenditures plus cost due to loss of earnings plus cost due to pain and suffering), multiplied by the probability of accomplishing successful research and of applying it. The probability of successful outcome in research, in turn, depends on what is already known and on the availability of trained scientific manpower to exploit it.

The large difference in cost between dialysis at the center and at home suggests that it may be worthwhile to explore the factors conducive to an expansion of home dialysis. It is obvious that one limitation on the performance of dialysis at home is the condition of housing. Accordingly, it may be desirable to consider alternative ways to improve the housing of patients with chronic renal disease and their families.

note — did not carefully check sensitivity of his assumptions!

Chapter Ten

ECONOMIC GROWTH AND HEALTH

M ANY OBJECTIVES of economic policy coexist in any country. Economic growth, reasonable price stability, elimination of poverty, low unemployment, and a positive environment are some of the broadest goals. The growth objective, if achieved, facilitates the realization of all the others, as economic growth implies the subsequent production of more goods and services that can be used for raising low incomes, increasing employment, and decreasing pollution, among other things.

The relationships between the health field and economic growth are complex. The health of the members of the labor force affects their ability to work and hence to produce. Nutrition and sanitation services further enhance the productive capacities of the workforce and directly affect the rate of economic growth. The size of the population and labor force of any given country are also affected by the existence and application of medical knowledge and technologies, as the quality and quantity of medical resources available effect both birth and death rates.

The presentation in this chapter begins with a definition of economic growth and a discussion of a theoretical model of economic growth (the neoclassical model). The second section focuses on the various relationships between the health field and economic growth. The third section contains a discussion of the nature of planning, and its role in fostering economic growth. The final section reviews some of the economic techniques that have been adopted in or proposed for use in health planning.

ECONOMIC GROWTH

Economic growth is defined as an increase in some measure of the amount of economic activity over time. The measure can be any national income concept, but Gross National Product (GNP), the total of all goods and services produced in a year, is most commonly used. For example, the Gross National Product of the United States in 1970 was 974 billion dollars and in 1971 it rose to 1,000 billion dollars in constant 1970 prices. Thus the growth, in constant dollars, over the year was 26 billion dollars. This represents a GNP growth rate of 2.7 per cent as determined by the following formula:

$$\frac{\text{Change in GNP}}{\text{GNP in first period}} = \text{GNP growth rate}$$

$$\frac{\$26 \text{ billion}}{\$974 \text{ billion}} = 2.7\%$$

Economic growth, as it has been defined, does not necessarily mean an improvement in the well-being of the average man, although the presumption is that hc will benefit from growth. The distribution of the extra produce resulting from economic growth among the various consumption options determines the correlation between economic growth and well-being. For example, the benefits of economic growth can be earmarked for increased public health expenditures or for increased government public relations expenditures. It is clear that the average individual will not benefit as much from the second option as from the first. Secondly, the effect on any individual of economic growth is dependent on the subsequent distribution of the increase in resources. If the entire increase in GNP went to any one individual or some small group of people, the average person would observe no improvement in his economic well-being. Such a situation could be contrasted to one wherein the entire increase in GNP was evenly distributed among the poorest 10 per cent of the households in the country, thereby increasing their incomes substantially. Finally, it is necessary to have an increase in *per capita* income to increase average well-being. If the population grew by the same percentage amount as GNP the entire increase in GNP would just suffice to give the new population an average income. Thus, while GNP increased, the increase in GNP per capita would have been zero so that the average person would be no better off. The distribution of the increase in goods and services implied by the economic growth is an important factor which has only recently begun receiving a great deal of attention from the economics profession.

As was seen in Chapter Two, national income accounts statistics have many conceptual and statistical problems built into them. Since these statistics form the base of growth measurement, one might be led to question the validity of growth statistics. Actually, economic growth statistics are more accurate than most others. A growth statistic is derived from the comparison of two different GNP levels, each of which has similar imprecisions embodied within it. As long as the GNP figures are derived in the same manner each year and the economy does not undergo radical institutional change, the effect of the imperfections is cancelled out. For example, if GNP is underestimated by the same proportion in each of two years, the measured growth rate will not be affected *at all,* as is demonstrated below:

	Year		
	1	*2*	*Growth*
Actual GNP	100	110	10%
Measured GNP (error of 5%)	95	104.5	10%

From a historical perspective, sustained economic growth has been rare. Only in the last few centuries and in a limited number of countries has income per capita been steadily expanding. About half the world's population is still living at or below a subsistence level, the level of income just sufficient to maintain life.

The industrial revolution, which began in Great Britain in the eighteenth century, is the watershed that marked the beginning of sustained economic growth. A number of major developments occurred during this period: new inventions appeared and new power sources were uncovered; a large export market arose resulting from the combination of colonialism and free trade; new supplies of labor that had been freed from agriculture appeared; new monetary institutions were created; and others. The manufacturers who appeared on the industrial scene in response to these developments typically reinvested their profits from their initial endeavors creating more and more capital. Together these events had the revoluntionary result of steadily increasing income per capita. While all the factors enumerated above contributed to this growth cycle, the key element was the savings and investment of the owners of capital as it enabled the continued productive utilization of the available labor, capital, and technology.

While a historical presentation explains what did happen, it does not constitute a theory or model of how or why economic growth occured. In order to guide policy, it is necessary to understand the processes that underlie and tie together events. One of the most prominent and versatile models of economic growth which highlights how the growth process occurs is the neoclassical model.

THE NEOCLASSICAL MODEL

In the neoclassical model, economic growth results from increases in any of the factors of production. This process can be illustrated with reference to a standard two factor production function [1] represented by equation (1).

$$Y = f(K,L) \qquad (1)$$

Where Y is output, K is capital, and L is labor. Growth in output could then be represented by

$$\Delta Y = f(\Delta K, \Delta L) \qquad (2)$$

where Δ represents the term *change in*. Division of equation (1) by equation (2) yields

$$\frac{\Delta Y}{Y} = f\left(\frac{\Delta K}{K}, \frac{\Delta L}{L}\right) \qquad (3)$$

[1] The concepts relating to production functions are developed in detail in Chapter Six.

Since the definition of the rate of growth is the change divided by the original amount, equation (3) can be transformed into

$$G_y = f(G_k, G_l) \qquad (4)$$

where G is a symbol representing the growth rate.

The growth of output in the neoclassical model is thus dependent on the growth of the factors of production, capital and labor. But how and why do the factors of production grow? Capital grows through net investment, that is, investment in addition to that which is necessary to replace depleted capital. In all modern industrial economies, net investment occurs because most individuals prefer to increase their future consumption at the expense of present consumption. (As will be noted in the next section, health has an impact on the rate of capital accumulation through its influence on the population growth rate.)

The growth of labor is a net result of several elements. First is the rate of population increase, since population is the base from which labor is derived. However, as a nation becomes richer, fewer hours of labor per worker tend to be offered. In addition, the labor force participation rates [2] of different groups change over time. In most industrialized countries the proportion of teenagers and elderly persons in the labor force has decreased steadily while the participation rate of women has increased. The increase in the labor input is a result of the balancing of these and other factors.

Equation (4) can be changed from a functional to a specific form as follows:

$$G_y = aG_k + bG_l \qquad (5)$$

where a represents capital's share in total output and b represents the share of labor in total output.[3] Thus, the growth of output is equal to the growth of capital times capital's share of

---

[2] Labor force participation is defined as the proportion of individuals who are either employed or seeking employment, relative to the entire civilian, non-institutional population.

[3] The share of a factor of production in total output can be determined by noting what proportion of total output (GNP) is paid in the form of wages and salaries, rent and interest, etc.

total output plus the growth of labor times labor's share of total output, so that capital and labor independently contribute to output. In this model a + b must equal 1 (one) in order to account for the entire growth of output.

As was suggested earlier, the objective of economic growth is not merely to increase the output of the economy but rather to increase the well-being of the population. Consequently it is the growth of income per capita that is important. A simple manipulation of equation (5) yields a formula for the rate of growth of income per capita. Since a + b = 1, it follows that a = 1 − b, and 1 − b can be substituted for a in equation (4) to yield

$$G_y = (1 - b)G_k + bG_l \qquad (6)$$

Subtracting the growth rate of labor from both sides results in

$$G_y - G_l = (1 - b)G_k - bG_l - G_l \qquad (7)$$

A rearrangement of terms yields:

$$G_y - G_l = (1 - b)(G_k - G_l) \qquad (8)$$

Since $G_y - G_l$ is the growth rate of income per capita (under the implicit assumption that the growth rate of labor and of population are equal), equation (8) indicates that the lower the growth rate of labor, the greater will be the growth rate of income per capita for a given growth rate of capital.[4]

For the neoclassical model a representation of the production function would look like the isoquant map shown in Figure 15. Such isoquants represent a production function that allows for substitutability between capital and labor. With L_a labor and K_a capital, production would be at the level represented by isoquant R. An increase of capital to K_c with no change in labor would increase output to the level represenetd by isoquant S. Similarly, if only labor had been increased to level L_b for exam-

----

[4] For example, if b = ¾, the following would hold

G_k	G_l	G_y	$G_y - G_l$
4%	0%	1%	1%
4	1	1¾	¾
4	2	2½	½

ple, production also would have been increased to the level of isoquant S. If both labor and capital are increased, to L_b and K_c, output would be increased even more, to isoquant T. Thus, the neoclassical model recognizes that added capital is a possible substitute for added labor and vice versa and that increases in either result in economic growth.

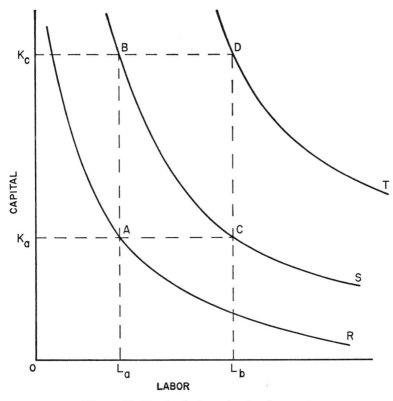

Figure 15. Neoclassical production isoquants.

When the actual data for the United States is inserted into the growth equation of the neoclassical model, it is seen that something is amiss. Historically, the value of the share of capital in national income, a, has been about one-quarter and the share of labor, b, has been about three-quarters. Capital has been growing at about 3 per cent per year, and labor has been growing by about 1 per cent per year. Therefore, the neoclassical

growth model would predict that the growth rate of income
would have been about 1.5 per cent:

$$G_y = aG_k + bG_l$$
$$= .25 \cdot 3\% + .75 \cdot 1\%$$
$$= 1.5\%$$

The United States economy has actually been growing at about
3 per cent per annum. Hence, there is a discrepancy of 1.5 percentage points between the actual growth rate and that which
the model attributes to the growth of labor and capital.[5] This
discrepancy has led to what has become known as the *residual
factor* controversy. One possible answer to the problem is that
some factor or factors of production were left out of the production function which account for the missing 1.5 percentage points
of growth. Some researchers suggest that this residual factor is
simply a measure of our ignorance; it includes not only missing
production but also any errors in the measurement of growth of
the relative shares in output of labor and capital. Another view
is that the residual 1.5 percentage points are accounted for by
technological progress.

Technological progress is a term that is utilized to describe
the fact that the inputs into the production process itself have
improved over time so that the same nominal quantity of inputs
yield more output in succeeding time periods. Technological
progress can be divided into two types for analytical purposes:
disembodied and embodied. *Disembodied technological progress* is defined as technological progress that is not embodied in
some factor of production. That is, its occurrence is entirely
independent of the amount or growth of the factors of production. Examples of disembodied technological progress include
the idea of interchangeable parts, time-motion study improvements, and discovery of better travel routes. Each of these leads
to greater output from the existing factors of production and
requires no new capital, labor, nor any other factor of production. Disembodied technological progress could be entered into

[5] A per cent and a percentage point are not identical concepts. In this case 1.5
percentage points is 50 per cent of the total growth rate—3 percentage points.

the neoclassical growth model, equation (5), by simply adding a parameter, δ

$$G_y = aG_k + bG_l + \delta$$

where δ represents disembodied technological progress. A value of 1.5 per cent for δ would bring the growth equation up to the required equality.

Embodied technological progress can be defined as improvements in the quality of the factors of production that lead to greater productivity. By definition these improvements are inexorably tied to the factors of production without which embodied technological progress could not exist. Better educated, better trained, and healthier laborers are examples of what might be considered technological progress embodied in labor. Examples of embodied technological progress in capital include any new machine that does the same job costing less or a larger job costing the same: electric typewriters, the newest movie projectors, automatic telephone switching systems, and "jumbo" jets. These also can be integrated into the basic neoclassical model as follows:

$$G_y = aG_n + bG_j$$

where n is *effective* capital, $G_n = f(G_k, \phi_1)$, ϕ_1 is the rate of embodied technological progress of capital, j is *effective* labor, $G_j = f(G_l, \phi_2)$, and ϕ_2 is the rate of embodied technological progress of labor. Thus, the effect of increasing the health level of the labor force is brought into the production function through ϕ_2.

Technological progress can be embodied not only in those new factors of production representing an increase in the total stock, but also in those replacing the factors being retired from production each year. That is, additional labor and capital that both replace retiring labor and capital and represent increases in the total of these factors of production are more productive due to improved technology embodied in them, for example, greater health and new machines.

The methods employed to date for attempting to measure the values of ϕ_1 and ϕ_2, the rates of embodied technological progress in capital and labor, have utilized the growth of expenditures on research and development and expenditures on education and health, respectively. No one has yet succeeded in attributing all of the growth of output to specific changes in the economy. Edward Denison's [6] attempt has come closest, but he still ends up with a residual which he attributes to changes in knowledge of 0.53 per cent out of 2.93 per cent or 18 per cent of the total growth of output for the period he was studying.

HEALTH AND ECONOMIC GROWTH

The importance of population growth for determining the welfare impact of economic growth has already been demonstrated. It is the impact of health levels on the rate of population growth that is undoubtedly the most important influence of health on economic growth and individual well-being, as health affects both the birth and death rates, the two determinants of the rate of population growth.

Steady population growth, like economic growth itself, has been a fairly recent occurrence in world history. Unlike economic growth, however, population growth has been almost universal and has slackened off only in most of the industrialized nations.[7] Historically, a pattern of population change over time has emerged which has been labelled the *demographic transition,* pictured in Figure 16. Through the end of the middle ages, the pattern of birth and death rates was a fairly constant one. Both were at high levels and both showed some variation. The death rate would increase in response to famines, epidemics, and, to a lesser extent, wars. Following such periods, the death rate would fall below normal because so many of the most vulnerable members of the society had recently died. The birth rate remained fairly steady. As seen in Figure 16, the net effect was a balance between births and deaths leaving no population growth.

[6] Denison, Edward F.: *The Sources of Economic Growth in the United States and the Alternatives Before Us.* New York, Committee for Economic Development, 1962.

[7] Even within industrialized nations there are often subgroups of the population that exhibit much higher rates of population growth than the nation as a whole. The factors typically associated with higher population growth rates are having a rural residence, a low level of education, and a low income.

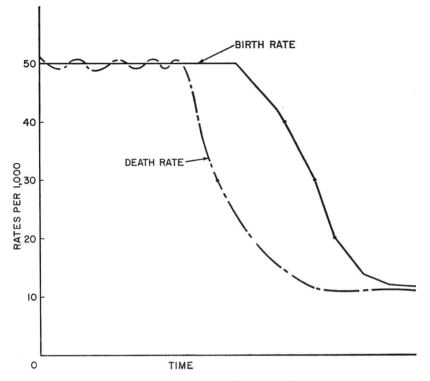

Figure 16. Demographic transition.

The emergence of food surpluses and new distribution methods which made it possible to ease famines, new medical techniques (the smallpox vaccination, developed in 1798, was the first of the preventive vaccines) and knowledge (especially sanitation), led to a decline in the death rate at the end of the 18th century. But the birth rate remained steady. This combination resulted in the population explosion in which, from a worldwide perspective, we remain today. For the industrialized nations, the birth rates eventually fell in a lagged response to higher levels of education, urbanization, income, and, contraceptive knowledge. In any case, most industrialized nations are in positions described by the last part of Figure 16; low birth and death rates with a low but positive rate of population growth.

Less developed countries in the world are characterized by a middle position in Figure 16. Medical advances have cut the death rates drastically in these countries but the birth rates are only beginning to respond to the changed education and urbanization levels, which have generally increased in most less developed countries, and to increased income per capita which is somewhat rarer. Indeed, in many less developed countries the situation is likely to get worse over the short run since the fall in the death rate will probably continue to exceed the fall in the birth rate. A typical death-birth pattern for a less developed country is to have 50 births per thousand per year and 20 deaths per thousand population per year implying a population growth rate of 3 per cent. In the industrialized nations a death rate of 10 per thousand is common, one half as much as the typical less developed country rate. Consequently the population growth rate could increase even more before it falls.

The implications of high rates of population growth are similar for less developed countries and poverty areas of developed nations. In either case a high dependency ratio [8] results, savings are probably depressed, and investment in education, health, and capital are all spread over more people. The dependency ratio reflects directly on the impact of population growth on economic growth. To attain economic growth it is necessary to accumulate and improve capital and labor. Accumulation of capital depends on savings. The larger the family size for a given income, the more difficult it is to save. With respect to less developed countries where average annual income per capita is as little as 75 dollars or families in the United States with family income of less than 3,000 dollars it is obvious that a large family makes it extremely difficult if not impossible to save. Similarly, the

[8] The dependency ratio is the ratio of the number of individuals who are *not* in the age group thought of as being appropriate for the labor force, relative to those who are in the labor force age group. It is usually measured as the population below 15 years of age plus those over 65 divided by the population 15 to 65 (times 100). Industrialized nations have low dependency ratios: 68 for the United States, 47 for Japan, 52 for Italy. For less developed countries the dependency ratio is higher than the highest industrialized countries in effectively every case: typical examples are 100 for Jordan, 79 for India, 102 for Costa Rica, and 83 for Nigeria. The difference between dependency ratios of 102 and 68 is that in the former country each adult has to support 50 per cent more dependents than in the latter.

quality of labor suffers when large families are the norm and income is low. Less can be spent on medical care and nutrition, and less education can be afforded. All of these affect the quality of the labor supplied to the productive process and hence negatively influence economic growth.

The role of health in determining the population growth rate is a major one. Vaccines alone have had a great impact on death rates all over the world. Perhaps more important has been the development of the knowledge of how to deal with pre-natal, child birth, and post-natal problems. The development of modern birth control devices such as the inter-uterine device, techniques such as safe and relatively accessable sterilization procedures, and drugs such as birth control pills, have all contributed to a significant improvement in the technology of reducing the birth rate. However, in spite of these technological advances, the impact of population control devices has not been great. First, many people are not able to make use of the technologies because they are too expensive, not available in sufficient quantity in their locale or not available at all. Secondly, people have to *want* to utilize the new technology of birth prevention. As long as the cultural mores are supportive of large families, large families will continue to predominate in such societies. For generations large families were the norm; large families that can support the parents in their old age, that will be fairly certain of yielding survivors to carry on the family traditions in spite of the high infant mortality rates, and that will supply labor for the family farm in countries where typically 85 to 95 per cent of the population is in agriculture. The birth rate tends to fall as societies become more urbanized, with the concomitant result that child labor becomes less important as they become richer, and experience a decline in infant mortality.

The level of morbidity in a country also affects both the quality and quantity of the work performed. The output per worker or per hour worked is the productivity of labor. The productivity is affected by the number and severity of chronic and acute health problems. In less developed countries the typical chronic problems include schistosomaisis, diarrhea and dysentery, malaria, and tuberculosis. All of these, in mild forms, allow the individual to work but any of them can reduce the productivity of the worker. In addition, the chronic effects of poliomyelitis and other permanently handicapping diseases severely limit the lifetime productive capacity of persons they affect.

Malnutrition is another health problem that affects the productive capacity of the labor force, since undernourished people are not likely to work at peak efficiency. Malnutrition can be a result of some of the other diseases mentioned, in particular diarrhea, causing malabsorption of the food that is consumed, as well as insufficient intake of calories and/or nutrients. Similarly, fevers from malaria or other diseases can burn up calories which cannot then serve a nutritional purpose. The less developed a country and/or an area, or the poorer the people, the greater is the number of calories required for work because of the availability of less capital and mechanical power with which to work. Finally, malnutrition can lead to permanent damage to the brain and/or body through such diseases as Kwashiokor (acute protein deficiency).

The potential effects of health on the quantity of work are based on similar considerations. When various chronic diseases flair up, the individual may be forced to stay away from work, thus directly reducing the quantity of work undertaken in a given year. In addition, an acute attack of any of the diseases may lead to the inability to work at all for short periods. On the other hand, certain diseases and medically related disabilities may lead to permanent withdrawal from the work force. When someone is removed from the work force, all the investment in his health and education in the past are lost to the economy from the point of view of production, thereby negatively affecting growth potential.

The extreme of morbidity is, of course, mortality. Mortality always implies a loss of human resources in addition to the emotional loss to the family. Even the death of a newborn baby means the loss of the nutrition that the mother invested in the child, the loss of the health services received by the mother, and the loss of some or all of the mother's productivity during the pre- and post-natal periods. When an older individual dies, a much greater investment is lost.

PLANNING

Planning is a technique frequently utilized to achieve economic growth. Planning is particularly important for less developed countries and less developed areas of developed countries. For several reasons less developed areas do not seem to be able to rely on the market to produce sustained growth to the extent that areas that developed in the past did. Of the two most important reasons, the first is the growth rate of population, which, as has been discussed, is at an unprecedented height in most less developed areas. No country that is now highly developed accomplished its development while its population was growing rapidly. The second factor is that the less developed areas are in a world that includes highly developed ones. Competition from developed areas cuts off for the less developed areas the very same routes the now highly developed areas followed in their successful attempts at development. In addition developed areas provide patterns of high consumption which, when copied by poor areas leave little for investment purposes. Finally, most less developed countries have a large government sector, a sector that does not have the full range of market forces affecting it. It is because of these difficulties that economic planning has been accepted as a rational supplement to the free market in most less developed areas. Although planning could be discussed in terms of mathematical models employed in the planning process,[9] the ensuing presentation will entail only a discussion of planning in general and an overview of several types of planning techniques.

In the health field, planning has an additional rationale. Health care by its very nature has many attributes that affect both the direct consumers of health care and many of the consumer's neighbors. This is especially true with regard to preventive care in the realm of communicable diseases. Consequently, society is reluctant to rely solely on market forces to allocate

[9] See for example, Nosta, Manohar and Shaprio, Robert: *Mathematical Models to Facilitate Management and Developmental Planning of a Hospital System,* Iowa City: Department of Industrial and Management Engineering, The University of Iowa, 1970.

health care services. Furthermore, it is frequently stated that no one should be denied health care because of lack of money to buy it.[10]

Planning can be defined as the process of specifying policy within the framework of a model with the objective of attaining some goal or goals at the lowest possible cost. This is a definition of formal planning; de facto planning of various degrees of sophistication is continuously undertaken in an economy. Examples of informal planning include the president of a company calling his sales managers together to plot out the sales campaign for the coming season or the hospital board meeting with the chiefs of service to discuss the type and number of medical and paramedical personnel to be hired for the coming year. Indeed, all activities implicitly have a planning element. Even when there are no changes, an implicit decision of no change is made.

To be most effective planning needs to involve, in the drafting process, all the agencies and individuals to be affected by the plan. There is a significant history of plans being completely sterile documents; lack of involvement of the operational agencies is often one reason for this. Not having been privy to the formulation of the plan, they have no direct interest in seeing it fulfilled. A second reason could be lack of machinery for following up the plan. To expect fundamental or even lesser changes in a large bureaucracy to develop from the mere publication of a document is unrealistic. A third reason could be that the plan may have been a purely political document to begin with, drafted with no expectation of implementation. With this overview of planning as background, a closer view of the benefits and costs of the planning process is in order.

The potential benefits derived from planning are several. First, there is the expectation of consistency.[11] Without planning,

---

[10] This objective is seldom realized because of its great potential cost. In less developed countries it is impossible to meet this objective and in those countries that could meet it (such as the United States) the necessary political decisions have not been made.

[11] Consistency is simply the piecing together of a whole program to make sure that it fits correctly.

there is a high probability that the set of policies adopted may be such that they conflict or overlap in some vital way. That is, the policies and goals may be such that the policies cannot achieve the goals due to internal contradictions.

An example of an inconsistency is a set of policies like the following: nurse's aide/registered nurse ratio is to remain constant; nurses' aides are to increase by 10 per cent; and number of registered nurses is to remain constant. Given the size and complexity of an economy or a health care system, there can be inconsistencies in programs which are not initially obvious. Such inconsistencies can lead to very costly errors.

Consistency may be a problem in any given year and also over time. Consistency over time is perhaps even more important than in any given year because of the greater chance of error. Usually it is not too difficult to see how pieces fit together in a given year. But over time, there is much less probability of a fit without a *formal* apparatus designed to assure a fit. For example, how can one assure that the number of nurse's aides, who require only a few weeks of training, and registered nurses, whose training encompasses a period of from 2 to 4 years will match without a plan in which to check the consistency of the policies regarding each of these items? Thus consistency, which may seem so obvious as to be trivial, but is far from trivial in its importance, is one benefit of planning.

A second benefit derived from planning is the specification and clarification of objectives and priorities. The process of planning for a period of one or several years necessitates the spelling out of ideas and desires on the part of planners and politicians (in the case of government programs). Such exercises cannot help but improve the ideas and the will and ability to carry them out. The process of achieving consistency from a plan which is not initially consistent will ideally employ priorities. It does not have to, however. De facto, priorities are always in effect in that certain things are done before others. The planning process implies specifying the objectives and weighing them against one another, thereby imposing a rational priority system on them rather than allowing a non-rational, or thoughtless priority system to prevail. Cutting the number of nurse's aides is one way of approaching the consistency problem above. But a decision on which is most important—more nurse's aides, a constant nurse's aide/registered nurse ratio, or no increase in the number of registered nurses—is a better approach to the problem.

Closely related to this second benefit is the determination of what information is needed to operate the system rationally. In the setting of objectives and priorities, certain information which is not available but necessary is identified. The amount of data that is possible to collect is infinite. Because data collection has a positive time and resource cost, it is a real benefit to determine what kind of data are needed and will be useful.

Third, planning leaves one with a structure in which evaluation can be systematically undertaken. With a plan consisting of specified objectives, policies, and a model of the system, the actual events that occur can be juxtaposed against the plan to determine whether policies were the right ones for meeting the objectives, what should be considered, and so forth. All of these can lead to better plans in the future. Without a plan, evaluation can still take place, but it is much more difficult due to the lack of a base against which to measure the results, and therefore is much less likely to occur. Planning does not assure evaluation—bureaucrats and politicians seldom feel that they have time or money for such action—but it does ease the task if there is an inclination to evaluate.

The fourth benefit from planning is a psychological one. There are two aspects of this benefit, one general and one rather narrow. Generally, the specification of objectives can have a psychological effect on the people affected by the plan, an effect that helps lead to the fulfillment of those objectives. The setting of goals can lead to the striving to meet them. More narrowly, for economic or health planning in less developed regions there is a greater likelihood of external aid coming in to assist planned than unplanned growth, which is a benefit from the perspective of the area engaged in planning.

The first cost of planning is the resources used in the process. A tremendous amount of manpower can be taken up in the planning process. Manpower is not required only in a planning office but in all areas and at all levels of the system since people need to communicate and be communicated to.

A second cost (or is it a benefit?) of planning is that it necessitates centralization. Centralization is a cost in that policy makers and planners are, by their nature, not involved with the day-to-day minutia of economic or health care production. They cannot know the problems peculiar to each town and hamlet, hospital, and physician. Therefore, centralization can lead to abstractions that are not workable when the actual forms of the problems are confronted. On the other hand, decentralized decision making can also be ineffective. For example, two hospitals may duplicate expensive, specialized equipment if there is complete decentralized decision making. These are events much better seen from an aggregate or centralized viewpoint.

Another cost of planning is a political one. The publication of a plan means that the priorities of the policy makers are opened to attack. Any action that even seems to be inconsistent with the plan is likely to be political fodder for the opposition. Stated objectives not met are even more explosive political tinder.

A final cost is the effect of a planner making a mistake. If an individual physician or hospital attempts something new that fails, the cost is limited because the weight of one project in an area is slight. However, if a planner with jurisdiction over a larger area errs, there can be a great loss.

Two general comments about planning follow. The idea of a rolling plan is the first. A *rolling plan* is one that is specified for a given number of years, say five, and periodically reevaluated and revised. For example, a five year plan for 1973–77 would be revised in 1974 and changed to a five year plan for 1974–78. The next year it could be changed to a 1975–79 five year plan, and so on; each year a new five year plan based on the last would be promulgated. Such a system has the advantage of keeping the goals realistic and relevant and of bringing new conditions into the plan. On the other hand, it has the disadvantage of being even more costly in terms of the resources necessary to undertake such frequent changes. There is a real danger with a rolling plan of a planning office spending all of its time repeatedly rewriting the plan rather than seeing that it is carried out. Generally, a plan that is rolled annually is not as efficient as one that is rolled every two or three years.

Second, it should be noted that it is possible to have both micro and macro planning in the sense of either geography or size. One can have planning on any geographic basis: neighborhood, city, subnational region, nation, international region, world. Planning can also be on a project or subject basis either by an individual firm or a government agency.

HEALTH PLANNING

Health planning has been undertaken to various degrees in different political and geographic jurisdictions. In the United States there is presently a great deal of interest in health planning and rational health care schemes and, probably as a consequence thereof, a great deal of research is underway on models and methodology for planning in this field. At present, however, planning in the health care field at the national level is very limited and even in smaller units the activity is minute.

One of the greatest difficulties with planning for an economically rational health care system is measuring the value of the benefits. What is the worth of a life saved, or an hour of pain alleviated, are questions often asked in this regard. However, it is not necessary to answer those questions to make a case for planning in the health field. The type of question that *can* be answered that makes health planning viable and necessary is: What are the relative health impacts of an additional 100,000 dollars spent on anti-polio vaccine versus an additional 100,000 dollars spent on the rehabilitation of children or adults who have been affected by the disease? And it is not sufficient to say that we have to have both, because there is only a limited number of dollars that can realistically be made available for health in a geographic area at a point in history given the political and economic situation. Choices must be made. And they are made every time a child receives or does not receive an anti-polio vaccine and every time a child visits or does not visit a physician to be treated for a cold.

The methodology of planning in the health field is rather

limited but developing quite rapidly. Several approaches to the whole or parts of the problem exist. These include the rate of return approach, utilization of aggregate demand forecasts, utilization of manpower planning techniques, and combinations of these three.

The rate of return approach has not been used as an exclusive methodology for the planning of any entire medical system. It has been used in planning of medical education and in planning for the treatment of various diseases.[12] The rate-of-return approach to overall medical planning suggests that various programs be ranked according to their rates of return. The programs yielding the highest returns, assuming they are greater than the return on other investments in the economy, should be increased relative to other programs.

The difficulties with this approach are many. First, with medical activities, it is extremely difficult to measure the monteary value of benefits. Second, there are large externalities in the health area. The prevention of a communicable disease in one man has a potentially great impact on his neighbor's personal health and well-being. Finally, there are a large number of technical problems associated with the calculation and meaning of an internal rate of return.[13]

Aggregate demand forecasts have also been receiving a great deal of attention in the realm of health planning. Presently a number of models for forecasting demand for health services in the aggregate and/or by type are under development. Many

---

[12] See Burton Weistrod's article in Chapter Nine for an illustration of this approach.

[13] The first problem with this approach is that it is based on a concept dealing with averages, and what is really needed is one dealing with marginals. That is, the rate of return is the average earned by all those with a given amount of education. The real question is: What did the last or marginal man earn—not the average man. If average earnings are different from marginal earnings, as they undoubtedly are, decisions based on the average could easily be incorrect. In addition, future rather than past rates of return are what are needed for planning. Finally, the rate-of-return analysis does not give any quantitative answers for planning. It suggests in which direction to move but not how far. For example, if the return to water fluoridation is 20 per cent and the return to mosquito control is 5 per cent, planning on the basis of rate-of-return analysis would prescribe an increase in the utilization of water fluoridation, but it cannot specify the size of the increase.

of these use an identity such as the following for estimating
purposes:

$$\text{GNP} \times \frac{G_i}{\text{GNP}} \times \frac{H_i}{G_i} \times \frac{H_s}{H_i} \times \frac{H_m \text{ (or } H_c)}{H_s} = H_m \text{ or } H_c$$

where GNP = gross national product; G_i = proportion of GNP
received as income by the various income groups from the poorest to the richest; H_i = health care services purchased by various
income groups; H_s = the types of services purchased by various
income groups; H_m = the health manpower necessary to provide
given services; and H_c = the cost of a given health service. Depending on the last term of the left hand side of the equation,
this may be used for projecting the manpower needed to furnish
the health care services demanded or for projecting the expenditures that will be made on health care.

The first step of this projecting process is to acquire a projec-
tion for GNP at the target date and a breakdown of how that
GNP will be divided among the population, that is, the proportion of income that the top decile and all other deciles of the
population receive. Such projections may already exist or have
to be developed. Then an estimation of the health services required by people at each income level is made. Next, the types
of services demanded by the various income groups is specified.
Finally, the type and number of medical personnel and/or the
aggregate expenditure necessary to provide the types of services
demanded is estimated. As can be seen, all of the factors of the
left side of the equation cancel out leaving either the total
health manpower or the total health expenditures implied by
the GNP projections. The art and the science of planning are in
the estimation of the various fractions on the left side of the
equation. These are done with econometric methods based on
sample surveys, national census, and other questionnaires and
data.

Using similar procedures, projections can be made of the
supply of manpower that will be trained at a given date in
various medical and related activities as well as the financial resources that will be available to support the system. With these
two elements, the fit or projected supply and demand yield

valuable insights for the planner to follow-up on.[14] For example, policies can be shifted to eliminate potential shortages or surpluses which become evident. All of this is part of the planning process.

One of the great difficulties with aggregate demand projections is that all of the estimation procedures are based on data from the past. To the extent that new technologies are discovered and new perceptions of need are developed, the methodology is bound to fall short of yielding accurate projections. Similarly, to the extent that it is felt that past emphases or policy decisions were incorrect, the projections will carry forward these errors. Furthermore, a decision to institute a new financing method or policy such as national health insurance or Medicare would require alterations in the projections.

All methods of planning suffer from the difficulty of dealing with the question of quality of health care. Whether speaking of the rate of return approach where the quality of life is a benefit to be measured or dealing with manpower needs for health where the question might be the quality of the training of one doctor versus that of another, or the quality of the services of a doctor versus those of a nurse in administering a shot of penicillin or in amputating an arm, the difficulty is obvious.

Planning in the health field in the next decade is likely to lead to a greater emphasis on preventive medicine, on health education, on sanitation, and on nutrition. The cost of the curative approach to medicine is bound to prove inefficient when compared to these other activities. The development of comprehensive planning models should help to clarify these points to increasing numbers of policy makers and the public. With the public's ever higher standard of living as well as educational level, these programs become potentially easier and more effective since all of them require a greater input from the public than does curative medicine.

[14] For an example of this technique see, Fein, Rashi: *The Doctor Shortage: An Economic Analysis*. Washington, D.C., The Brookings Institution, 1967.

Chapter Eleven

FINANCING HEALTH CARE

O NE OF THE basic problem areas confronting both health care administrators and planners is the financing of health care services. Concern is being expressed over whether the health care sector is receiving a large enough share of the nation's resources to insure the provision of basic health care services to all. The provision of health care services, and other services wholly or partially provided by government, is further affected by the distribution of governmental revenue among the federal, state, and local units. The governmental units with the major responsibility for providing direct health care services, states and localities are increasingly confronted with dire fiscal problems leading in some cases to a cutback in the provision of public services.

A second aspect of the financing issue that has been receiving increasing attention is the need for devising a more comprehensive and efficient reimbursement scheme. An adequate and effective system of reimbursement is needed to insure both the smooth operation of the myriad of existing health care institutions and the access of all people to the acquisition of their perceived health and medical needs. The method of reimbursement adopted, however, not only finances the purchase and provision of services but also determines to a significant extent the degree of utilization and the production method by which the health care services are provided.

This chapter addresses itself to both the macro and micro aspects of the financing of health care. The first section presents a statistical overview of recent trends and developments in the financing of health care services at the federal, state, and local levels. The fiscal woes of state and local government units as they affect the provision of health care services are briefly noted, the underlying reasons for this predicament are analyzed, and possible courses of action are outlined. The second section adopts a micro approach and focuses on an analysis of current reimbursement schemes, highlighting the economic consequences of the prevailing reimbursement formulas. Alternate reimbursement plans that seek to insure, reimburse, and stimulate more efficient behavior on the part of the providers and consumers of health care are presented and discussed in the last section of the chapter.

FINANCING: MACRO ASPECTS

National health expenditures have increased from 12,130,-000,000 dollars in fiscal year 1950 to 75,012,000,000 dollars in fiscal year 1971, an increase of 62,882,000,000 dollars (approximately 518 per cent) in a twenty-two year period. In real terms, an increase of 33,766,000,000 dollars (approximately 137 per cent) occurred over this period.[1] Health expenditures have increased not only absolutely but also relatively to other expenditure areas; the per cent of GNP accounted for by health expenditures rose from 4.6 per cent in 1950 to approximately 7.4 per cent in 1971. A complete listing of the various types of health expenditures and the amounts spent on each category during the period 1950–1970 is presented in Table XIX.

An important development affecting the aggregate financing of health care services is the relative distribution of public and private expenditures. As can be seen from the last five entries in Table XIX and from Table XX, the *relative* share of private expenditures (individual consumers and philanthropic institutions) has declined since 1965 even though actual private dollar expenditures continued to increase. Public expenditures (expenditures by government), however, have increased significantly in the post-1965 era. This substitution in the relative burden of paying for health expenditures is primarily attributable to the

[1] The *Medical Care Price Index* for 1950 and 1971 was used to adjust the gross dollar expenditures.

TABLE XIX

NATIONAL HEALTH EXPENDITURES, BY TYPE, SELECTED YEARS 1950–1970
(in millions of dollars)

Type of Expenditure	1950	1955	1960	1965	1968	1969	1970[1]
Total	12,130	17,924	26,367	38,912	53,651	59,905	67,240
Private expenditures	9,064	13,503	19,972	29,366	33,728	37,125	42,258
Health and medical services	8,812	13,123	19,327	28,036	32,218	35,382	39,647
Direct payments	7,146	9,448	13,087	17,590	19,100	20,278	22,909
Insurance benefits	879	2,344	4,698	8,280	10,444	12,333	13,813
Expenses for prepayment	274	596	792	1,212	1,558	1,581	1,667
Other	513	735	750	954	1,116	1,190	1,258
Medical research	37	55	121	162	185	192	195
Medical-facilities construction	215	325	524	1,168	1,325	1,551	2,416
Public expenditures	3,065	4,421	6,395	9,546	19,923	22,780	24,982
Per cent of total	25.3	24.7	24.3	24.5	37.1	38.0	37.2
Health and medical services	2,470	3,862	5,346	7,647	17,469	20,231	22,275
Health insurance for the aged	(2)	(2)	(2)	(2)	5,347	6,598	7,149
Temporary disability insurance (medical benefits)[3]	2	20	40	51	55	58	60
Workmen's compensation (medical benefits)[3]	193	315	420	580	790	875	970
Public assistance (vendor medical payments)	51	212	493	1,367	3,581	4,423	5,042
General hospital and medical care	886	1,298	1,973	2,516	2,928	3,010	3,132
Defense Dept. hospital and medical care	336	745	820	858	1,483	1,531	1,650
Military dependents' medical care	(2)	(2)	60	78	165	218	250
Maternal and child health programs	30	93	141	223	337	409	429
School health (educational agencies)	31	66	101	142	205	231	263
Other public health activities	351	384	401	671	1,001	1,195	1,429
Veterans' hospital and medical care	583	721	879	1,121	1,372	1,434	1,599
Medical vocational rehabilitation	7	9	18	34	102	125	152

TABLE XIX (continued)

Type of Expenditure	1950	1955	1960	1965	1968	1969	1970[1]
Office of Economic Opportunity (OEO) health and medical care	(2)	(2)	(2)	6	104	126	149
Medical research	73	139	471	1,229	1,616	1,600	1,695
Medical-facilities construction	522	419	578	669	839	949	1,013
Defense Department	1	33	40	31	27	72	52
Veterans Administration	161	34	60	81	46	54	78
Other	360	352	478	557	766	823	883
Personal health care expenditures, total[4]	10,549	15,865	23,236	33,505	46,552	52,149	58,048
Private expenditures	8,447	12,396	18,307	26,551	30,319	33,425	37,586
Per cent of total	80.1	78.1	78.8	79.2	65.1	64.1	64.7
Public expenditures	2,102	3,469	4,930	6,954	16,233	18,724	20,462
Per cent of total	19.9	21.9	21.2	20.8	34.9	35.9	35.3

[1] Preliminary estimates.
[2] Not applicable.
[3] Includes medical benefits paid under public law by private insurance carriers and self-insurers.
[4] Includes all health and medical services except (a) expenses for prepayment, (b) philanthropic expenditures of private agencies, (c) other public health activities, and (d) administrative expenses for "health insurance for the aged," "maternal and child health programs," and "veterans; hospital and medical care."

Source: U.S. Bureau of the Census: *Statistical Abstract of the United States, 1971* (92nd Edition). Washington, D.C.: U.S. Government Printing Office, 1971, p. 62.

TABLE XX

NATIONAL HEALTH EXPENDITURES,
BY SOURCE: 1950 to 1969 [1]

Expenditure	Amount (in millions of dollars)				
	1950	*1960*	*1965*	*1968*	*1969*
Total	12,867	27,973	40,591	56,577	63,812
Spent by:					
Consumers	8,501	18,911	28,174	32,484	36,528
Government	3,578	6,637	10,075	21,382	23,790
Philanthropy and other	788	1,428	2,343	2,711	3,494

Expenditure	Per cent				
	1950	*1960*	*1965*	*1968*	*1969*
Total	100.0	100.0	100.0	100.0	100.0
Spent by:					
Consumers	66.1	70.1	69.4	57.4	57.2
Government	27.8	24.6	24.8	37.8	37.3
Philanthropy and other	6.1	5.3	5.8	4.8	5.5

[1] Calendar year data; therefore, differ from Table XIX which is based on fiscal year data.

Source: U.S. Bureau of the Census: *Statistical Abstract of the United States, 1971* (92nd Edition). Washington, D.C., U.S. Government Printing Office, 1971, p. 63.

impetus of Public Law 89–97 enacted in July 1965, containing the historic provisions for Medicare and Medicaid.

The increase in public expenditures for health care did not occur uniformly over all levels of government. As can be seen in Table XXI, the share of state and local government's social welfare expenditures earmarked for health care has been rather constant. On the federal level, a dramatic increase is noted in the post-1966 period. The increase in federal health expenditures came primarily in the form of grants-in-aid to state and local governments rather than in direct expenditures, as can be seen from the data presented in Table XXII. An analysis of Table XXIII indicates that the increased funding stemming from federal grants-in-aid have been used primarily for manpower training, provision of comprehensive health care, support of health educational facilities, and medical assistance welfare payments.

Federal grants-in-aid for the provision of health care services, however, are allocated unequally among the states. On a per capita basis, some states receive more than twice as much support as others. The data appearing in Table XXIV indicate that states such as Alaska, Arizona, Colorado, Hawaii, New Mexico, and Vermont received more than 8 dollars per capita in federal

TABLE XXI

HEALTH CARE EXPENDITURES AS A PER CENT OF TOTAL SOCIAL WELFARE EXPENDITURES, BY LEVEL OF GOVERNMENT, SELECTED YEARS, 1935–1970

Year	Total Social Welfare (in millions of dollars)			Health Care [1] (in millions of dollars)			Per cent		
	Total	Federal	State & Local	Total	Federal	State & Local	Total	Federal	State & Local
1935	6,548	3,207	3,341	543	103	440	8.3	3.2	13.2
1940	8,795	3,443	5,351	782	178	604	8.9	5.2	11.3
1945	9,205	4,339	4,866	2,579	1,909	670	28.0	4.4	13.8
1950	23,508	10,541	12,967	3,065	1,362	1,704	13.0	12.9	13.1
1955	32,640	14,623	18,017	4,421	1,948	2,473	13.5	13.3	13.7
1960	52,293	24,957	27,337	6,395	2,918	3,477	12.2	11.7	12.7
1963	66,766	32,675	34,091	8,304	4,103	4,201	12.4	12.6	12.3
1964	71,491	34,928	36,563	8,971	4,462	4,509	12.5	12.8	12.3
1965	77,121	37,720	39,401	9,546	4,635	4,910	12.4	12.3	12.5
1966	87,949	45,387	42,562	10,822	5,390	5,432	12.3	11.9	12.8
1967	99,694	53,244	46,449	15,878	9,773	6,106	15.9	18.4	13.1
1968	112,044	60,548	51,497	19,711	13,022	6,689	17.6	21.5	13.0
1969	126,306	68,294	58,012	22,780	15,148	7,632	18.0	22.2	13.2
1970 [2]	143,046	76,755	66,290	24,982	16,667	8,315	17.5	21.7	12.5

[1] Includes "health and medical programs" with medical services provided in connection with social insurance, public aid, veterans and other social welfare programs.

[2] Preliminary estimates.

Source: U.S. Bureau of Census: *Statistical Abstract of the United States, 1971* (92nd Edition). Washington, D.C., U.S. Government Printing Office, 1971, p. 271.

TABLE XXII
FEDERAL GOVERNMENT HEALTH CARE
EXPENDITURES, SELECTED YEARS,
1950–1970

Year	Per Capita Health and Medical Program Expenditures	Grants to State and Local Governments for Health Purposes (in millions of dollars)
1950	$13	$ 123
1955	19	119
1960	25	214
1965	32	346
1966	35	365
1967	39	436
1968	42	823
1969	44	866
1970 [1]	47	1,043

[1] Preliminary estimates

Source: U.S. Bureau of the Census: *Statistical Abstract of the United States, 1971*, (92nd Edition). Washington, D.C., U.S. Government Printing Office, 1971, p. 273.

grants-in-aid during 1969, while other states such as California, Illinois, Indiana, New Jersey, Washington, and Wisconsin received less than 4 dollars per capita. The distribution of grants does not appear to conform to patterns of urbanization or industrialization as can be seen by a comparison of grants received by Vermont and New Hampshire or Pennsylvania and New Jersey. A geographic pattern, however, does emerge; in general, mid-western and southern states seem to have received greater per capita amounts than northern and eastern states.

Distinct interstate and intercity differences are also discernable in expenditures for health care, as can be seen from the data reported in Tables XXV and XXVI. On the state level, per capita expenditures in 1969 ranged from a high of $43.20 for New York to a low of $10.04 for Arizona. Direct state and local expenditures were totally unrelated to relative federal grants-in-aid patterns; the Spearman's rank correlation between the two is − 0.12.[2] State per capita health expenditures were also unrelated to per capita expenditures by nongovernmental health institutions located within states.[3] A small but positive relation-

[2] Refer to Appendix II for a discussion of rank correlation.

[3] A statistically insignificant Spearman rank correlation of 0.07 exists between 1969 state per capita health and hospitals expenditures, and state nongovernmental hospital expenditures (i.e. expenditures by individual voluntary and proprietary hospitals).

TABLE XXIII

FEDERAL AID TO STATE AND LOCAL GOVERNMENTS FOR HEALTH CARE, 1965 to 1971 [1]
(in millions of dollars)

Category	1965	1966	1967	1968	1969	1970	1971 [4]
Total grants-in-aid and shared revenue	10,906	12,962	15,245	18,599	20,255	23,955	30,297
Health [2]	644	1,244	2,105	2,706	3,193	3,831	4,383
Hospital Construction	193	196	205	253	255	272	241
Health Manpower	—	7	32	33	35	45	68
Comprehensive Health	—	—	(3)	87	119	122	181
Health Educational Facilities	2	—	—	107	133	186	182
Mental Health	11	92	11	192	62	146	147
Environmental Health	5	44	89	16	33	10	17
Maternal Health	70	84	139	152	199	236	204
Medical Assistance	272	770	1,173	1,806	2,285	2,727	3,250
Health as a per cent of total grants-in-aid and shared revenue	5.9	9.6	13.8	14.5	15.8	16.0	14.5

[1] For years ending June 30.
[2] Includes programs not shown separately.
[3] Less than $500,000.
[4] Preliminary estimates.
Source: U.S. Bureau of the Census: *Statistical Abstract of the United States, 1971* (92nd Edition). Washington, D.C., U.S. Government Printing Office, 1971, p. 401.

TABLE XXIV
FEDERAL PER CAPITA GRANTS FOR HEALTH PURPOSES
TO STATE AND LOCAL GOVERNMENTS, 1970

State	Per Capita Grant	State	Per Capita Grant
Alabama	$ 7.57	Montana	$ 6.22
Alaska	8.16	Nebraska	5.53
Arizona	8.58	Nevada	4.43
Arkansas	5.52	New Hampshire	4.41
California	3.56	New Jersey	3.14
Colorado	8.19	New Mexico	10.55
Connecticut	4.80	New York	4.46
Delaware	4.47	North Carolina	6.81
Florida	4.81	North Dakota	6.17
Georgia	5.87	Ohio	4.35
Hawaii	11.38	Oklahoma	4.88
Idaho	5.36	Oregon	4.93
Illinois	3.46	Pennsylvania	5.36
Indiana	3.78	Rhode Island	4.71
Iowa	4.82	South Carolina	5.84
Kansas	5.24	South Dakota	5.62
Kentucky	6.45	Tennessee	6.41
Louisiana	5.68	Texas	4.45
Maine	5.06	Utah	7.33
Maryland	5.38	Vermont	9.28
Massachusetts	5.44	Virginia	4.40
Michigan	5.35	Washington	3.56
Minnesota	4.10	West Virginia	5.81
Mississippi	6.17	Wisconsin	3.88
Missouri	6.09	Wyoming	7.32

Source: U.S. Bureau of the Census: *Statistical Abstract of the United States, 1971* (92nd Edition). Washington, D.C., U.S. Government Printing Office, 1971, p. 274.

ship does prevail, however, between federal grants-in-aid to states and localities and state expenditures adjusted for effort and ability, as measured in Chapter Three.[4] Per capita health care expenditures in the three largest cities—New York, Chicago, and Los Angeles—in 1969 also exhibited noticeable expenditure variations ($89.73 to $1.42). Not only did cities located in different states exhibit noticeable expenditure differences but even within a state expenditure differences were also quite significant, as can be seen by comparing health and hospital expenditures for

---

[4] The Spearman rank correlation coefficient between federal grants-in-aid to states and localities and adjusted state expenditures is 0.28. One bias inherent in this analysis is that the adjusted state expenditures exclude expenditures by localities. Had they been included, the correlation between these two expenditure variables would probably have changed. On an *a priori* basis, the direction of change can not be predicted.

TABLE XXV

PER CAPITA STATE AND LOCAL GOVERNMENT
HEALTH AND HOSPITALS EXPENDITURES, 1969

State	Per Capita Expenditure State & Local [1] Gov't	State Gov't
Alabama	$36	$17.59
Alaska	42	31.91
Arizona	27	10.04
Arkansas	29	18.05
California	50	19.50
Colorado	44	27.14
Connecticut	38	35.00
Delaware	39	38.90
Florida	45	18.60
Georgia	55	22.00
Hawaii	46	36.52
Idaho	33	16.71
Illinois	37	23.63
Indiana	37	20.32
Iowa	35	19.10
Kansas	36	22.00
Kentucky	29	16.71
Louisiana	40	29.64
Maine	24	19.43
Maryland	49	31.10
Massachusetts	49	30.73
Michigan	48	26.01
Minnesota	46	25.95
Mississippi	31	15.70
Missouri	40	22.80
Montana	26	17.30
Nebraska	39	22.80
Nevada	68	15.32
New Hampshire	29	25.71
New Jersey	33	18.20
New Mexico	33	17.10
New York	84	43.20
North Carolina	29	20.60
North Dakota	21	19.51
Ohio	29	13.80
Oklahoma	30	20.64
Oregon	31	19.20
Pennsylvania	28	23.60
Rhode Island	36	35.13
South Carolina	36	22.30
South Dakota	19	13.70
Tennessee	39	17.31
Texas	29	14.93
Utah	28	18.20
Vermont	24	22.80
Virginia	31	27.20
Washington	36	20.90
West Virginia	27	20.34
Wisconsin	39	23.90
Wyoming	68	21.90

[1] Reported to nearest whole number only.

Source: State and Local Data: U.S. Bureau of the Census. *Statistical Abstract of the United States: 1971* (92nd Edition) Washington, D.C., U.S. Government Printing Office, 1971, p. 4.

State Data: Expenditures—*Ibid.*, p. 441. Population—U.S. Bureau of the Census: *Statistical Abstract of the United States: 1970* (91st Edition). Washington, D.C., U.S. Government Printing Office, 1970, p. 12.

TABLE XXVI
PER CAPITA HEALTH AND HOSPITALS
EXPENDITURES, TWENTY-FIVE
LARGEST CITIES, 1969 [1]

City	Per Capita Expenditure
New York	$ 89.73
Chicago	8.76
Los Angeles	1.42
Philadelphia	21.70
Detroit	21.05
Houston	3.57
Baltimore	39.51
Dallas	2.13
Washington, D.C.	124.57
Cleveland	4.80
Milwaukee	7.81
San Francisco	59.80
San Diego	0.07
San Antonio	3.36
Boston	62.40
Memphis	30.45
St. Louis	51.45
New Orleans	3.54
Seattle	9.23
Pittsburgh	0.10
Denver	38.64
Atlanta	0.10
Buffalo	0.86
Cincinnati	50.80
Honolulu	7.38

[1] As 1969 population by city data were not readily available, 1970 population data were utilized to transform total expenditures into per capita expenditures.

Source: U.S. Bureau of the Census: *Statistical Abstract of the United States, 1971* (92nd Edition). Washington, D.C., U.S. Government Printing Office, 1971, pp. 21–23, 416.

New York and Buffalo; Los Angeles, San Francisco, and San Diego; Philadelphia and Pittsburgh; Houston and Dallas; and Cleveland and Cincinnati.[5]

The expenditure data presented highlight both the geographic disparity in expenditures for health care services, symptomatic of the geographic inequalities in the provision and availability of health care services, and the recent increase in aggregate health care expenditures emanating at the federal level. A third dimension of the macro financing picture, one frequently pub-

[5] Among the possible explanations for these intrastate difference are the unequal distribution of voluntary and proprietary health care facilities, and the possible inclusion of county health care expenditures in some cases but not in others.

licized in newspapers,[6] is the fiscal plight of health care institutions at the state, and especially the local, level. Even though state and local health care expenditures have been increasing, the financial needs of health care institutions exceed the resources earmarked for them. The underlying causes of this problem are of a dual nature: costs that are rising rapidly and tax revenues that are not.

The cost of operating health care institutions has been increasing at a rapid pace and will probably continue to do so for the foreseeable future. This phenomenon can be attributed to two primary factors. First, the provision of health care, as is true of many services, is highly labor intensive and labor productivity appears to have been increasing at a slower rate in the health field than in other sectors of the economy. Successful unionization attempts, worker militancy, and large wage settlements have been characteristic of the dominant institution in the health field, the hospital, during the last decade. Second, new technological innovations are constantly being introduced and applied to the health field resulting in a rapid rate of capital obsolescence and a steady stream of large capital outlays. The sacredness with which health care is regarded by a majority of the population and the common desire for human attention in the administering of medical care prompt the prediction that the rate of cost increases, as mirrored in the Medical Care Cost Index reported in Chapter Three, will not be easily contained, even if productive efficiency is dramatically improved.

The problems surrounding insufficient tax revenues are traceable directly to the prevailing allocation of tax revenues among the federal, state, and local levels of government. As can be seen from the data reported in Table XXVII, the primary types of taxes levied in the United States are: individual and corporate income taxes, sales and gross receipts taxes, and property taxes. Since the early 1900's the individual and corporate income tax have been earmarked primarily as federal taxes, sales and gross receipts taxes and licenses have been primarily as-

---

[6] See for example, Hospitals here face financial emergency, *New York Times,* March 25, 1971, pp. 1, 43.

TABLE XXVII

DISTRIBUTION OF TAX REVENUE BY SOURCE, SELECTED YEARS, 1942–1969

Year	Total Tax Revenue	Individual Income	Corporation Income	Sales, Gross Receipts, and Customs	Property	Other Taxes, including Licenses
1942	20,793	3,481	4,999	5,776	4,537	2,000
1950	51,100	16,533	11,081	12,997	7,349	3,140
1955	81,072	29,984	18,604	17,221	10,735	4,527
1960	113,120	43,178	22,674	24,452	16,405	6,411
1965	144,953	52,882	27,390	32,904	22,583	9,191
1967	176,121	67,352	36,198	36,336	26,047	10,188
1969	222,708	96,157	39,858	44,345	30,673	11,675
Per cent						
1942	100.0	16.7	24.0	27.8	21.9	9.6
1950	100.0	32.3	21.8	25.4	14.4	6.1
1955	100.0	37.0	22.9	21.2	13.3	5.6
1960	100.0	38.2	20.0	21.6	14.5	5.7
1965	100.0	36.5	18.9	22.7	15.6	6.3
1967	100.0	38.2	20.5	20.6	14.8	5.8
1969	100.0	43.2	17.9	19.9	13.8	5.2

Source: U.S. Bureau of the Census: *Statistical Abstract of the United States, 1971* (92nd Edition). Washington, D.C., U.S. Government Printing Office, 1971, p. 398.

signed as state revenue raisers, and property taxes have been left to the localities as their primary revenue source. Although there has been a growing tendency for states and localities to levy payroll, income, and sales taxes (the latter pertaining primarily to localities) in an attempt to equilibrate revenue with the rapidly increasing needs for additional public services, the tax tricotomy enumerated above still prevails.

All tax sources, however, are not equivalent in their revenue raising capacity as can be seen by utilizing elasticity measures. Tax elasticity can be defined as follows: [7]

Elasticity of Tax	*Attributes of Tax*
Elastic	Tax revenue increases proportionately more than the tax base.
Unitary Elasticity	Tax revenue increases proportionately with the tax base.
Inelastic	Tax revenue increases less than proportionately with the tax base.

The *tax base* is that which is being taxed: income, sales, or property. The *tax rate* is the rate applied to the designated base. A 2.5 per cent sales tax is a tax on sales whose rate is 2.5 per cent.

An example of an income elastic tax is the individual income tax as levied at the federal level. As national income increases by 1 per cent, tax revenue increases by more than 1 per cent because as people earn additional income they move into tax brackets in which the tax rate is higher. Some state income taxes and some forms of sales taxes approach the unitary elasticity level. State income taxes are not as progressive as the federal income tax; they have fewer tax brackets, the tax rate does not increase as steeply between brackets, and the maximum tax rate is reached at lower income levels.

Property taxes and sales taxes based on staples rather than

[7] In the public finance literature an alternate schema exists for classifying different taxes; taxes are often categorized as either progressive, proportional, or regressive. While there is no theoretical correspondence between this trichotomy and an elasticity schema, in the United States economy progressive taxes are usually revenue elastic, proportional taxes usually display unitary revenue elasticity, and regressive taxes are usually revenue inelastic.

luxuries are income inelastic. These taxes have but one rate and as income increases, the amount spent on these items, the tax base, does not increase as fast. Property values are reassessed intermittently, often only at the time of resale. Since assessment partially determines the tax payment, property tax revenues do not increase as rapidly as increases in income and property values. Compounding the revenue inelasticity of the property tax is the fact that property tax rates, in contrast to rates on other tax bases, are locally determined and susceptable to a high degree of voter leverage. While tax rates are seldom central issues in state elections and almost never in national elections, they are quite often the determining factor in local contests, thereby deterring many politicians from supporting or initiating necessary tax increases.

The different revenue elasticities of the major tax sources telegraph their revenue raising potential. The elastic personal and corporate income taxes are the major revenue raisers as can be seen from Table XXVII and these sources are by convention federal taxes.[8] States have typically depended on selected sales taxes and licenses,[9] which at best are of unitary elasticity; while localities are heavily dependent on the revenue inelastic property tax.[10]

To compound the problem, the unequal distribution of tax revenue is not only a present phenomenon, but the dynamic implications of the relevant revenue elasticities indicate that the revenue inequality will widen with time. In a nutshell, the problem is that localities, and to a lesser degree states, utilize tax sources which are neither responsive nor adequate to the rising needs of these areas. The levying of additional taxes by these governmental units has not yielded sufficient revenue to bridge the ever increasing gap between needs and available resources.

Two lines of attack other than the assumption of a greater

[8] Over 90 per cent of revenues raised by the personal income and corporate income tax go to the federal government.

[9] Over 50 per cent of the taxes raised by these means go to state governments.

[10] Over 95 per cent of the revenues raised by property taxes go to local governments.

degree of the social welfare burden by the federal government are open for ameliorating the revenue bind of states and localities: tax restructuring, and tax revenue sharing. Tax restructuring would, by changing the tax base and/or the tax rate, attempt to give lower levels of government a share of aggregate tax revenues commensurate with the increasing cost of providing public services such as health care and education which have traditionally been their responsibility. In the absence of major tax revisions, or possibly in conjunction with future revisions, tax revenue sharing either in the form of returning tax money to state and local governments or federal grants-in-aid can be instituted. Federal health expenditures in the post-1967 period, as reported in Table XXII, indicate that a start has already been made in this direction. The continuing plight of the localities indicates that the measures adopted to date are inadequate. Unless more drastic steps are taken in tax restructuring and tax sharing, the only alternate to a drastic curtailment in service is an even greater assumption of financial responsibility by the federal government.

FINANCING: MICRO ASPECTS

The importance of third party (private health insurance, government, and philanthropy) reimbursement in the financing of personal health care consumption is highlighted by the statistics reported in Table XXVIII. Whereas 35.1 per cent of personal health care expenditures were covered by third party payments in 1950, 60.5 per cent were covered in 1969. It is highly likely that this percentage will increase even further with the continued proliferation of employee collective bargaining victories and with the advent of some form of national health insurance.

Currently, reimbursement for incurred health care expenditures takes the following form. Individuals purchase, either directly or through their employers, hospital and medical insurance from among a host of insurance companies. These policies provide stated coverage for various illness episodes including physician fees and hospitalization costs. Although the precise

TABLE XXVIII

PERSONAL HEALTH CARE: THIRD PARTY PAYMENTS AND PRIVATE CONSUMER EXPENDITURES, SELECTED YEARS, 1950–1969

Item	1950	1955	1960	1965	1966	1967	1968	1969
Personal health care expenditures [1]	11,109	15,933	23,758	34,942	38,794	44,202	49,895	55,296
Third Party Payments								
Total	3,900	6,662	10,690	16,771	19,420	24,860	29,550	33,427
Per cent of total health care	35.1	41.8	45.0	48.0	50.1	56.2	59.2	60.5
Private health insurance	992	2,536	4,996	8,729	9,142	9,545	11,310	13,068
Per cent of total health care	8.9	15.9	21.0	25.0	23.6	21.6	22.7	23.6
Government	2,588	3,705	5,157	7,345	9,534 [2]	14,550 [2]	17,455 [2]	19,520 [2]
Per cent of total health care	23.3	23.3	21.7	21.0	24.6	32.9	35.0	35.3
Philanthropy and others	320	421	537	697	744	765	785	839
Per cent of total health care	2.9	2.6	2.3	2.0	1.9	1.7	1.6	1.5
Private Consumer Expenditures								
Total [3]	8,201	11,807	18,066	26,902	28,516	28,887	31,658	34,939
Per cent met by private health insurance	12.1	21.5	27.7	32.4	32.1	33.0	35.7	37.4
Hospital care	1,965	3,244	5,188	8,251	8,890	8,612	9,916	11,729
Per cent met by private health insurance	34.6	51.8	63.7	70.2	67.4	71.2	73.7	71.2
Physicians' services	2,597 [4]	3,433 [4]	5,309	8,184	8,362	8,302	9,040	9,458
Per cent met by private health insurance	12.0	25.0	30.0	32.7	33.9	35.7	38.4	42.6

[1] All expenditures for health services and supplies except expenses for prepayment and administration, government public health activities, and expenditures of private voluntary agencies for other health services.
[2] Includes benefit payments under the health insurance for the aged program.
[3] Includes other expenditures not shown separately. Excludes expenses for prepayment.
[4] Includes small amounts for other types of professional services.

Source: U.S. Bureau of the Census: *Statistical Abstract of the United States, 1971* (92nd Edition). Washington, D.C., U.S. Government Printing Office, 1971, p. 64.

provisions vary by contract, the modal policy provides for a specified number of hospital days by type of accomodation and for total or partial payments of physician fees. Physician reimbursement is usually determined based on a chart of average or reasonable charges per illness, while reimbursement for hospitals and other health care institutions is based on the particular institution's cost of operation. Whereas a uniform list of reasonable charges usually exists for physician reimbursement by services rendered category in any geographic area, institutions are usually reimbursed on the basis of their *individual* cost profiles. The reimbursement formula for institutions is based on audited allowable costs, *with almost all costs being considered allowable.* Reimbursement by governmental agencies for services provided for the elderly (Medicare) or the poor (Medicaid) follow a similar pattern although the precise formulas and forms used for reimbursement differ.

Reimbursement formulas are not merely neutral financial formulas for paying the bills incurred, although this may be considered to be their primary objective. For better or worse they also affect patterns of service, cost of service, and the quality of service. From an economic perspective, the prevailing pattern of reimbursement is defective on three primary counts.

First, the prevailing form of reimbursement favors the aged regardless of their financial ability, the non-aged who can afford the significant cost of medical insurance, and those employed by institutions providing some form of medical insurance as a fringe benefit. Those excluded from these three categories who cannot afford to pay for their medical care are forced to rely on the state or charity for the payment of their medical needs. Recent cutbacks in Medicaid payments and the long known but often neglected fact of low quality of care received by the charity patient prevents the realization of equal accessibility of all to elementary medical care based on perceived need.

Second, the prevailing reimbursement arrangements offer no incentive for economic efficiency within health care institutions. The reimbursing parties fail to seek the lowest price for medical care within geographic areas where more than one provider of care exists, thereby eliminating a competitive incentive among institutions. Within institutions, as practically all costs and cost increases can be passed on to insurance companies or governmental agencies, cost consciousness is minimized and the incentive for managerial discretion and autonomy is dramatically curtailed. The payoff for attempting to institute cost saving techniques is a lower reimbursement in a future period at the expense of alienating the institution's medical and nonmedical staff. Neither the institution nor any member of it's staff benefits directly from any cost savings that accrue to the reimbursing agency. Similarly, there is a reduced incentive to resist the demand of employees for wage increases, additional fringe benefits, and for the acquisition of expensive equipment whose main function may be enhancing either the institution's or its staff's prestige among peer groups and within the community. Furthermore, the existence of more than one reimbursing channel creates extra administrative costs due to the multiplicity of forms that must be completed for reimbursement.

Cost consciousness is not only minimized at the administrative level but also at the level where care is dispensed. For many purposes it is useful to view the physician as the patient's contractor.[11] He (the physician) chooses both the nature and the content of the prescribed treatment and the means by which it will be administered. At present most physicians are part of the profit making sector of the economy. It is quite reasonable to assume that cost minimization considerations do enter the manner in which they organize and manage their own private practices. However, under current reimbursement formulas, a physician's choice of patient care is influenced by the knowledge that his patient's insurance plan will absorb all or most of the costs stemming from any hospital stay. Thus, for example, there is an incentive to hospitalize patients thereby concentrating a large proportion of the population he treats at any one time in a single locale, order costly diagnostic procedures which may have a marginal impact on patient care but which significantly reduce the chance of a successful malpractice suit, and conceivably even

---

[11] For a detailed exposition of this viewpoint see, Rice, Robert: Analysis of the hospital as an economic organism, *Modern Hospital, 106* (4) :87, 1966.

prolong or acquiese in the prolonging of a patient's length of stay to insure a critical mass of hospital activity for him thus financially justifying his direct and indirect (time) costs in making hospital calls. There is no incentive under the current reimbursement schema to carry over the degree of cost consciousness that influences the physician's personal practice to the choice he makes as his patient's contractor.

The gross effect of the absence of cost minimization considerations is the overutilization of facilities within health institutions on the mistaken ground that comprehensiveness is synonomous with quality, and the needless duplication of facilities and even entire health institutions within geographic area leading to inefficiencies on a societal level. Superimposing a *cost free* atmosphere on an industry with a strong eleemosynary tradition has created a totally noneconomic environment. As noted by Herman and Anne Somers, "In no other realm of economic life today are payments guaranteed for costs that are neither controlled by competition nor regulated by public authority, and in which no incentive for economy can be discerned." [12]

A third major defect of the current method of reimbursement is the distortion of the demand for medical care. Although the consumer pays for his health insurance, either directly or via his employer,[13] he usually correctly views these payments as either forced expenditures or sunk costs that are unaffected by his individual behavior. Having paid for the insurance the consumer then tends to view the cost of medical care as his out-of-pocket and time costs at the time of consumption of the services. In many cases, the direct, out-of-pocket cost is zero or minimal due to the insurance coverage, thereby creating an increase in the use of medical services. Furthermore, current insurance coverage prompts consumers to demand the *best,* i.e. most expensive, care regardless of its effect on the chances of

[12] Somers, Herman M., and Somers, Anne R.: *Medicare and The Hospitals.* Washington, D.C., The Brookings Institution, 1967, p. 192.

[13] Employees often fail to realize that employers agree upon contract terms and allow the employee's representatives to allocate the gains among direct wage payments and fringe benefits. As any fringe benefit package can usually be converted into direct wage payments, workers receive fringe benefits at the expense of direct wage gains.

their recovery. Quality is often confused with comprehensiveness and the possession of the most modern equipment. While it is beyond our scope to hypothesize whether the increased demand for medical services and equipment eventually leads to better health care, it is clearly within our scope to note that the partial or total elimination of price as a rationing device on the demand side of the medical market has distinct economic effects.

A second dimension of the distortion in consumer demand is that the prevailing reimbursement plans cover a much larger proportion of medical costs incurred within hospitals as opposed to a physician's office or a private laboratory. Similarly, in-patient costs are covered to a greater extent than out-patient (ambulatory) costs. Pursuing the natural incentive of choosing the mode of treatment with the lowest net cost to the consumer, however, leads to the choice of a mode of treatment with the highest gross costs—hospitalization. In addition to influencing the mode of treatment chosen, most current insurance plans also influence the type of care demanded since they do not reimburse for preventive care costs, thereby often postponing the consumption of medical services until the actual onset of an illness when treatment is more expensive.

A third area of distortion in demand is that current reimbursement plans, by subsidizing only medical care and not other components of health care such as nutrition, housing, or environmental control, distort consumer choice within the health field and in general among all consumption options. Although the consumption of medical care may be desirable, its subsidization is far from harmless. The following analogy with automobile production illustrates both the subsidy effect and the other noneconomic aspects of current methods of reimbursement mentioned above.

> Making an expensive good 'free' to consumers will not necessarily make them better off; in fact, it will, in general, make them worse off. Suppose that the government decreed that all automobiles would henceforth cost 100 dollars and that it would make up the difference between 100 dollars and the automobile's real cost. Most consumers would demand Cadillac-quality cars, because a Cadillac would be no more expensive than a Volkswagen to any individual consumer. We would

also expect the cost of producing Cadillac-quality cars to rise if only styling, convenience, and quality concerned the consumers, not the cost of these features. Producers would therefore have little reason to control costs or to strive for greater efficiency. Consumers in the aggregate would be worse off for two reasons. First, as demand for Cadillacs rose, society's resources would flow from production of other goods and services into automobile production, reducing the amount of other goods and services. Since aggregate demand for Cadillacs would not be disciplined by the 'true' cost trade-offs, more of society's resources would be used in automobile production than consumers would truly desire. And second, the cost of producing high quality automobiles would rise because the cost of production would be unimportant to consumers and, therefore, to the producers.[14]

A REVIEW OF SELECTED ALTERNATE REIMBURSEMENT PLANS

Having noted the economic objections to the prevailing method of reimbursement—inclusiveness, internal efficiency, and external efficiency—we now turn to a selective presentation of reimbursement alternatives which attempt to overcome some, or all, of these objections. For the purpose of this presentation the alternate plans are grouped into two categories: those that focus initially on the providers of medical care and those that focus initially on the consumers of medical care.

Two general reimbursement incentive proposals have been advanced that focus initially on the providers of care. One focuses on the hospital and seeks to affect only its efficiency. The other is directed at the physician, the person who generally controls the medical services provided to a patient upon his entry into the health care system, and seeks to affect both internal and external efficiency. Neither proposal focuses directly on increasing access to care; these proposals could, however, be incorporated into any system of national health insurance.

[14] Newhouse, Joseph P., and Taylor, Vincent: How shall we pay for hospital care?, *The Public Interest, 23*:85, 1971. Newhouse and Taylor note that the objection to an automobile analogy on the grounds that low income individuals need medical care but not automobiles is not valid as it ignores the fact that under current insurance schemes *everyone* is given a price subsidy, not just low income individuals. They can find no justification for removing the economic barrier to medical care for upper income people.

Economists generally argue that the formula adopted for hospital reimbursement should be based on an estimate of *average*
cost of operation with specific geographic and case-mix adjustments. Hospitals that are more efficient than the average would
then find themselves with extra funds at the end of the reimbursement period. These funds could then be used at the discretion of each individual institution. Hospitals that are less efficient
than the average will experience a deficit at the end of the
reimbursement period and will either have to institute measures
to increase efficiency or begin to contract their services.

An interesting variant of this general proposal is that advanced
by Kong-Kyun Ro and Richard Auster. The primary features
of their proposal are the following:

1. Hospital product is defined as the number and categories
   of episodes of illness given adequate treatment.
2. The standard of efficiency toward which the incentive is
   to be directed is set by defining the 'standard cost' of each
   episode of illness for the area (determinable at the end of
   the designated accounting period) plus or minus a number
   of standard deviations chosen on the basis of the level of
   efficiency desired.
3. The amount of reimbursement is determined by a
   weighted average of the actual cost of the case to the hospital
   and the 'standard cost' as defined above, the weighting factor
   being chosen to produce the desired degree of incentive.[15]

Under this general formula, rewards will go to hospitals whose
average cost is less than the stated standard cost, and penalties to
those whose average cost exceeds standard costs. Assume a hospital's cost for a designated illness episode is 300 dollars, average
cost among a group of hospitals in a designated area for this illness
episode is 470 dollars with a standard deviation of 40 dollars, and
two standard deviations and weighting factor of $\frac{1}{2}$ are chosen as
efficiency/incentive parameters. Under the Ro and Auster proposal the hospital would receive an incentive reward to 45 dollars

[15] Ro, Kong-Kyun, and Auster, Richard: An output approach to incentive reimbursement for hospitals, *Health Services Research*, 4:178, 1969. (See Appendix II,
for a definition and discussion of standard deviations.)

for that illness episode or a total reimbursement for that illness episode of 345 dollars.[16] Alternately if the hospital's actual cost was 750 dollars, a penalty of 100 dollars would result as total reimbursement for that illness episode would only be 650 dollars.[17] Using the efficiency/incentive parameters assumed above, any hospital with actual costs below 390 dollars is rewarded and any with actual costs above 550 dollars is penalized. Hospitals with actual costs between these two boundary points are reimbursed at cost. Choosing a lower number of standard deviations to define the efficiency boundary widens the range of actual costs that can be rewarded or penalized and choosing a higher weighting factor increases the dollar value of the incentive or penalty; the reverse also applies.[18]

In support of their proposal the authors note that their choice of disease episodes as a measure of output allows the reimbursing agency to adopt any degree of refinement deemed appropriate. Although the proposed plan could prompt all hospitals in a given area to enter into a collusive agreement to jointly increase costs and make life more comfortable for all, such agreements can usually be detected and dealt with. On an individual basis each hospital would have an incentive to adopt the cheapest mode of treatment subject to quality conditions decreed by the reimbursing agency. A further merit of this proposal is that it does not seek to alter existing institutional arrangements such as physician payment on a fee-for-service basis and direct hospital payment by the reimbursing agency. Insurance can continue to be purchased along current lines, with the savings accruing from the induced increase in efficiency being passed along to the consumer in the form of reduced premiums.

A second type of reimbursement formula proposes a radical

[16] Standard Cost (E) $= \$470 - 2\,(40) = \$390$
Reimbursement (R) $=$ (1-weighting factor [W]) Actual Cost (A) $+$ W (E)
$= \frac{1}{2}\,(300) + \frac{1}{2}\,(390) = \$345$
[17] $E = \$470 + 2\,(40) = \$550$
$R = \frac{1}{2}\,(750) + \frac{1}{2}\,(550) = \$650$
[18] For example if 3 standard deviations were used the range below (above) which rewards (penalties) would be realized would be: 350 dollars (590 dollars). If a weighting factor of $\frac{3}{5}$ were used a reward of 54 dollars (total reimbursement being 354 dollars) and a penalty of 120 dollars (total reimbursement being 630 dollars) would have been incurred.

change in prevailing institutional arrangements by adopting a capitation system of physician payment and making the physician financially responsible for the *total* treatment he prescribes for the patient. Typical of such a reimbursement plan is the proposal advanced by Paul Feldstein.[19] Although Feldstein's proposal is focused directly only upon Medicare reimbursement and on physicians engaged in group practice, the thrust of his proposal is equally applicable to all physicians regardless of mode of practice and to all reimbursement situations.

Under this type of reimbursement formula the physician is paid a lump sum per patient, with the actual payment determined primarily by the patient's age.[20] The physician is then held financially responsible for the *entire* medical care of the patient —hospital care, nursing home care, physician care, medication, etc.—during a designated period and will therefore have a direct financial interest in the provision of all medical care. Under such a proposal patients would be able to choose their own physicians and would be allowed to switch physicians at specified intervals but not during a major illness episode. The rationale underlying this proposal is that the physician is the most knowledgeable consumer of medical care, is in the best position to exert the required influence within hospitals for more efficient operation, and should be held financially responsible for any of his actions that lead (directly or even indirectly) to an inefficient use of resources.

The intent of such a proposal is to create an economic atmosphere conducive to: less duplication and overutilization of medical facilities by prompting physicians to purchase care from the lowest cost institution; efficient operation of institutions;

---

[19] Feldstein, Paul J.: A proposal for capitation reimbursement to medical groups for total medical care, in, U.S. Department of Health, Education, and Welfare: *Reimbursement Incentives for Hospital and Medical Care*. Washington, D.C., U.S. Government Printing Office, 1968.

[20] Payments can be made directly by the individual or by some third party in his behalf. It is entirely feasible that physicians will determine this payment based on recognized patient characteristics. The proponents of a basic capitation proposal envision a degree of competition among physicians which will be reflected in their annual rates. In the absence of such competition, rate setting by an outside agency would be required to prevent collusion.

more effective use of outpatient facilities, generic rather than proprietary drugs, and more skilled personnel who can increase physician productivity; an emphasis on preventive care; and the fostering of an active interest in innovations in the organization and delivery of medical care. Quality of care need not be sacrificed under such a scheme since patient choice of physicians should provide the necessary incentive to insure patient satisfaction with the service dispensed. Concurrently, the physician's financial stake in the provision of care would motivate a general reeducation of patients to recognize the limits of medical care and of "quality" frills. Failure to act along these lines would entail financial penalties.

Another group of reimbursement proposals focus initially on the consumer in an attempt to create an economic climate for the purchase of health care services by making consumers assume a significant degree of financial responsibility for their use of medical resources even though they have insurance coverage. Under these proposals the function of health insurance is primarily to *protect* against sudden, unexpected, expensive illness episodes rather than to just reimburse. Two broad proposals have been advanced along these lines: one focusing on total medical care and the other primarily on hospital care.

Martin Feldstein's proposal of *major risk insurance,* similar to existing "major medical" policies, and government guaranteed loans for the payment of noninsured medical bills adopts a global focus of health care. He proposes that:

> Every family would receive a comprehensive insurance policy with an annual direct expense limit (i.e. deductible) that increased with family income. A 500 dollar 'direct expense limit' means that the family is responsible for the first 500 dollars of medical expenses per year but pays no more than 500 dollars no matter how large the year's total medical bills. Different relations between family income and the direct expense limit are possible. For example, the expense limit might start at 300 dollars per year for a family with income below 3000 dollars, be equal to 10 per cent of family income between 3000 dollars and 8000 dollars, and be 800 dollars for incomes above that level. The details of the schedule are unimportant at this point. The key feature is an expense limit that is large in comparison to average family spending on health care but low relative to family income. The availability in addi-

tion of government guaranteed loans for the postpayment of medical bills would allow families to spread expenditures below the expense limit over a period of a year or even more.[21]

Feldstein's proposal would be universal (national) in coverage, thus providing increased access to medical care and would be financed through existing tax sources. It would discriminate in favor of the poor, protect against large risks, and would give consumers a direct incentive to demand and choose preventive as opposed to therapeutic care, and less expensive and more efficiently produced medical care, as the vast majority of payments for physicians and hospitals would not be insured. Furthermore, the administrative costs of maintaining a reimbursement scheme would be minimized as only one claim per year need be submitted by each family although loans could be applied for more frequently. Adjustments in the "direct expense limit" could easily be made to reflect family size, age composition, geographic location, or any other factor affecting the family's expected medical expenses.

A second proposal directed at consumer behavior but focusing only on hospital care has been advanced by Joseph Newhouse and Vincent Taylor. They propose a system of *variable cost* hospital insurance (VCI) whose basic features are:

1. An insurance organization (either the government or a private company) offering VCI would determine an expense class for each hospital in a community or area by examining the history of its costs and charges.

2. Subscribers would designate, in consultation with their physicians, their preference in hospitals.

3. In private plans, the insurance premiums charged subscribers would be proportional to the expense class of their preferred hospital(s). In government–sponsored plans, premiums would be charged only for coverage in excess of a 'standard benefit plan.'

4. The insurance organization would pay hospitals on the basis of either billed charges or costs, whichever is mutually agreed upon.

[21] Feldstein, Martin S.: A new approach to national health insurance, *The Public Interest, 23*:99, 1971.

5. In the event that the subscriber enters a hospital, the proportion of the bill paid by VCI would vary inversely with the expense class of the hospital used.[22]

Newhouse and Taylor stipulate that in emergencies and when special services available only at more expensive hospitals are required, the subscriber would be reimbursed at full cost. They further note that coinsurance provisions could be attached, if desired, to a basic VCI scheme. Under this proposal individual consumers would have to bear the cost of any "frills" that they desire both in terms of their insurance premiums and the insurance payments that are inversely related to the expense class chosen. If, for example, a hospital bill were 2,000 dollars and the hospital used was 30 per cent more expensive than the subscriber's coverage, 30 per cent (or more depending on the actual formula adopted) of the bill would not be met by the insurance plan. The premiums for a poor family's insurance under a VCI plan can easily be payed for through government sponsored plans funded through taxation.

The proponents of this scheme realize that only a small proportion of the population live in areas where a choice among hospitals is feasible and only a small proportion of prospective patients may choose a low expense class policy. But they argue that "if only 10 per cent of the patients of a high-cost, low-quality hospital decide to go elsewhere, the management of the hospital will be under considerable pressure to improve its performance." [23] They further assert that although physicians exert a strong influence on which hospital a patient chooses by virture of his own staff appointments, if only a few physicians are motivated to seek additional or primary appointments in lower cost hospitals in response to patient demand a definite impact on hospital management will have been made.

Although the four alternate reimbursement proposals differ in terms of scope and thrust, it should be evident that each one is an improvement over the existing pattern of medical and hospital reimbursement in that economic considerations are rein-

---

[22] Newhouse and Taylor, *op. cit.*, p. 88.
[23] *Ibid.*, p. 90.

troduced into an industry where resources are scarce and where the need to improve productive and allocative efficiency is universally recognized. The ultimate choice among plans which embody different levels of access, and structural and institutional change belongs in the political realm.

MATHEMATICAL TOOLS

MODELS AND THEIR COMPONENTS

The tools of mathematics[1] are generally used in economics in the process of building, testing, and quantifying models. A *model* is defined as *an abstraction of reality*. Models can be either dynamic or static. That is, they can be concerned with change over time or a description of some actual or potential event at a point in time. It is the quality and relevance of the abstraction embodied within a model which determines its usefulness. Models are useful tools of analysis as reality is often too complex and includes too much data to be easily studied directely.

Equations, Constants, Parameters, and Variables

A mathematical model consists of a system of one or more equations and/or functions, expressing the relationship between two or more factors. An *equation expresses an equality* between two or more factors such as

$$25 = 10 + 10 + 5$$

while an *inequality* represents unequal relationships such as

$$50 > 40 \qquad or \qquad 40 < 50$$

where the symbols $>$ and $<$ mean *greater than* and *less than* respectively.

Three major types of equations are used in economic models:

---

[1] For elaboration and further discussion of the topics discussed here see, Lewis, J. Parry: *An Introduction to Mathematics for Students of Economics*, Second Edition. New York, St. Martin's Press, 1969; or Brennan, Michael J.: *Preface to Econometrics*, Second Edition. Cincinnati, South-Western, 1965, Parts I and II.

identities, technological equations, and behavioral equations. *Identities specify a definitional relationship* such as net expense equals total cost minus reimbursable items, or the physician-population ratio equals the number of physicians divided by the size of the population. *Technological equations describe technological facts:* 5 units of labor, 3 units of assorted raw material, and 2 units of machine time produce one stethoscope $(5L + 3RM + 2M = 1S)$. *A behavioral equation describes human behavior.* A demand equation (which postulates an inverse relationship between price and quantity demanded) is a behavioral equation, as it hypothesizes how people react to price.

Equations may contain constants and/or variables. A *constant* is a *number which is invariant.* Within the category of constants, there are two types: absolute constants and parameters. An absolute constant is one whose value is always the same regardless of the model or context within which it is used. The mathematical terms pi (π) and e (the base for natural logarithms) are examples of absolute constants.[2] *Parameters* are constants within a particular model but may vary between models. A *variable,* as its name implies, is *a datum which does not have a fixed value even within a particular model.* Any datum may be a parameter in one model and a variable in another model, depending on the time frame adopted and the activity which the model attempts to symbolize. Thus, salary costs for administrative personnel may be a parameter in a model describing weekly hospital costs, but a variable in a model describing annual personnel costs.[3] Similarly case-mix could be a variable in a model of hospital reimbursement but a parameter in a model of hospital dietary costs.

There are several groupings into which variables can be classified: independent and dependent, exogenous and endogenous, and policy and target. These three pairings are not, however, necessarily mutually exclusive. The distinction between an *independent* and a *dependent* variable usually entails a decision of which variable influences the other. The *influencing variable is described as the independent variable* and the *influenced variable*

---

[2] The values of these two terms are 3.1417 and 2.718, respectively.

[3] This illustration assumes that administrative personnel are salaried and must be considered fixed factors in any short run analysis.

as the dependent variable, as its value is determined (influenced) by that of the independent variable. For example, one could construct an equation relating the number of physicians (MD), the physician-population ratio (R), and the size of the population (P), as:

$$R = MD/P$$

In this equation, MD and P are the independent variables and R is the dependent variable. The physician-population ratio, R, is dependent on the variation in the number of physicians, MD, and on population size, P; as the number of physicians increases or as the size of the population decreases, the physician-population ratio increases. Conversely, a decline in the number of physicians or an increase in population would result in a decline of the physician-population ratio.

Variables can alternately be classified as exogenous or endogenous. An *exogenous variable is one which is not affected by the system or model* under consideration. The number of physicians and the size of the population are exogenous in the equation of the physician-population ratio noted above; they are assumed to be a cause and not an effect of the other variables in the equation. *Endogenous variables are ones whose values are affected by the system or model.* The physician-population ratio is determined by the independent variables and is therefore endogenous.

Alternately, variables can be dicotomized as policy or target, if the discussion is within a planning context. Depending upon the goals of the planner and the nature of his control over that which is being planned, the designation of variables as target or policy is circumscribed. *A policy variable is one whose value can be affected directly by the decision making body* which is undertaking the planning. Referring to the previous example, a licensing commission may have control over the number of physicians licensed. The number of licensed physicians is then considered a policy variable. But the licensing board does not have control over the number of people living in any geographic area.[4] That number will vary with time and demographic conditions and

---

[4] From a short run planning perspective, population size can be considered a parameter.

cannot be considered a policy variable by the licensing commission. A *target variable* is simply *a variable whose value is set at some target or desired level.* The physician-population ratio may be considered a target variable and set at some value such a 1/750. Setting a target puts constraints on other variables such as the number of physicians. The nature of these constraints can then be studied. Alternately, or concurrently, the effect of changes in various policy variables on the target variable can be investigated.

The above discussion demonstrates that any given variable can be classified in a variety of manners. The number of physicians was seen to be an independent variable, a policy variable, and an exogenous variable under different schema. Similarly, the physician-population ratio was classified as dependent, target, and endogenous. The choice of variable title to be employed is usually dictated by the type of analysis being conducted.

Consistency

Given these various types of variables and constants, certain limitations on the manner in which they can be entered into a model exist. In order to come up with a unique value for each of the variables, there have to be as many equations in the model as there are variables. If the number of variables is greater than the number of equations, the model is said to be underdetermined and there will be an infinite number of values which will fulfill the conditions of the model, thereby extremely limiting the model's usefulness. For example, for the single equation system with three variables relating the physician-population ratio (R) to the number of physicians (MD) and to population size (P)

$$R = MD/P$$

there are an infinite number of combinations of values of R, MD, and P, which will fulfill the equation. For any value of P (500, 800, 1,000) and MD (10, 100, 500) there will be a resultant value of R fulfilling the equation ($\frac{1}{50}$, $\frac{1}{8}$, $\frac{1}{2}$).

If two equations with no new variables are added to the model, such as

$$P = 120,000$$
$$MD = 250$$

thereby enlarging the system to one of three equations and three variables, the possible solutions are reduced to one, which in this case is $R = 1/480$. When the number of equations equals the number of variables, the system is said to be determined. However, if there are more equations than variables, the system is overdetermined. For example, if a fourth equation is added to the model

$$R = 1/450$$

a situation with four equations and only three variables results; not all of the equations can be solved as the equations are inconsistent with one another.

Functions

A *function* such as

$$Y = f(X)$$

which is read Y equals f of X, *indicates that the value of one variable, Y, depends upon* (is a function of), *the value of another variable, X*.[5,6] Furthermore the functional relationship may include more than two variables such as a hypothesized functional relationship between an institution's cost (C), and its size (S), age (A), and number of employees (E). Such a functional relationship could be represented as

$$C = f(S, A, E)$$

In its abstract form, functional notation does not indicate precise quantitative relationships. Functions can, however, be specified more precisely, as for example

$$C = \frac{S}{a} + bA + dE$$

---

[5] The variable (or variables) inside the parentheses of any functional notation are called *arguments* of the function. The functional notation should not be confused with a multiplicative relationship such a Y equals f times X. Unfortunately, no hard and fast rule exists for avoiding such confusion. Whether a function is intended can only be determined from the context of the analysis.

[6] Other notations are also employed for a functional relationship such as $g(X)$, $F(X)$, and $f_1(X_1)$.

where a, b, and d are parameters. Whereas the first functional equation specified only the direction of the relationship, the second equation specifies the form of the relationship. For example, the effect of A or E on C is equal to the value of A or E (or the value of a change in A or E) times some parameter b or d, whereas the effect of S on C is equal to the value of S (or the value of a change in S) divided by some parameter a. Additional precision can be introduced into functional relationships by specifying the precise values of a, b, and d. Once the numerical values of these parameters are known, one can predict institutional cost (C), given data on size (S), age (A), and number of employees (E). The principal statistical tool used for determining the actual values of parameters in any functional relationship is regression analysis. (This technique is defined and described in Appendix II).

DERIVATIVES

A derivative is used when it is of interest to know the change in one variable associated with the change in another variable. This concept, taken from calculus, is utilized extensively in economics. It is used, for example, in calculating elasticities in demand theory and in ascertaining the optimal combination of factor inputs to maximize output under a budget constraint in production theory. The information embodied in a derivative could also be found by graphing a relationship between two or more variables; however, the use of derivatives does away with the time consuming and often inaccurate process of drawing graphs.

Simple Derivatives

A simple derivative, represented mathematically as $\dfrac{dY}{dX}$, describes, in quantitative terms, the relationship between two variables, X and Y. It can be defined in two different but equivalent terms. A *derivative is the value of the slope of a line tangent to a curve.* Alternately, it is the *limit of the change in the dependent variable divided by the change in the independent variable,* $\dfrac{\Delta Y}{\Delta X}$ (where the symbol Δ is called "delta" and represents the term "change in"), *as the change in the independent variable, ΔX, approaches zero.*

A *tangent is a line which touches a curve at a particular point but does not intersect it,* such as the line aa in Figure 17. The *slope* of a straight line is a number which indicates its steepness. It is defined as *the ratio of the change in Y to the change in X between any two points on the line.*

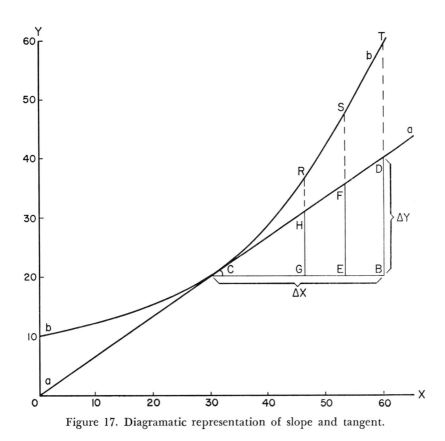

Figure 17. Diagramatic representation of slope and tangent.

Referring to Figure 17, the slope of line aa between points C and D (or any other two points) is 2/3. In this case Y changes from 20 to 40, a change of +20; while X changes from 30 to 60, a change of +30. The ratio of this change is +20/+30, or 2/3. Since 2/3 is the value of the slope of line aa and aa is tangent to curve bb at point C, 2/3 is the derivative of the curve at that point.

The second definition of the derivative, the limit of $\frac{\Delta Y}{\Delta X}$ as ΔX approaches zero, i.e., $\lim_{\Delta X \to 0} \frac{\Delta Y}{\Delta X}$, is the one which best describes the derivative but it is also the hardest to grasp. It states that the derivative is the value of $\frac{\Delta Y}{\Delta X}$ as ΔX approaches zero. That is, it is the value of $\frac{\Delta Y}{\Delta X}$ as ΔX is made smaller and smaller. The value of the slope of the tangent does not describe the actual change in the *curve* bb for all changes in X. If the value of X on curve bb increases by 30 units (from point C to point B), the value of Y on the curve bb is 60 (point T). Thus, a $+30$ unit change in X is associated with a $+40$ unit change in Y, or $\frac{\Delta Y}{\Delta X}$ is actually 40/30 or 4/3 rather than the value previously found for the slope of the tangent, 2/3. It is because of this difference between the slope of a *curve* and that of a *line* that the definition of the slope specifies the existence of two terminal points. As can be seen by looking at line CB in Figure 17, as the value of the change in X becomes smaller and smaller (BC to EC to GC), the corresponding change in Y along the tangent line aa gets closer and closer to the actual change on the curve bb (DB versus TB, FE versus SE, and HG versus RG).

As ΔX becomes very small, approaching but never quite reaching zero, ΔY as seen on the tangent line comes closer and closer to the change in Y as seen on the curve.[7] At the limit, when the change in X is so small as to be effectively zero, the change in Y as seen on the tangent *line* and as seen on the *curve* are equal so that the value of the slope of the tangent is the derivative.

For any functional relationship, the derivative indicates the value of the slope of the tangent at any point on the curve representing the function. For example, suppose the relationship between institutional cost (C) and number of employees (E) is expressed by the following function:

$$C = 4 + E + E^2$$

[7] The change in X can only approach but not reach zero because at ΔX equal to zero, $\frac{\Delta Y}{\Delta X}$ is undefined.

The graph of this function appears in Figure 18. The derivative $\dfrac{dC}{dE}$ would indicate the effect of an increase of one employee (E) on institutional cost. Graphically, the derivative at any point can be found by drawing a tangent to that point. Thus, at E = 5, the value of the slope of the tangent is equal to 11.[8] This means that if an

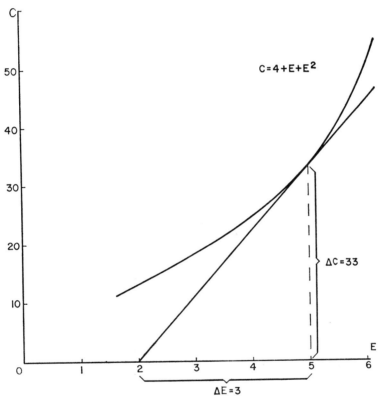

Figure 18. Graph of equation $C = 4 + E + E^2$.

institution had 5 employees, the rate of change (increase) in institutional cost for adding an additional employee is $11. This procedure could be duplicated to find the value of the slope of the tangent at any point along a curve.

A simpler, more generalized method, however, exists for obtain-

[8] At E = 5, $\dfrac{\Delta C}{\Delta E} = \dfrac{33}{3} = 11$

ing the value of the slope of the tangent. By employing a few simple rules of differentiation, a derivative indicating the value of the slope of the tangent at any point is immediately ascertainable. These rules, accompanied by simple illustrations, are:

1) *The derivative of a constant term is zero.*

$$Y = 50 \qquad\qquad Y = \pi$$

$$\frac{dY}{dX} = 0 \qquad\qquad \frac{dY}{dX} = 0$$

2) *The derivative of a variable is a term whose coefficient is the original exponent times the original coefficient and whose exponent is the original exponent minus 1.*[9] The derivative of $Y = aX^b$ is baX^{b-1}. That is, the new coefficient (b·a) of the variable X is the old coefficient (a) times the original exponent (b) and the new exponent (b − 1) of the variable is the old exponent (b) minus 1.

$$Y = 25X^1 \qquad\qquad\qquad Y = 3X^5$$

$$\frac{dY}{dX} = 1 \cdot 25X^{1-1} \qquad\qquad \frac{dY}{dX} = 5 \cdot 3X^{5-1}$$

$$= 25 \cdot X^0 \qquad\qquad\qquad = 15X^4$$

$$= 25 \text{ (since } X^0 = 1)$$

3) *The derivative of a series of factors is equal to the sum of the derivatives of each of the factors.*

$$Y = 4X^2 + 2X + 7 \qquad\qquad Y = \frac{1}{a}X^5 + 76X + 9$$

$$\frac{dY}{dX} = 2 \cdot 4X^{2-1} + 1 \cdot 2X^{1-1} + 0 \qquad \frac{dY}{dX} = 5 \cdot \frac{1}{a}X^{5-1} + 76X^{1-1} + 0$$

$$= 8X^1 + 2X^0 \qquad\qquad\qquad = \frac{5}{a}X^4 + 76X^0$$

$$= 8X + 2 \qquad\qquad\qquad\quad = \frac{5}{a}X^4 + 76$$

[9] In the term aX^b, a is a coefficient of variable X and b is the exponent of X. A coefficient is a number by which the variable is multiplied. An exponent is the power to which a variable is raised. Raising a variable to a power entails multiplying the variable times itself a given number of times (e.g. $X^4 = X \cdot X \cdot X \cdot X$).

All that is necessary to find many derivatives is the ability to utilize these three simple rules.[10]

By applying rules 2 and 3 one can determine mathematically the value of the slope of the tangent at point $E = 5$ for the cost function $C = 4 + E + E^2$ by calculating $\dfrac{dC}{dE}$ and substituting 5 for E. The derivative $\dfrac{dC}{dE}$ is equal to $1 + 2E$; at $E = 5$ this derivative equals 11 $(1 + 2(5))$. Using the same formula one can also determine the value of $\dfrac{dC}{dE}$ at $E = 7, 10, 3$, or any other value.

Second Derivatives and Maximization

Simple derivatives allow one to calculate rates of change. They do not indicate the direction of change. That is, simple derivatives do not indicate whether the algebraic value of the derivative is increasing, decreasing, or constant. This is found by calculating the derivative of the derivative, or the *second derivative*. For any function

$$Y = aX^b$$

the second derivative, written $\dfrac{d^2Y}{dX^2}$ or $d\dfrac{\frac{dY}{dX}}{dX}$, is found by treating the first derivative as if it were a function and differentiating it. The first derivative of this function, $\dfrac{dY}{dX}$, is $b \cdot a X^{b-1}$; its second derivative is: $(b - 1) b \cdot a X^{b-1-1}$ or $(b - 1) ba X^{b-2}$. For all values of X, the second derivative indicates the rate or direction of change of the first derivative. A positive second derivative indicates that the algebraic value of the first derivative is increasing, a negative sec-

---

[10] Two additional rules which are not generally needed in understanding health economics research are: the derivative of a product of two functions $Y = UV$ where $U = f_1(X)$ and $V = f_2(X)$ is given by $\dfrac{dY}{dX} = U\dfrac{dV}{dX} + V\dfrac{dU}{dX}$; and the derivative of a quotient of two functions $Y = \dfrac{U}{V}$ is given by $\dfrac{dY}{dX} = \dfrac{U\dfrac{dV}{dX} - V\dfrac{dU}{dX}}{V^2}$.

ond derivative indicates that the algebraic value of the first derivative is decreasing, and a zero second derivative connotes a first derivative whose algebraic value is constant.

Ascertaining the rate of change of the first derivative is a crucial step in any problem of maximization or minimization. It is used in solving such production problems as: What is the optimal (minimum cost) size of an institution? What is the optimal combination of inputs required to achieve a designated production (output) level at minimum cost? What is the maximum output that can be obtained given a designated budget and input restraints? The methodology employed in such calculations can be illustrated by solving the following hypothetical function relating cost (C) to size (S):

$$C = aS^2 + bS + d$$

for its minimum cost point. The first derivative of this equation indicates the change of costs relative to a change in size, which is the interpretation of the tangent to the curve at any point. As can be seen in Figure 19, the lowest C value occurs at the point where the tangent is horizontal. Determining the value of S where the tangent is horizontal, is the first step in solving the cost minimization problem. By definition a horizontal tangent signifies that there is no change at all in C for a small change in S along the tangent line. Therefore, the value of a tangent must be zero when it is horizontal. Thus in order to find the minimum cost point, the first derivative is set equal to zero and solved for S; that is, one finds the value of S for which the derivative is zero. The derivative of $C = aS^2 + bS + d$, $\frac{dC}{dS} = 2aS + b$, equals 0 when $2aS + b = 0$. Solving for S yields, $S = \frac{-b}{2a}$.

One does not initially know whether this is a maximum cost point, as in Figure 19A or a minimum cost point as in Figure 19B. Solving for the second derivative answers this question. The second derivative of the equation is the derivative of $\frac{dC}{dS} = 2aS + b$, which is 2a. If a is negative, the second derivative is negative for all values of S. That is, the slope or tangent of the function is always decreas-

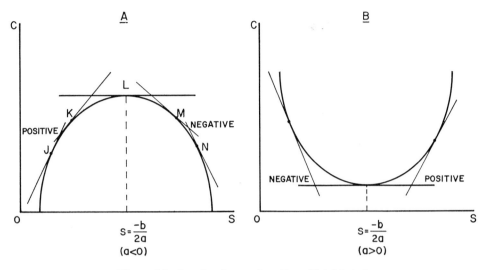

Figure 19. Graph of equation $C = aS^2 + bS + d$.

ing in value as S increases, as seen in Figure 19A. The tangent starts at a very high value at J, decreases but is still positive at K, is zero at L, becomes negative at M, and is even more negative at N. In such a case, a maximum rather than a minimum point has been attained. However, if a is positive, the second derivative is positive and therefore always increasing which implies, as seen in Figure 19B, that a minimum cost point has been reached. Thus, the second derivative being positive means that when the tangent is equal to zero the equation is at a minimum. As was noted earlier, one can determine this information from a graph, namely, whether the equation is at a minimum or maximum point. However, the use of the first and second derivatives eliminates the need to graph the equation at all.

Partial Derivatives

When a variable, say institutional cost (C), is dependent on two or more variables, say number of employees (E), and size (S):

$$C = f(E,S) \quad \text{or} \quad C = 50E + 20S$$

one must calculate *partial derivatives* rather than derivatives. Partial derivatives determine *the change in the dependent variable for a small change in only one of the independent variables,* assuming that the other independent variable(s) are held constant (i.e. *ceteris paribus*). For all equations, as many partial derivatives exist as there are independent variables. In this case two partial derivatives can be found: $\frac{\partial C}{\partial E}$ and $\frac{\partial C}{\partial S}$, where the symbol ∂ represents the partial derivative. These are, respectively, the change in costs for a change in the number of employees, all other variables (size) held constant, and the change in cost for a change in size holding all other variables (number of employees) constant. The terms $\frac{\partial C}{\partial E}$ and $\frac{\partial C}{\partial S}$ could also be read as the partial derivative of C with respect to E and the partial derivatives of C with respect to S. The same rules used for calculating regular derivatives apply also for partial derivatives with the understanding that variables other than the one whose partial derivative is being calculated are treated as constant. Thus, $\frac{\partial C}{\partial E} = 50$, since for a change in E, 20S is a constant just as 200 would be; $\frac{\partial C}{\partial S} = 20$ for similar reasons. These partial derivatives indicate that total costs increased by 50 for each additional employee (holding size constant) and by 20 for each additional unit increase in size (holding number of employees constant). In solving for maximum or minimum values for a function consisting of two variables, an additional test must be performed. For both maximum and minimum values the following condition must prevail:

$$\frac{\partial^2 C}{\partial E^2} \cdot \frac{\partial^2 C}{\partial S^2} > \left(\frac{\partial^2 C}{\partial E \partial S} \right)^2$$

The example appearing in the appendix to Chapter Six illustrates both a situation where partial derivatives are used and the method of solving the derivatives.

Appendix II

STATISTICAL TOOLS

PROBABILITY AND SAMPLING

Probability is the base on which statistical analyses are built.[1] While several approaches to the concept of probability are available, an intuitive approach is expounded here. *Probability, simply defined, is the expected average occurrence when an action is repeated many times.* For example, the probability of a tossed coin landing with its tail side up is one half, or the probability of an even number turning up on any one toss of a die is $1/2$, as there are six possible outcomes to a toss of a die, 1, 2, 3, 4, 5, and 6, and three of the outcomes (2, 4, and 6) are even numbers.

The probability of any event occurring does not, however, necessarily describe the outcome of any one particular event. What it does describe is the proportion of the expected outcome in a large number of trials of the experiment. For example, the following hypothetical results may represent the outcome of tossing a die 1,000 times.

Number of Tosses	Number of Even Numbers
10	0
30	9
50	20
70	30
100	52
1,000	500

While no even numbers resulted from the first 10 tosses, 9 even numbers were obtained in 30 tosses, and 20 even numbers were

[1] For elaboration and further discussion of the topics presented here see, Freund, John E.: *Modern Elementary Statistics,* Second Edition. Englewood Cliffs, N.J., Prentice-Hall, Inc., 1960; or Brennan, Michael J.: *Preface to Econometrics,* Second Edition. Cincinatti, South-Western Publishing Co., Inc., 1965, Part IV.

273

obtained in 50 tosses. As additional tosses occurred, however, the number of even numbers begins to approach the expected probability. If a sufficient number of tosses are undertaken, the results of the experiment will conform to the mathematical probability of the outcome.[2]

Many events about which a probability figure is quoted cannot be repeated. A rat either turns left or right at his first exposure to a given wall; a person either chooses a career in the health field or he does not; a baby is either a boy or a girl. While these experiments cannot actually be repeated many times to find the average occurrence, one can perform the experiment with many different subjects and in that manner approximate a set of exact replications.

Many statistical procedures deal with estimating probabilities when an experiment is not repeated an infinite number of times. To establish the conditions where probability estimates are valid, random samples are utilized. *A sample is a subgroup of some population,* where a population is any group. While one could find an average value of some characteristic of a population by measuring that characteristic for each member of the population, one can also estimate the value of a characteristic through statistical methods utilizing only a small portion of the entire group. Since the process of measurement entails time and resource costs, there is a distinct gain derived from alleviating the necessity of measuring every member of the population.

A *random sample* is simply *a sample which is selected so that every member of the population has an equal chance of being included.* This can be accomplished by a blind chance drawing

---

[2] Probability can be symbolically defined as:

$$P = \lim_{n \to \infty} \frac{x}{n}$$

Where P is the probability, x is the number of occurrences of the desired event (an even number), n is the number of trials of the experiment (toss of a die), and limit symbolizes the value of $\frac{x}{n}$ as n becomes very large, approaching infinity.

Probability is found by calculating the ratio of the number of possible ways an event being considered can occur to the number of possible occurrences, provided that each outcome is equally likely.

or consulting a table of random numbers which can be found in most volumes of mathematical or statistical tables. Insuring randomness is very important. If, for example, one wanted to find the average height of a group of 50 people, and asked them to line up according to age, a sample consisting of the first 10 people would not be random at all but according to some predetermined attribute (in this case age) of the population group.

In order to minimize the required sample size *stratified random samples* are often utilized. That is, the population is divided according to certain attributes, say age and sex, and the same proportion is selected from each of the subgroups. It has been found that one can achieve good estimates of the desired attribute of a population utilizing a stratified random sample of a much smaller size than with a simple random sample. Of course, the attributes upon which one stratifies must be ones which are hypothesized to have some influence on the variable whose value is being estimated. If one is estimating the incidence of an illness among a specified population group, it would probably not help to stratify on the basis of hair color.

CHARACTERISTICS OF DISTRIBUTIONS

The results of a sample are often diagrammed in what is known as a *frequency distribution, a plotting of the number of cases of each value found in the sample* and a connection of these points. For example, a sample of the number of beds occupied on any given day in an 80 bed health care institution may consist of the following observations:

66	67	68	69	72
67	67	68	70	73
67	68	69	71	74
67	68	69	71	

Plotting these observations on a conventional two axis diagram yields the frequency distribution appearing in Figure 20A. If instead of connecting the series of points appearing in Figure 20A, a bar were drawn from each point to the horizontal axis, (Figure 20B) the resulting diagram would be known as a *histogram* or *bar diagram*.

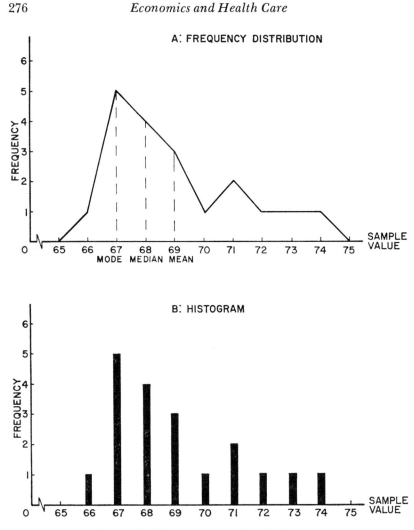

Figure 20. Characteristics of a distribution.

Many different statistics can be employed to describe a sample. These can be classified as measures of central tendency, dispersion, and skewness. Each presents a different picture of the group. Measures of *central tendency* include the mean, the median, and the mode. *They describe what are loosely called "average" values.* The *mean* is defined as the *sum of the values of*

each member of a group divided by the number in the group.[3]
A median is computed by first grouping the observations in a
sample in ascending (or descending) order. The *value which
has as many observations below or equal to it as above or equal
to it* is the *median.* If there are an even number of observations,
the median value is the average of the two middle observations.[4]
The *mode is the value which occurs most frequently.* In the
occupancy example noted above, the mean is 69, the median 68,
and the mode 67. The mean value is determined by dividing
the total number of occupied beds, 1311, by the number of
observations, 19. Since there are 19 observations in the sample,
the tenth highest observation, 68, is the median value, as there
are nine observations which are lower and nine observations
which are higher. One value, 67, appears more frequently in the
sample of observations than any other, and is therefore the modal
value. Depending on the precise configuration of any sample,
the mean, median, and mode may all be equal or, as seen above,
different. Similarly two samples may have identical mean, median,
or mode values but display great variation in the values of each
observation.[5]

In most studies, the mean is the most often employed and
useful measure of central tendency. When people speak of an
average value, they generally are referring to the mean. There
are some cases, however, when the median or the mode is a better
representation of the central tendency. For example, the median
puts much less weight on extreme values than does the mean.
Since one very high or very low value can drastically affect the

[3] The formula for calculating the mean is $\dfrac{\sum_{i=1}^{n} X_i}{n}$ where X_i is the value of each individual observation, n is the total number of observations, and Σ denotes the summation
of all values of the term that follows it.

[4] If, for example, there are eight observations in a sample, the median value
would be equal to the sum of the fourth and fifth values divided by two.

[5] The following two samples have identical medians and modes but differ in all
other respects.

        SAMPLE A: 75   75   75   80   80
        SAMPLE B: 71   74   75   75 100

mean but not the median, the median is often a better indication of the middle item in a distribution. The mode is the statistic that, for example, a pharmacist would be most interested in since it is the drug with the largest amount of sales which requires the largest stock.

Two additional statistics which are often utilized for describing a sample or a population are the *variance* and the *standard deviation*. Both of these are *measures of the dispersion of the observations*. That is, they indicate how closely the sample is grouped around the mean. For example, two samples, A and B

| Sample A | 75 | 75 | 75 | 75 | 75 | 66 | 57 | 57 | 57 | 57 | 57 |
| Sample B | 68 | 67 | 67 | 67 | 66 | 66 | 66 | 65 | 65 | 65 | 64 |

may both have means of 66 but otherwise are quite different from one another. The variance is found by squaring the value of the deviations from the mean (if the value of the observation is 75, and the mean is 66, the deviation is 9), summing these squared deviations, and dividing the sum of the squared deviations by the number of observations minus one.[6] The standard deviation, which is utilized more often than the variance, is the square root of the variance. The standard deviation of samples A and B are 8.22 and 1.08, respectively.

A third statistical description of a sample or distribution is its symmetry. If a distribution is *symmetrical*, its mean, mode, and median coincide as shown in Figure 21A. On the other hand, the distribution may be skewed to the left, as in Figure 21B, or the right, as in Figure 21C. One particular symmetrical distribution is extremely important in statistics: the *normal distribution*. The normal distribution is a theoretical frequency distribution which accurately describes the actual distribution of many different things such as, height, weight, the number of heads of ten coins tossed repeatedly, several estimates of the size of a room, and many, many other distributions. It is derived from the theory of

[6] The formula for the variance is $\dfrac{\sum_{i=1}^{n} (X_i - \bar{X})^2}{n-1}$ where X_i represents each individual observation and $\bar{X}$ the group mean.

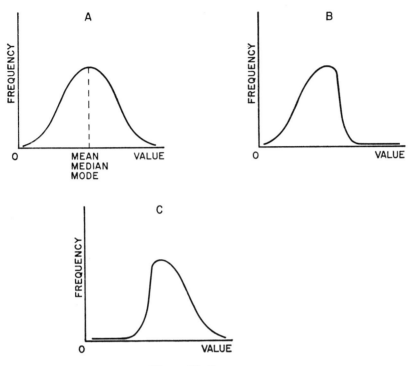

Figure 21. Symmetry.

probability and because of that, it is extremely useful in probability problems.

The normal distribution's usefulness is a result of its property
of having a specific proportion of its area within a given number
of standard deviations from its mean. Since the area under the
normal curve represents all of a sample whose observations are
normally distributed, the area between any two values represents
the proportion of the sample lying between those two values,
which is equivalent to the probability of any random observation
falling between the two selected values. For example, 68.26 per
cent of the area under the normal curve is within one standard
deviation on either side of the mean, 95.44 per cent within two
standard deviations on either side, and 99.74 per cent within
three standard deviations. This is true for all normal curves regardless of their means or standard deviations. Taking a more
concrete case, for the sample of occupancy, the mean is 69 beds

and the standard deviation is 2.2. Therefore, one could predict that 68.26 per cent of the observations would be between 66.8 and 71.2 (69 ± 2.2) beds occupied if the distribution of beds occupied for the population sampled were normal.[7] This attribute of the normal curve makes it possible to determine whether observed relationships are real or merely due to chance as will be noted below when the testing of significance is discussed.

MEASURES OF ASSOCIATION

Two tools of statistics which are frequently used in the health economics literature to denote association between variables are correlation and regression. Both are based on probability and are often applied to samples. A correlation or regression is known as *simple when two variables are involved* and *multiple when there are more than two variables*. While correlation and regression analyses can be executed on functions containing linear or non-linear variables, the discussion here will only consider the linear case.

The statistical tools of correlation and regression do not intrinsically demonstrate causality between variables. By themselves these tools can only indicate whether there is a relationship between the variables. Causality can only be inferred from a statistical analysis when the formulation of the relationship is based on a theoretical foundation. The distinctive attribute that differentiates regression from correlation is that the former provides a measure of the quantitative effect of one variable on another, in addition to a measure of the degree of association.

Simple Correlation

A correlation coefficient (r) measures the degree of linear association between two variables. A linear association is one which, when graphed on a four quadrant diagram yields a straight line. The general equation for any straight line is

---

[7] In fact, 79 per cent of that sample was within the specified one standard deviation from the mean. The difference between 68.26 per cent and 79 per cent is due either to chance variations of samples or to the actual distribution being non-normal.

$$Y = a + bX$$

where X and Y are any two variables and a and b are parameters.[8] The plot of that equation is a straight line with an intercept (the value of Y when X is equal to zero, that is, the point where the line crosses the Y-axis) equal to a and a slope (the change in Y, ΔY, for a given change in X, ΔX, or the angle at which the line cuts the Y-axis) of b as seen in Figure 22A.

The requirement of linearity is not as restrictive as it may initially appear. Many nonlinear relations can be transformed

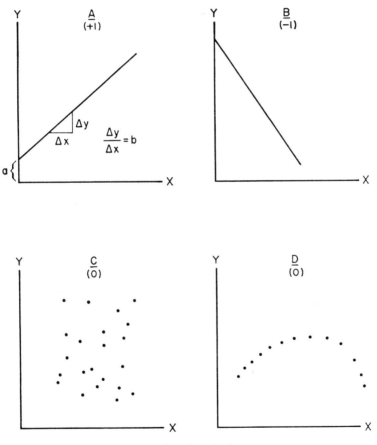

Figure 22. Correlation.

8 See Appendix I for a definition of the terms variable and parameter.

into linear form. For example, an equation such as $Y = aX^b$ can be transformed into linear form by taking the logarithms of both sides, which yields, $\log Y = \log a + b \cdot \log X$. That is, if one makes the following transformations—$Y' = \log Y$; $a' = \log a$; and $X' = \log X$—the equation would be exactly like the model for a linear equation, $Y' = a' + bX'$. Similarly, a relation such as $Y = a + bX^2$ can be converted to a linear form by calculating the value of X^2 for each value of X, calling it X^*, and substituting X^* for X^2 so that the equation reads $Y = a + bX^*$.

A *perfect correlation* exists when the plotting of pairs of values for any two variables yields a straight line, as in Figures 22A and 22B. A perfect *positive correlation* yields a straight line with a positive slope, as in Figure 22A, and indicates that as one variable increases by a given amount, the other increases by a specific amount determined by the slope. A perfect *negative* correlation yields a straight line with a negative slope, as in Figure 22B, and indicates that as one variable increases by a given amount, the other decreases by some specific amount determined by the slope. Alternately, there may be no relation at all between any two variables, as seen in Figures 22C and 22D. While a relationship between the two variables does exist in Figure 22D, no correlation exists as the relationship lacks linearity in that when X increases Y just as often decreases as increases.

The coefficient of correlation (r) for a perfect positive correlation has a value of $+1$, the correlation coefficient for a perfect negative correlation is -1, and the absence of any linear relationship is denoted by a correlation coefficient of 0. Positive and negative correlations that are not perfect have absolute values greater than 0 but less than 1.[9]

The evaluation of the degree of correlation utilizes the cri-

The formula for calculating r is:

$$r = \frac{\sum_{i=1}^{n} (X_i - \bar{X})(Y_i - \bar{Y})}{\sqrt{\left[\sum_{i=1}^{n} (X_i - \bar{X})^2\right]\left[\sum_{i=1}^{n} (Y_i - \bar{Y})^2\right]}}$$

where X_i and Y_i are the two variables being correlated, and $\bar{X}$ and $\bar{Y}$ are the respective means of these variables.

terion of *least squares.* Since correlation measures the degree that two variables are linearly related, the coefficient of correlation is determined by comparison of the actual scatter of points to a straight line which most closely fits the points on a graph. The choice from the infinite number of straight lines which could be drawn is based on minimizing the square of the vertical errors, which are called deviations.[10] Other criteria could be employed in making such a choice; however this one has proven to be quite versatile in its implications and it is used as the basis of

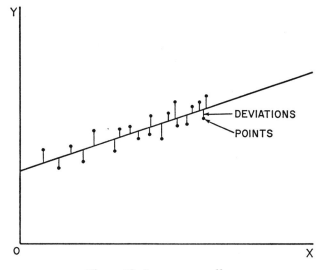

Figure 23. Least squares line.

many statistical tests. Thus, the straight line which minimizes the squares of the vertical errors (as seen in Figure 23) is found and the coefficient of correlation is a measure of how close the actual points (in the scatter diagram) match that line. The closer the points are to a straight line, the nearer the correlation coefficient is +1 or −1.

In addition to correlation between the actual values of variables, one can also find the correlation between the rankings of variables. This procedure is known as *rank correlation* and is frequently

---

[10] The square of the deviations is used to make all values positive, a procedure which prevents positive and negative deviations from cancelling each other out.

used when great confidence cannot be put in the exact values of the data as they are deemed to be gross estimates, or when the data are not in quantitative form (e.g. very high, high, medium, low, and very low). Under such circumstances, the data are ranked and the rankings, rather than the original data, are correlated.[11]

Multiple Correlation

Multiple correlation measures the degree of linear association between three or more variables. Two statistics are associated with multiple correlation: partial correlation coefficients and the coefficient of multiple correlation. *Partial correlation is the correlation between two variables net of* (that is, after account has been taken of) *the influence of other variables.*[12] The partial correlation coefficient reflects the portion of the variance of one variable associated with the variance of a second variable holding some other variable or variables constant. For example, one might want to correlate the number of physician visits with a measure of health status in various years. But a more revealing investigation would result if the effect of income level were held constant (netted out) while undertaking that correlation. Since income is most likely correlated with both physician visits and health, it is quite useful to eliminate, or hold constant, this effect on the number of physician visits when finding the correlation between health status and number of physician visits. Such a correlation would be represented by the partial correlation coefficient: $R_{12.3}$ (the correlation between variables 1 and 2 holding

[11] A frequently used rank correlation coefficient is Spearman's Rho (r_s) whose formula is:

$$r_s = 1 - \frac{6 \sum_{i=1}^{n} d_i}{n(n^2 - 1)}$$

where d_i is the numerical difference between the two ranks of any one observation and n is the total number of observations being correlated.

[12] The formula for calculating a partial correlation coefficient in a three variable case is:

$$R_{ij \cdot k} = \frac{R_{ij} - (R_{ik})(R_{jk})}{\sqrt{1 - R_{ik}^2} \ \sqrt{1 - R_{jk}^2}}$$

where i, j, and k are any three variables. For an extension of this formula to a situation involving more than three variables see, Blalcock, Hubert M.: *Social Statistics*, New York, McGraw-Hill Book Co., Inc., 1960, pp. 335–336.

variable 3 constant). If more than one variable is being held constant, the notation would be: $R_{12.34}$, $R_{12.345}$, etc.

In addition to partial correlations, one can also calculate the *coefficient of multiple correlation* (R).[13,14] This is the degree to which one variable is correlated with a whole set of other variables. That is, using the above example, R would be the degree of correlation between the number of physician visits, health status, and income.

Simple Regression

Simple regression analysis (only two variables involved) is closely related to the simple correlation analysis discussed above. The basic difference is the objective: *correlation analysis is designed to find the degree to which the pairs of X and Y observations fit a straight line, while regression analysis is designed to define the straight line,* (by finding the value of the parameters of the linear equation, that is, finding the values of a, the intercept, and b, the slope, in the equation for a straight line, $Y = a + bX$). Through the regression procedure, estimates are made of the parameters of an equation such as

$$Y = a + bX + u$$

where Y is designated the dependent variable (the variable whose variation is to be explained), X is designated as the independent (explaining) variable and u is the error term, that is, the vertical distance between the actual points and the line which minimizes the squares of those errors.[15] For example, if Y is

---

[13] The difference in notation for the partial correlation coefficient and the coefficient of multiple correlation is that the former is subscripted.

[14] The formula for calculating R in a three variable case ($R_{1.23}$) is

$$R_{1.23} = \sqrt{r^2_{13} + r^2_{12.3} (1 - r^2_{12})}$$

See, Blalcock, *Op. Cit.*, pp. 349–350, for an extension of this formula to a case of four or more variables.

[15] The solution for a simple regression equation is as follows:

$$b = \frac{\sum_{i=1}^{n} (X_i - \bar{X})(Y_i - \bar{Y})}{\sum_{i=1}^{n} (X_i - \bar{X})^2} \quad \text{and}$$

$$a = \bar{Y} - b\bar{X}$$

health care expenditures and X is family income, the values of a and b might be calculated to be 100 and 0.05 respectively. In such a case, the regression analysis would predict that a family with an 8,000 dollar income would have health care expenditures of 500 dollars $(100 + 0.05 \cdot 8,000)$. If the family actually had health care expenditures totaling 532 dollars, the error term, u, would be equal to 32 dollars. In actual research the error term is rarely reported. Its magnitude, however, can be partially estimated from the value of the coefficient of determination.

The degree that the regression line fits the actual sample is summarized by the *coefficient of determination*, (r^2).[16] Mathematically, r^2 is the square of the coefficient of correlation, r. As such, its value also ranges from a low of 0 to a high of 1. Conceptually, *it is the portion of the variance in the dependent variable "explained" by the independent variable.* Thus a relatively high r^2 indicates that the independent variable is a good explanator or predictor, and vice versa. Low r^2 values imply the existence of large error term (u) values as much of the variation in the dependent variable has not been explained or accounted for by the independent variable.

Multiple Regression

The regression procedure can be extended to cases with many independent variables such as that represented by

$$Y = a + b_1X_1 + b_2X_2 + \cdots + b_nX_n + u$$

Here too, one can estimate the values of all the b's and a, thereby completely estimating the relationship between the independent variables and the dependent one.[17] Each of the *partial regression coefficients* (b's) estimated through the multiple regression analysis *represents the relationship between the de-*

---

[16] This statistic is often written as R^2. However, here the use of R and R^2 are reserved for multiple relationships in order to emphasize the distinction between simple and multiple correlations and regressions.

[17] The conventional solution of a multiple regression model entails the use of matrix algebra. For a detailed description of the formulas involved see, Johnston, J.: *Econometric Methods*, New York, McGraw-Hill Book Co., Inc., 1963, Chapter 4. As is true for most statistical computations, many computer programs are readily available to perform the required calculations for correlation and regression analysis.

*pendent variable and an independent variable, holding all other
independent variables constant.* If, for example, the relationship
to be estimated is that between health care expenditures, income, and educational attainment for each individual, it could
be formulated as:

$$E = a + b_1Y + b_2S + u$$

where E is health care expenditures, Y is income, S is number of
years of schooling completed, and u is an error term. Given the
values of the variables for a group of people, the values of the
b's and a can be estimated. Then to predict an expenditure
level, one need merely substitute the values of each of the independent variables into the equation which has been estimated.
For example, if $a = 25$, $b_1 = 0.04$, and $b_2 = 1.2$ then persons with
an income of 7,000 dollars and a high school education (12 years
of schooling) would be predicted to spend $319.40 on health care
$(25 + 0.04 \cdot 7000 + 1.2 \cdot 12)$. If they actually spent 325 dollars, u,
the error term, would be $5.60. The b's represent the effect of each
of the variables taken separately. That is, b_1 is the effect of income
holding education level constant, and b_2 represents the effect of
educational attainment holding income constant.

There are two tests, in particular, which help in the interpretation of the "goodness" of the hypothesized relationship as a
representation of the actual relationship between the variables
considered. The first is the R^2 or *coefficient of multiple determination,* which is derived by squaring R, the coefficient of multiple
correlation. The R^2 coefficient indicates what proportion of the
variance in the values of the dependent variable is explained by
the independent variables. That is, referring to the previous
example, it tells how much of the difference in health care
expenditures is explained by the independent variables, income
and education, and how much is not explained. Thus, the higher
the R^2 the better the equation predicts the value of the dependent variable from information on the independent variables.

In addition, one can test whether or not each independent
variable's coefficient, b_i (where i represents any variable) is significantly different from zero. If a given b_i is not significantly
different from zero, then the variable of which it is the coefficient

is not a significant explanatory variable. This is, if that variable were excluded, the amount of the variance in the dependent variable explained would not be significantly reduced. Several times in this discussion the term *significance* has been employed. In statistics, significant has a specific technical meaning. *Whether a coefficient is significantly different from zero is determined by a t-test. The t-test analyzes the standard error of b_i and determines whether a coefficient of that size with a standard error of the given amount is different from zero merely because of chance quirks of the given sample or due to an actual difference.*[18] Most statistical research adopts a significance level of .05 or .01, meaning that if significance is achieved, the chance of a coefficient of that size and standard error not being different from zero is 5 or 1 in 100, respectively.[19]

Dummy Variables

Regression analysis is quite versatile in spite of the requirement of a linear relationship between the dependent and independent variables. A variable may be non-linear but be entered into a relationship in linear form as was noted in the discussion of simple correlation. In addition non-quantitative variables can be utilized. For example, race, sex, health status, place or type of residence, and type of institution, are all variables which cannot be easily represented by numbers.

One could conceivably represent male by 1 and female by 2 or 10 but what does the one or nine units that separate male and female represent? Is a female twice or nine times as much as a male? To handle such variables a system known as *dummy*

[18] The standard error of a regression coefficient is a measure of the standard deviation of the coefficient's variable relative to the coefficient of multiple determination. In practice, the standard error of any statistic is usually corrected for *degrees of freedom*. Degrees of freedom are calculated by subtracting the number of independent restrictions placed upon the calculation of the statistic from the actual number of observations in the sample.

In regression analysis, the number of observations minus the number of constants (intercept plus regression coefficients) constitute the degrees of freedom. The fewer the number of constants, the greater the freedom left for additional inferences.

[19] T values for the .05 and .01 significance levels are 1.96 and 2.57, respectively. If t-values equal to or greater than these values are obtained, the coefficient is judged to be significant at the designated significance level.

variables has been developed. *A dummy variable is one which is evaluated at either 1 or 0 depending upon whether some particular condition is fulfilled.* For example, one might have a variable for sex, S, which is equal to 1 when the individual is a male and 0 when it is a female. Including such a variable in the regression equation would determine the effect of sex on the dependent variable. Thus, if the value for its coefficient were 5.2 the interpretation would be that males had, other things being equal, 5.2 more units of the dependent variable than do females ($5.2 \cdot 1 = 5.2$ versus $5.2 \cdot 0 = 0$).

In addition to one dummy variable representing some qualitative factor, there are cases when a set of dummy variables may be employed if a comparison among categories is of interest. For example, if it were hypothesized that the type of hospital one chooses has an effect on hospital expenditures, more than one dummy variable would be required since three types of hospitals can be specified: government, voluntary, and proprietary. In such a case two variables (X_1, and X_2) could be specified, where X_1 would equal 1 if the person chose a government hospital but would be 0 in any other case, and X_2 would be 1 if the person chose a proprietary hospital and 0 otherwise. This dummy variable specification can be summarized as

	Variable	
Type of Hospital	X_1	X_2
Government	1	0
Proprietary	0	1
Voluntary	0	0

Within this formulation there are three types of hospitals but only two variables. This is because the coefficient of each variable is being compared to the situation of being in the omitted category, voluntary hospitals. Just as in the earlier example of a sex dummy variable the coefficient showed the effect of being male compared to being female, so here, the coefficients of X_1 and X_2 show the effect of being in that category (a government or proprietary hospital) compared to being in the omitted category (a voluntary hospital).[20]

[20] See Suits, Daniel: Use of dummy variables in regression equations, *American Statistical Association Journal, 52*:547, 1957 for a more detailed discussion of the use of dummy variables.

For example, an equation for predicting hospital cost per day might be:

$$C = a + b_1X_1 + b_2X_2 + u$$

where the variables X_1 and X_2 are defined above and the values of a, b_1, and b_2 might be 110, $+5$, and -10. If the regression equation were used to predict cost per day in a voluntary hospital, the values of X_1 and X_2 would be zero so that the predicted value of C would be 110 dollars, the value of a. If costs in a government hospital are to be predicted, the estimate would be 115 dollar (since in this case X_1 is 1, X_2 is 0, and $C = a + b_1$ or 115). Similarly, if interest focuses on a propriety institution, the predicted cost would be 100 dollars (since X_2 is now 1, X_1 is 0, and $C = a + b_2$).

One can have a series of dummy variables and ordinary variables in the same regression equation. For example, the regression relating health care expenditures to income and education could include a series of dummy variables signifying the purchase of physician services under three different schemes: solo practice, single specialty group, and multi-specialty group. Regression coefficients of $+10$ and -20 associated with a dummy variable comparing multi-specialty and single specialty groups respectively to solo practice would imply that the predicted expenditures would be 10 dollars higher (20 dollars lower) if the person consumed physician care provided through a single specialty (multispecialty) group rather than through solo practice, income and education being held constant.

SELECT BIBLIOGRAPHY

General Economics Texts

Eckaus, Richard S.: *Basic Economics*. Boston, Little, Brown and Co., 1972.

Fusfeld, Daniel R.: *Economics*. Lexington, Mass., D. C. Heath, 1972.

Lipsey, Richard G. and Steiner, Peter O.: *Economics*. Third Edition. New York, Harper and Row, 1972.

McConnell, Campbell R.: *Economics: Principles, Problems, and Policies*. Fifth Edition. New York, McGraw-Hill, 1972.

Samuelson, Paul A.: *Economics: \An Introductory Analysis*. Eighth Edition. New York, McGraw-Hill, 1970.

General Economics of Health

Axelrod, S. (ed.) : *The Economics of Health and Medical Care*. Ann Arbor, Bureau of Public Health Economics, University of Michigan, 1964.

Klarman, Herbert: *The Economics of Health*. New York, Columbia University Press, 1965.

Klarman, Herbert (ed.) : *Empirical Studies in Health Economics*. Baltimore, The Johns Hopkins Press, 1970.

Use of National Income Concepts in Health Research

Anderson, Odin W.; Collette, Patricia; and Feldman, Jacob: *Changes in Family Medical Care Expenditures and Voluntary Health Insurance*. Cambridge, Harvard University Press, 1963.

Craft, Edward M.: Consumer income and expenditures for health care. *Journal of the American Medical Association, 207*:139, 1969.

Muller, Charlotte: Income and receipt of medical care. *American Journal of Public Health, 55*:510, 1965.

The Medical Care Price Index

Berry, William and Dougherty, James: A closer look at rising medical costs. *Monthly Labor Review, 91* (11) :1, 1968.

Commission on the Cost of Medical Care. The medical care price index, in, *General Report*, Volume I. Chicago, American Medical Association, 1964, pp. 39–56.

Craft, Edward M.: Health care prices, 1950–1967—Discussion of trends and their significance. *Journal of the American Medical Association, 205:* 231, 1968.

German, Jeremiah J.: Some uses and limitations of the Consumer Price Index. *Inquiry, 1:*137, 1964.

Greenfield, Harry and Anderson, Odin W.: *The Medical Care Price Index.* New York, Health Information Foundation, 1959.

Scitovsky, Anne: Changes in the costs of treatment of selected illnesses, 1951–1965. *American Economic Review, 57:*1182, 1967.

Demand Studies

Bailey, Richard M.: An economist's view of the health services industry. *Inquiry, 6:*3, 1969.

Feldstein, Martin S.: Hospital cost inflation: A study of nonprofit price dynamics, *American Economic Review, 59:*853, 1971.

————: The rising price of physicians' services. *Review of Economics and Statistics, 52:*121, 1970.

Feldstein, Paul J.: Research on the demand for health services. *The Milbank Memorial Fund Quarterly, 44* (3) :128, 1966.

————: The demand for medical care, in, Commission on the Cost of Medical Care: *General Report,* Volume I, Chicago, American Medical Association, 1964, pp. 57–76.

Fuchs, Victor and Kramer, Marcia: Expenditures for physicians' services in the United States, 1948–1968. New York, National Bureau of Economic Research, 1971 (mimeographed) .

Jeffers, James R.; Bognanno, Mario F.; and Bartlett, John C.: On the demand versus need for medical services and the concept of shortages. *American Journal of Public Health, 61:*46, 1971.

Leveson, Irving: The demand for neighborhood medical care. *Inquiry, 7* (4) : 17, 1970.

Weisbrod, Burton A.: Anticipating the health needs of Americans: Some economic projections. *Annals of the American Academy of Political and Social Science, 337:*137, 1961.

Wirick, Grover: A multiple equation model of demand for health care. *Health Services Research, 1:*301, 1966.

Production Studies

Bailey, Richard M.: A comparison of internists in solo and fee-for-service group practice in the San Francisco Bay area. *Bulletin of the New York Academy of Medicine, 44:*1293, 1968.

Berry, Ralph E.: Product heterogeneity and hospital cost analysis. *Inquiry, 7* (1) :67, 1970.

————: Returns to scale in the production of hospital services. *Health Services Research, 2:*123, 1967.

Brown, Max: An economic analysis of hospital operations. *Hospital Administration, 15*:60, 1970.

Carr, W. John, and Feldstein, Paul J.: The relationship of cost to hospital size. *Inquiry, 4* (2) :45, 1967.

Feldstein, Martin S.: *Economic Analysis for Health Service Efficiency.* Chicago, Markham, 1968.

Hefty, Thomas: Returns to scale in hospitals: A critical review of recent research. *Health Services Research, 4*:267, 1969.

Ingbar, Mary Lee and Taylor, Lester D.: *Hospital Costs in Massachusetts: An Econometric Study.* Cambridge, Harvard University Press, 1968.

Lave, Judith R. and Lave, Lester B.: Estimated cost functions for Pennsylvania hospitals. *Inquiry, 7* (2) :3, 1970.

Rafferty, John: Hospital output indices. *Economic and Business Bulletin, 24* (2) :21, 1972.

Ro, Kong-Kyun: Determinants of hospital costs. *Yale Economic Essays, 8*:185, 1968.

Ruchlin, Hirsch S. and Levey, Samuel: Nursing home cost analysis: A case study. *Inquiry, 9* (3) :3, 1972.

Investment Studies

Bellante, Donald M.: A multivariate analysis of a vocational rehabilitation program. *Journal of Human Resources, 7* (2) :139, 1972.

Berkowitz, Monroe and Johnson, William G.: Towards an economics of disability: The magnitude and structure of transfer and medical costs. *Journal of Human Resources, 5* (3) :271, 1970.

Conley, Ronald W.: A benefit-cost analysis of the vocational rehabilitation program. *Journal of Human Resources, 4* (2) :226, 1969.

Crystal, Royal A. and Brewster, Agnes W.: Cost-benefit and cost-effectiveness analysis in the health field: An introduction. *Inquiry, 2* (4) :3, 1966.

Fein, Rashi: *Economics of Mental Illness.* New York, Basic Books, 1958.

Hallan, Jerome B.; Harris, Benjamin, S., H.; and Alhadeff, Albert V.: *The Economic Cost of Kidney Diseases and Related Diseases of the Urinary System.* Washington, D.C., U.S. Government Printing Office, 1968.

Klarman, Herbert E.: Syphilis control programs, in, Dorfman, Robert (ed.) : *Measuring Benefits of Government Investments.* Washington, D.C., The Brookings Institution, 1965, pp. 367–414.

LeSourd, David A.; Fogel, Mark E.; and Johnston, Donald R.: *Benefit-Cost Analysis of Kidney Disease Programs.* Washington, D.C., U.S. Government Printing Office, 1968.

Mushkin, Selma J. and d'A. Collings, Francis: Economic costs of disease and injury. *Public Health Reports, 74*:795, 1959.

Rice, Dorothy: *Economic Costs of Cardiovascular Diseases and Cancer, 1962.* Washington, D.C., U.S. Government Printing Office, 1964.

————: *Estimating the Cost of Illness.* Washington, D.C., U.S. Government Printing Office, 1966.

Smith, Warren: Cost-effectiveness and cost-benefit analysis for public health programs. *Public Health Reports, 83:*899, 1968.

Weisbrod, Burton A.: *Economics of Public Health.* Philadelphia, University of Pennsylvania Press, 1961.

Wiseman, Jack: Cost-benefit analysis and health service policy. *Scottish Journal of Political Economy, 10:*128, 1963.

Economic Growth, Planning, and Health

Barlow, Robin: ʼThe economic effects of malaria eradication. *American Economic Review, 57* (2) :130, 1967.

Enke, Stephen: The gains to India from population control: Some money measures and incentive schemes. *Review of Economics and Statistics, 42:* 175, 1966.

Feldstein, Martin S.: An aggregate planning model of the health care sector. *Medical Care, 5:* 369, 1967.

————: Health sector planning in developing countries. *Economica, 16:*139, 1970.

Malenbaum, Wilfred: Progress in health: What index of what progress," *Annals of the American Academy of Political and Social Science, 393:*109, 1971.

Newman, Peter: Malaria control and population growth. *The Journal of Development Studies, 6:*133, 1970.

Schultz, T. Paul: An economic model of family planning and fertility. *Journal of Political Economy, 77:*153, 1969.

Yett, Donald E.; Drabek, Leonard; Intriligator, Michael D.; and Kimbell, Larry J.: A macroeconomic model for regional health planning. *Economic and Business Bulletin, 24* (1) :1, 1971.

Financing Health Care

Baird, Charles W.: A proposal for financing the purchase of health services. *Journal of Human Resources, 5* (1) :89, 1970.

Berki, Sylvester: Economic effects of national health insurance. *Inquiry, 8* (2) : 37, 1971.

Burns, Eveline: A critical review of national health insurance proposals. *HSMHA Health Reports, 86:*111, 1971.

Eilers, Robert D. and Moyerman, Sue S. (eds.) : *National Health Insurance: Proceedings of the Conference on National Health Insurance.* Homewood, Ill., Richard D. Irwin, 1971.

Klarman, Herbert E.: Reimbursing the hospital: The differences the third party makes. *Journal of Risk and Insurance, 34:*553, 1969.

Pauly, Mark V.: An analysis of government health insurance plans for poor families. *Public Policy, 19:*489, 1971.

————: Efficiency, incentives, and reimbursement for health care. *Inquiry, 7:* 114, 1970.

Rothenberg, Jerome: Welfare implications of alternate methods of financing medical care. *American Economic Review, 45:*666, 1951.

U.S. Department of Health, Education, and Welfare, Social Security Administration. *Reimbursement Incentives for Hospital and Medical Care: Objectives and Alternatives.* Washington, D.C., U.S. Government Printing Office, 1968.

Weiss, Jeffrey H. and Brodsky, Lynda: As essay on the national financing of health care. *Journal of Human Resources, 7:*139, 1972.

Other Studies of Interest

Arrow, Kenneth J.: Uncertainty and the welfare economics of medical care. *American Economic Review, 53:*941, 1963.

Auster, Richard; Leveson, Irving; and Sarachek, Deborah: The production of health: An exploratory study. *Journal of Human Resources, 4* (4) :411, 1969.

Berki, Sylvester: *Hospital economics.* Lexington, Mass., D. C. Heath, 1972. The Brookings Institution, 1967.

Culyer, A. J.: The nature of the commodity "health care" and its efficient allocation. *Oxford Economic Papers, 23:*189, 1971.

Davis, Karen: Economic theories of behavior in nonprofit, private hospitals. *Economic and Business Bulletin, 24* (2) :1, 1972.

Dunlop, John T.: The capacity of the United States to provide and finance expanding health services. *Bulletin of the New York Academy of Medicine, 41:*1325, 1965.

Fein, Rashi: *The Doctor Shortage: An Economic Analysis.* Washington, D.C., The Brookings Institution, 1967.

Feldstein, Martin S.: An econometric model of the medicare system. *Quarterly Journal of Economics, 75:*1, 1971.

————: Economic analysis, operational research, and the National Health Service. *Oxford Economic Papers, 15:*19, 1963.

————: *The Rising Cost of Hospital Care.* Washington, D.C., Information Resources Press, 1971.

Fuchs, Victor R.: The contribution of health services to the American economy. *The Milbank Memorial Fund Quarterly, 44* (4) :65, 1966.

Kaitz, Edward M.: *Pricing Policy and Cost Behavior in the Hospital Industry.* New York, Frederick A. Praeger, 1968.

Lee, Maw Lin: A conspicious production theory of hospital behavior. *Southern Economic Journal, 38:*48, 1971.

Mushkin, Selma J.: Toward a definition of health economics. *Public Health Reports, 73:*785, 1958.

Newhouse, Joseph P.: Toward a theory of nonprofit institutions: An economic model of a hospital. *American Economic Review, 60:*64, 1970.

Pauly, Mark V.: *Medical Care at Public Expense: A Study in Applied Welfare Economics.* New York, Frederick A. Praeger, 1971.

Rice, Robert: An analysis of the hospital as an economic organism. *Modern Hospital, 106* (4) :87, 1966.

Ro, Kong-Kyun: Patient characteristics, hospital characteristics, and hospital use. *Medical Care, 7:*295, 1969.

Ruchlin, Hirsch S. and Levey, Samuel: The economics of long-term care, in, Sherwood, Sylvia (ed.) : *Long Term Care Research: A Review and Analysis of the Literature.* Washington, D.C., National Center for Health Services Research and Development, 1973.

Somers, Herman M.: Economic issues in health services, in, Chamberlain, Neil W. (ed.) : *Contemporary Economic Issues.* Homewood, Ill., Richard D. Irwin, 1969, pp. 109–144.

NAME INDEX

A

Abbe, L. M., 87
Abel-Smith, B., 87
Ackley, Gardner, 15, 16
Alhadeff, Albert V., 293
Anderson, Odin W., 88, 291, 292
Arrow, Kenneth J., 295
Auster, Richard, 252, 295
Axelrod, S., 51, 173, 291

B

Bailey, Richard M., 292
Baird, Charles W., 294
Baligh, Helmy H., 124, 117, 144
Barlow, Robin, 294
Bartlett, John C., 292
Baumol, William J., 109, 196
Becker, Gary S., 66
Bellante, Donald M., 293
Berki, Sylvester, 294, 295
Berkowitz, Monroe M., 293
Berry, Ralph E., 292
Berry, William F., 47, 291
Bognanno, Mario F., 292
Brennan, Michael J., 259, 273
Brewster, A. W., 87, 293
Brodsky, Lynda, 295
Brown, Max, 125, 293
Buffa, Edward S., 116
Burns, Eveline, 294

C

Carr, W. John, 293
Chamberlain, Neil W., 296

Cohen, Harold, 123, 124, 125
Collette, Patricia, 291
Conley, Ronald W., 293
Craft, Edward M., 291, 292
Crick, Francis H. D., 189
Crystal, Royal A., 293
Culyer, A. J., 295

D

d'A. Colling, Francis, 293
Dales, Sophie R., 179, 196
Dantzig, G. B., 157
Davis, Karen, 295
Deasy, L. C., 88
Densen, P. M., 88
Denison, Edward, 216
Dickinson, F. G., 87
Donabedian, Avedis, 124
Dorfman, Robert, 195
Dougherty, James C., 47, 291
Dowling, William L., 125
Drabek, Lenard, 294
Dunlop, John T., 295

E

Eckaus, Richard S., 291
Eilers, Robert D., 294
Enders, John F., 190
Enke, Stephen, 294

F

Falk, I. S., 87
Fein, Rashi, vii, 71, 173, 176, 229, 293, 295
Feldman, Jacob J., 88, 291

297

Feldstein, Martin, vii, 144, 156, 157, 255, 256, 292, 293, 294, 295
Feldstein, Paul, 71, 254, 292, 293
Fogel, Mark E., 293
Francis, John O's., 177
Friedman, Milton, 17
Freund, John E., 273
Fuchs, Victor, vii, 71, 292, 295
Fusfield, Daniel R., 21, 291

G

Galbraith, John K., 17
German, Jeremiah J., 45, 292
Gottschalk, Carl W., 202
Greenfield, Harry, 292
Griliches, Zvi, 180, 191, 196

H

Hallan, Jerome B., 293
Hansen, W. Lee, 173, 180, 188, 196
Harris, Benjamin S., 293
Haveman, Robert, 180, 196
Hefty, Thomas, 293

I

Ingbar, Mary Lee, 293
Intriligator, Michael D., 294

J

Jeffers, James R., 292
Jones, Norman, 71
Johnson, William G., 203
Johnston, Donald R., 293
Johnston, J., 286
Jureen, L., 78, 98

K

Kaitz, Edward M., 295
Kimbell, Larry J., 294
Klarman, Herbert, vii, 177, 195, 291, 293, 294
Koos, E. L., 88
Kramer, Marcia, 71, 292
Kurtz, Richard A., 131, 132, 134, 138

L

Lancaster, Kevin J., 66
Langford, Elizabeth A., 47
Laughhunn, Danny J., 117, 124, 144

Lave, Judith R., 293
Lave, Lester B., 293
Lee, Maw Lin, 125, 295
LeSourd, David A., 293
Leveson, Irving, 292, 295
Levey, Samuel, 293, 296
Lewis, J. Parry, 109, 259
Lipsey, Richard G., 291

M

Malenbaum, Wilfred, 294
Mann, Judith K., 17
Mayerman, Sue S., 294
McConnell, Cambell R., 291
Moyerman, Sue S., 294
Muller, Charlotte, 291
Mushkin, Selma J., 293, 295

N

Newhouse, Joseph P., 125, 251, 256, 295
Newman, Peter, 294
Nosta, Manohar, 221

O

Odoroff, M., 87

P

Pauly, Mark V., 294, 295, 296
Peters, W. S., 157

R

Rafferty, John, 293
Rice, Dorothy, 293, 294
Rice, Robert, 248, 296
Ro, Kong-Kyun, 252, 293, 296
Robbins, Frederick C., 190
Roemer, M. I., 88
Rogers, Daniel C., viii, ix
Rosenthal, Gerald, 71, 72, 73, 74, 177
Roth, F. B., 87
Rothenberg, Jerome, 295
Ruchlin, Hirsch S., viii, ix, 293, 296

S

Saathoff, Donald E., 131, 132, 134, 138
Sabin, Albert Bruce, 179
Salk, Jonas, 179
Samuelson, Paul A., 21, 55, 291
Sarachek, Deborah, 295

Schultz, T. Paul, 294
Scitovsky, Anne A., 51, 52, 53, 63, 292
Shain, M., 88
Shanas, E., 87
Shaprio, Robert, 221
Sherwood, Sylvia, 296
Skolnik, Alfred M., 179, 196
Smith, Warren F., 177, 294
Somers, Anne, 249
Somers, Herman, 249, 296
Spivey, W. Allen, 116
Steiner, Peter L., 291
Suits, Daniel, 289
Sullivan, Daniel F., 103
Summers, G. W., 157

T

Taylor, Lester D., 293
Taylor, Vincent, 251, 256

Theil, H., 76, 78
Titmuss, R. M., 87

W

Watson, J. D., 189, 196
Weisbrod, Burton, 71, 175, 176, 182,
    183, 184, 186, 192, 193, 196, 227,
    292, 294
Weiss, Jeffrey H., 295
Weller, Thomas H., 190
Wilkens, Maurice H. F., 189
Wirick, Grover, 292
Wold H., 76, 77, 78, 98

Y

Yett, Donald E., 17, 173, 294

INDEX

A

Accreditation, medical
  control of, 9
Advisory Commission on Intergovernmental Relations, The, 33
Algebra, matrix, 116
American Economic Association, 10
American Hospital Association, 71, 73,
  74, 88, 127, 129, 138
American Medical Association, 47, 71,
  87, 189, 196
American Nurses Association, 26, 127
American Stock Exchange, 12
Analysis, correlation
  objectives of, 285
Analysis, cost-effectiveness
  application of, 197
  characteristics of, 198
  definition of, 177
  description of, 197
  procedures of, 177
  uses of, 198
Analysis, demand, 77
Analysis, economic
  fields of, 11
Association, linear
  definition of, 280
Analysis, linear multiple regression, 72,
  124
Analysis, linear programming, 124
Analysis, longitudinal, 24, 43
Analysis, regression, 77, 137, 264 (see
  also Parameters)
  estimations of, 286

Analysis, regression (Continued)
  objectives of, 285
  purposes of, 77
  uses of, 286
  versatility of, 288
Analysis, sensitivity
  techniques of, 156
Analysis, statistical
  basis of, 273
Analysis, time series (see Analysis, longitudinal)
Anguish, mental
  value of, monetary, 195
Arguments, theoretical, 15
Assets, monetary, 102 (see also Capital)

B

Bar diagram (graph), 276
  definition of, 275
Base
  definition of, 40
  percentage increase over, 41
  percentage of, 41
Benefit-cost ratio, 159
  discounting process applied, 168
  formula for computation, 168
  uses of, 168
Benefit-cost ratio calculations
  interest rate affecting, 168–169
  use of, 173
Birth control devices, 219 (see also
  Birth rate)
Birth rate, 216, 217
  decline, factors of, 217, 219

Birth rate (*Continued*)
  mores affecting, cultural, 219
  mortality rate compared with, 218
  urbanization affecting, 219
"Black markets", 64
Bonds, 162
  liquidity of, 161
Bonds, Corporate Aaa (graph), 162
Budget constraint
  formula for, 120
Budget line
  construction of, 108
Bureau of Labor Statistics, 40, 45

C

Calculus, differential, 101
Capital, 102 (*see also* Production, factors of)
  definition of, 102
  investments in, 218
  progress of, embodied technological, 215
  progress of, rate of embodied technological, measurement of, 215–216
  types of, 160
  use of, general, 165
  use of, specific, 165
  utilization of, 210
Capital, growth rate of, 213, 214
  investment affecting, net, 211
Capital, human
  definition of, 102
Capital inputs, 104, 105, 109, 110
Ceteris paribus assumption, 16
Competition, 11
  absence of, 14
  benefits of, 14
  definition of, 14
Competitive atmosphere, 14
"Constant dollars," 24
Constants
  definition of, 260
  types of, 260
Consumer Price Index, viii, 26, 38, 40, 53, 178, 182, 184
  basis of, 43
  components of, 46
  components of, weight of, 44–45

Consumer Price Index (*Continued*)
  computation of, 43–44 (*see also* Laspeyeres Index)
  functions of, 43
  indications of, 46
  interpretation of, 45–46
  limitations of, 45–46
  medical care percentage of, 46
  price quotations affecting, 45
    descriptions of, 45
    obtainment of, 45
  use of, 45–46
Consumer Price Index, 24 (*See also* Price indices)
Consumer Price Index base
  derivation of, 44
Consumer Price Index, 1971, The (table), 44
Corporate Aaa bonds (*see* Bonds)
Correlation (graphs), 281 (*see also* Analysis, Correlation)
  discussion of, 280
Correlation, multiple
  definition of, 284
Correlation, partial
  definition of, 284
Correlation, perfect
  definition of, 282
Correlation, perfect negative
  definition of, 282
Correlation, perfect positive
  definition of, 282
Correlation, rank
  definition of, 283
  uses of, 284
Correlation coefficient
  computation, formula for, 282
  determination of, 283
  function of, 280
Correlation coefficient, multiple
  computation of, 285
  computation of, formula for, 285
Correlation coefficient, partial
  computation of, formula for, 284
Cost, opportunity, 176
  definition of, 66
Cost, standard
  definition of, 252

Cost-benefit approach
  characteristics of, 197
  uses of, 198
Cost-benefit calculations
  cost affecting, opportunity, 176
Cost-benefit studies
  techniques of, 172
Cost curve, 124
  derivation of, 101
Cost curve, average (graph), 119, 120, 143
Cost curve, marginal, 143
  computation of, 137
  definition of, 137
Cost curve, total, 137
Cost-effectiveness analysis (*see* Analysis, cost-effectiveness)
Cost of Selected Illness Index, 51
  components of (table), 52, 53
  features of, 51–52
  limitations of, 53
  uses of, 53
Cost profiles, 168
Cost profiles, individual, 247
Cost solution, minimum
  derivation of, mathematical, 120–122
Crime
  affects of, economic, 27
Curricula, medical
  social science affecting, 3

D

Debt certificates, bank, 162
Debt certificates, commercial, 162
Demand
  changes in, 60
  characteristics of, fundamental, 57–58
  components of, 88
  concept of, 54–55
  definition of, 55
  influences affecting, 58–60, 68
  need compared with, 55
  price affecting, 57–58
  quantity affecting, 57–58
  shifts in (diagram), 59, 60
  time element affecting, 56
Demand, aggregate
  computation of, 55

Demand, arc price elasticity of
  computation of, 70
  formula for, 70
Demand, effective, 55–56
Demand, income elasticity of
  measurements of, 62
Demand, point price elasticity of
  computation of, 69
  formula for, 69
Demand, price elasticity of
  application of, 61
  computation of, 60, 68–69
  definition of, 60
  formula for, 69
  measurements of, 60
  ranges of, numerical, 60
  revenue, total
    relationships between, 61
Demand curve (diagram), 56 (diagram), 63, 68
  construction of, 55
  definition of, 55
  equation for, 70
Demand curve, aggregate (diagram), 57
Demand model, 72, 88
  criteria for, 75–76
  description of, 75
  discussion of, 78
  formula of, 76
  prediction and, 71
  type of, least-squares linear multiple regression, 76
  uses of, 76
Demand model, curvilinear multiple regression (table), 99, 100
  computation of, 100
Demand model, linear
  curvilinear demand model compared with, 100
  description of, 77
  limitations of, 98, 100
Demand relationship, elastic
  affects of, 61
Demand relationship, inelastic
  affects of, 61
Demand schedule, 70
  illustration of, 55

Demand theory
  prediction and, 54
  reformulation of, 65–66, 67
Demographic transition (graph), 217
  definition of, 216
Dental care
  income affecting, distribution of
    (table), 30
Dependency ratio
  definition of, 218
Derivatives
  capabilities of, 264
  change, determination of rate of,
    270–271
  computation of, 268–269
  computation of, graphic, 267
  definition of, 264–265, 266
  indications of, 266–267
  uses of, 264
Derivatives, partial
  computation of, 272
  uses of, 271–272
Derivatives, second
  computation of, 269
  indications of, 269–270
Derivatives, simple
  capabilities of, 264
  uses of, 269
Determination, coefficient of, 286
Determination, coefficient of multiple
  discussion of, 287–288
Deviations, standard, 252, 253
  computation of, 278
DI (*see* Disposable Income)
Dialysis (*see* Hemodialysis)
Diet
  income affecting, distribution of, 30
Differentiation, 108
Differentiation, rules of, 268
Discount rate
  function of, 198
Discount rate, gross, 178
Discount rate, net, 177, 178, 201
Disease, particular
  research, cost of, 181
  research in
    benefits, assessment of, 175
    costs, assessment of, 175–176

Distribution, normal
  characteristics of, 279–280
  derivation of, 278–279
Distribution, symmetrical (graphs), 279
  definition of, 278

E

Economic growth (*see* Growth, economic)
Economic index
  change, factors of, 23–24
Economic policy
  objectives of, 207
Economic Report of the President, 1972,
  25, 26
Economics
  discipline of, vii
  experimentation of, controlled, 16
  factors of, 10
  goals of, 14–15
  subareas of, 10–11
Economics, activity of
  guidelines of, 62
Economics, health
  approach to, humanistic, 3
  demand affecting, income elasticity of,
    61–62
  income affecting, distribution of, 28,
    30–31
  macro theory and, 11
  micro theory and, 11
  price-quantity relationship affecting,
    65–66
  research in, 3
    foundations of, 3–4
    methods of, 3
    techniques of, econometric, 3
    techniques of, managerial, 3
    techniques of, mathematical, 3
Economy
  goals, interpretation of, 176
Economy, United States
  growth rate of, annual, 214
Education (*see also* Investments, human beings, in)
  investments in, 172–173, 218, 220
  rate of return, internal, 180
Education, medical
  control of, 9

Elderly, the
  health care for, 4 (*see also* Health care
    industry)
Equation, regression
  solution, formula for, 285
Equations
  inconsistancy between, 263
  types of, 259–260
Equivallency classes
  revenue generated by, 152–153
Equivalence classes, patient, 146–147,
    148, 149
  requirements, levels of
    relationships between, 149–150
  resource absorption of, 152
  services provided, quantity of
    determination of, 151
  subsets corresponding to, 155
  values of, optimal, 156–157

F

Factor payment, 165 (*see also* Interest)
Federal Reserve discount rate (graph),
    162
Fiscal capacity
  definition of, 33
  measurement of, 33
Freedom, degrees of
  computation of, 288
Frequency distribution (graph), 276
  definition of, 275
Function
  arguments of, 263
  formulas representing, 263–264
Funds, loanable
  demand, determination of, 163
    interest rate affecting, 163
  rationing of, 163
  supply, determination of, 161–163
    interest rate affecting, 163
Future payment, series of
  value of, present
    formula for, 165, 166–167

G

GNI (*see* Gross National Income)
GNP (*see* Gross National Product)
GNP-deflator, 24 (*see also* Price indices)

Goods, complementary
  definition of, 60
  price increase affecting, 60
Goods, consumer
  groupings of, 158–159
Goods and services
  characteristics of, 158
Goods and services, consumer
  definition of, 158
Goods and services, investment
  definition of, 159
Gross National Income (table), 21 (*see
    also* Gross National Product)
  components of, 20
  computation of, 20
Gross National Product, 4 (table), 21
    (table), 25, 208, 211, 228 (*see also*
    Growth, economic)
  change, factors of, 24
  components of, 20, 28
  composition of, aggregate, 24
  computation of, 19–20
  definition of, 19
  distribution, discussion of, 208–209
  health expenditure percentage of, 231
  treatment and health, 183
Gross National Product, deflated
    (table), 25
Gross National Product, real (table), 25
  computation of, 25
Gross National Product deflator index,
    25
Gross National Product growth rate
  formula for, 208
Growth, economic
  attainment, factors of, 218
  competition affecting, international,
    221
  definition of, 208
  dependency ratio affecting, 218
  family size affecting, 218–219
  government affecting, 221
  health, influence of, 216, 220
  morbidity affecting, level of, 219–220
  objectives of, 212
  planning affecting, 221
  production affecting, factors of, 210
  theory of, vii

Growth model, neoclassical economic, 212–213
  formula for, 210
  growth included, embodied technological
    formula for, 215
  progress included, disembodied technological
    formula for, 214–215
  prediction of, 213–214
Growth, rate of
  definition of
    formula for, 211
Growth statistics, economic
  accuracy of, 209
  derivation of, 209
Growth, sustained economic
  history of, 209–210

H

Health
  investments in, 218, 220
Health care
  distribution of, unequal, 29–31
  expenditures for, 83–84
  expenditures for, per capita, 33–34
  income affecting, distribution of, 32–33
  quality of, 27, 50–51
Health care effort
  adjustments in, 35
  computation of, 34
  cost affecting, relative, 34
  fiscal capacity affecting, 34
  morbidity rate affecting, 34
  population affecting, 34
  population affecting, age of, 34
Health care effort, state (table), 36
  adjustments in (table), 36
  comparisons between, 35
Health care expenditures, 4
  aid to state and local governments, federal (table), 237
  distribution of, relative private, 231 (table), 233
  distribution of, relative public, 231 (table), 233, 234
  grants to state and local governments, federal per capita (table), 238

Health care expenditures *(Continued)*
  income affecting, per capita personal, 23
  types of, 231 (table), 232–233
  variations in, geographical, 234, 236, 238, 240
Health care expenditures, city per capita (table), 240
Health care expenditures, federal, 234 (table), 236, 240, 245
Health care expenditures, governmental, 234, 241
Health care expenditures, national, 231
  sources of (table), 234
Health care expenditures, nongovernmental
  distribution of, 236
Health care expenditures, state
  distribution of, 236, 238
Health care expenditures, state and local government per capita (table), 239
Health care expenditures, third party and private (table), 246
Health care facilities
  construction of, 54
  construction of, expenditures for, 4
  shortages of, 65
Health care facilities, regional, 125
Health care financing
  insurance affecting, health, 245, 247, 248, 249, 250
Health care industry
  advertisement and, 9
  competition and, 8–9
  components of, institutional, 6–7
  contributions affecting, philanthropic, 8
  costs of, lower, 101
  demand and, 54
  demand theory applied to, 71
  economic growth
    relationships between, 207
  economics of, vii
  economists affecting, vii
  expenditures of (table), 5, 6
  expenditures of, private, 4
  expenditures of, public, 4
  expenditures of, research, 6

Health care industry (*Continued*)
  gross national product, affecting, 4
  innovations in, technological, 241
  insurance arrangements affecting, 9,
    245, 247–250
  output of, definition of
    research in, 123
  output of, estimation of
    criteria for, 123
  output and, greater, 101
  output of, measure of, 123
  planning of, 221–222
  production inputs and, 103–104
  production models
    research in, 123
  profit motive and, 7, 8
  quality of, 8
  quality of, cost of, 8
  reimbursement philosophy affecting, 8
  research studies, vi
  scale, economics of
    research in, 123
  shortages of, personnel, 65
  size of, 4
Health care institution
  difficulties of, financial, 241
  operation, cost of, 241
  reimbursements, alternative, 251–258
    categories of, 251
    formula for, 252–254
  reimbursement, formula for
    basis of, 247
  reimbursement, patterns of
    limitations of, 247–248, 249, 250,
      251
Health care institution efficiency
  reimbursement affecting, alternative,
    251–255, 257
Health care labor
  training of, 54
  unionization of, 241
Health care services
  availability of, 98
  demand affecting, 65, 68
  expenditures for (*see* Health care ex-
    penditures)
  financing of, viii, 230–231, 245
  financing of, government, 230–231
  financing of, macro, 230–231, 240–241

Health care services (*Continued*)
  financing of, micro, 230–231
  financing of, public, 21–23
Health care services
  fiscal capacity affecting, 33, 34
  grants-in-aid, federal
    allocation of, 234, 236, 238
  income affecting, viii
  rationing of, 64, 65
  supply affecting, 65
  tax effort affecting, 33
  tax revenues affecting, 241, 243
  use of
    income affecting, distribution of, 66
Health care service, state
  funds for, federal, 35, 37
Health care service need, 68
Health care studies
  limitations, 67–68
Health index
  construction of, problems in, 103
Health Information Foundation, The,
  83, 87, 88, 98
Health occupations
  investments in, 173
Health profile
  components of, 7
"Heckscher-Ohin" result, 140
Hemodialysis
  application, cost of, 193
  capacity of, 200
  considerations of, economic, 177–178
  cost of, 201
  function of, 198
Hemodialysis, home, 197
  cost of, annual average, 197
  expenditures for, total (table), 205
Hemodialysis, hospital, 197
  cost of, annual, 197
  expenditures for, total (table), 205
Hemodialysis patient
  life expectancy of average, 204
  life years gained (table), 205
Hemodialysis patient, home
  life style of, 200
Hemodialysis patient, hospital
  life style of, 200
Hemodialysis program
  life years gained (table), 199, 202

Hill-Burton Act, 9
Hill-Burton program, 125
Histogram (graph), 276
  definition of, 275
Hospital
  modal pattern of control, 7, 8
  types of, 289
  utilization of (*see* Utilization, hospital)
Hospital care
  expenditures for, 6
Hospital construction
  funds for, federal, 9, 125
Hospital costs
  analysis, factors of, 128
  analysis, regression (graph), 131
  comparisons between, adjusted, 130–131
    formula for, 129
  measurement of, 132–133, 138
  studies of, 131
  urban and rural, comparisons between (table), 140
Hospital costs, average
  estimation of, 133
Hospital costs, relative, 135
Hospital costs, total, 135, 136
  percentages of, direct labor (table), 139
  regression equation for, 137
Hospital costs studies
  limitations of, 126
Hospital efficiency
  size affecting, 144
Hospital facilities
  size, optimal, 125, 138, 144
  size, unit, 138
  utilization of, 76, 77, 78, 80 (*see also* Utilization, hospital)
  utilization of, estimated, 73
Hospital facilities model
  budget constraint affecting, 152
    formula for, 153
Hospital operating resources
  categories of, 149–150
Hospital output
  measurement, formula for, 123–124
  policy decisions affecting, 153–154

Hospital output capacity
  concept of, economic, 157
  value of, optimal, 157
Hospital planning
  models, construction of, 144, 150–151
  objectives of, 148
Hospital planning model
  budgetary constraint
    formula for, 154
  patient constraint affecting
    formula for, 154
  policy constraints affecting, 153–154
    formula for, 155
  resource constraint affecting
    formula for, 154
Hospital planning model, linear
  limitations of, 156
  versatility of, 156
Hospital product
  definition of, 252
Hospital resources, variable
  cost of, formula for, 153
Hospital service units
  cost of, relative (table), 143
Hospital technology
  coefficients, formula for, 155
  discussion of, 150–151
Hospital technology, linear
  characteristics of, 151
Hospitals
  guide issue of, 129, 130, 133, 136, 138, 141, 142

I

Illnesses
  treatment of, increase in cost of (table), 52
Income
  distribution of, equal, 29
  distribution of, unequal, 28–29, (table), 29, (table), 32
  health care affecting, 32–33
Income, disposable, 21
Income, growth rate of
  formula for, 214
Income, national, 21 (*see also* National income accounts)
Income, per capita
  expansion of, 209, 210

Income, per capita (*Continued*)
  growth, rate
    formula for, 212
Income, per capita personal (table), 22–23
  computation of, 23, 28
Income, personal
  definition of, 21
Income, regional
  definition of, 23
Income, state
  definition of, 23
Income, total regional (table), 22–23
Income, total state (table), 22–23
Income accounting, national, vii
Income effect, 57–58
  definition of, 57
Income elasticity
  definition of, 162
Index number series
  construction of (table), 40, 41
Index numbers, 38
  construction of, 38–39
  definition of, 38
  uses of, 41
Indices
  changes, reflecting, 38–39
  construction of, 40
  types of, 41
  uses of, 38
  valuation of, 40
Indices, general
  construction of, 39, 43
Industrial revolution, 209
Industry consumption patterns, 11
Inefficiency (*see also* Competition, absence of)
  results of, 14
Infant mortality
  income affecting, distribution of (table), 30
  race affecting (table), 30
Inputs (*see* Production inputs)
Institute of Medicine, vii
Insurance, health, 9, 84, 245 (*see also* Variables, implicit price)
  function of, 255
  policy, model, 247
Insurance, hospitalization, 74, 86, 95, 96

Insurance, major risk, 255
Insurance, national health, 229, 245, 251
Insurance, variable cost hospital, 256–257
Insurance industry, 6 (*see also* Health care industry, components of)
Interest
  definition of, 102–103
Interest rate, 159, 172
  definition of, 160
  existence of, determination of, 160
  factors of, 160
  fluctuation of, 161
  inflation affecting, 160–161
  level of, 160
  level of, determination of, 161, 163
  liquidity affecting, 161
  risk premiums affecting, 160–161
  transaction costs affecting, 161
Interest rates, coexisting (graph), 162
Interest rate, pure, 160
Internal Rate of Return (*see* Rate of return, internal)
Investment
  costs of, transaction, 161
  factors of, 161
  human beings, in, 172
  inflation affecting, 160
  liquidity of, 161
  rational for, 160
  risk and, 160–161
  techniques of, 172
  value of, present
    computation of, 163–164
Investment opportunities
  discussion of, 163
  interpretation of, 163
Investment patterns, 11
Investment theory
  efficiency and, long-run, 158
Investment theory tools
  use of, 175
Isocontribution curve
  representation of, mathematical, 116
Isocontribution line, 114, 115, 116
Isocost, 108, 114
Isocost line
  definition of, 107

Isoquants, 108, 117, 118 (graph), 106
  (graph), 107, 212, 213
  definition of, 105
Isoquant map, 106, 107
Isoquants, neoclassical production
  (graph), 213
Issues, normative
  definition of, 17
Issues, positive
  definition of, 17
Iterative process
  discussion of, 170

K

Kidney failure
  distribution between dialysis and mor-
    tality (table), 202
  mortality rate from, annual (table),
    200
Kidney transplantation, 197, 198, 200
  cost of, 201
  cost of, average, 197
  considerations of, economic, 177
  expenditures for, total (table), 205
  life years gained, 202 (table), 203–204
Kidney transplantation patient
  life expectancy of, average, 204 (ta-
    ble), 205
  life style of, 200
  life years gained (table), 205
Kidneys
  preservation of, 206
  storage of, 206

L

Labor, 102 (*see also* Production, factors of)
  definition of, 102
  progress of, embodied technological,
    215
  progress of, rate of embodied techno-
    logical, measurement of, 215–216
  utilization of, 210
Labor, effective, 140
Labor, growth rate of, 211–212, 213, 214
Labor, productivity of
  definition of, 219
  health affecting, 220

Labor, productivity of (*Continued*)
  malnutrition affecting, 220
  morbidity affecting, level of, 219–220
Labor force participation
  definition of, 211
Labor inputs, 104–105, 109, 110–111
Lagrange multiplier method, 109
Land, 102 (*see also* Production, factors
  of)
  definition of, 102
Land inputs, 104
Laspeyeres Index, 41
  construction of (table), 43
Laspeyeres Index formula
  computation of, 41–42
  uses of, 43
Law of decreasing marginal returns,
  110–111
Least squares (graph), 283
Leisure time
  affects of, economic, 27
"Leontieff paradox," 140
Licensing, medical
  control of, 9
Line, straight
  equation for, 280–281
Linear association (*see* Association,
  linear)
Linearity
  discussion of, 281–282
Loanable funds (*see* Funds, loanable)
Lorenz curve
  definition of, 31–32
  illustration of, 32
Loss, net
  definition of, 176

M

Macroeconomics (*see also* Analysis, economic)
  definition of, 11
Malpractice suit, 248
Manpower training
  investments in, 172–174 (*see also* In-
    vestments, human beings, in)
Market, 11, 64
  activities of, corrective, 24
  definition, 12–14
  types of, 14

Market, buyer's, 64
Market, engineering
  mechanics of, 13
Market, export, 210
Market, Perfectly Competitive
  definition of, 14
Market, seller's, 64
Market equilibrium (diagram), 63
  discussion of, 64
Mathematics, tools of
  uses of, 259
Mean
  computation, formula for, 277
  definition of, 276–277
  uses of, 277
Median
  computation of, 277
  definition of, 277
  uses of, 277–278
Medicaid, 6, 234, 247
Medical associations, professional
  influences of, 9
Medical Care Cost Index, 241
Medical care costs
  measures of, 51
Medical care industry
  definition of, 6–7 (*see also* **Health care industry**)
Medical Care Price Index, viii, 38 (table), 48–49, 178
  Cost of Selected Illnesses Index compared with, 53
  description of, 46–47
  limitations of, 50–51
  measurements of, 46
  nature of, 52
  revisions in, 47
Medical care services
  prices of, overview of, 47–50
Medical occupations
  training, cost of, 8
Medical research
  efficiency, economic, 179
  expenditures for, federal, 178–179
Medicare, 6, 229, 234, 247, 254
Microeconomics (*see also* Analysis, economic)
  definition of, 11
Modal pattern, 7

Mode
  definition of, 277
  uses of, 278
Model
  definition of, 259
  types, description of, 259
  usefulness, determination of, 259
Model, determined
  definition of, 263
Model, economic
  description of, 15, 16
Model, mathematical
  components of, 259
Model, overdetermined
  definition of, 263
Model, underdetermined
  definition of, 262
Monetary measures
  convertion of, 25
Monetary unit
  adjustments of, 24
  changes in, 24
  deflation of, 24
  inflation of, 24
Monopoly, 102
Mortality
  implications of, economic, 220
  loss, economic
    estimation of, 176
Mortality rate, 216
  decline, factors of, 217, 218
  factors affecting, 219

N

National Academy of Sciences, vii
National Health Survey, 82
National income accounts
  expressions of, real term, 24
  limitations of, 26–28, 209
  measurement of, 24
  nature of, arbitrary, 28
  tax rates, affecting, 33
  use of, 18–20
Net National Product, 21
Net loss (*see* Loss, net)
NI (*see* National Income)
NNP (*see* Net National Product)
Nursing home, 92

Nursing home care, 254
  expenditures for, 6
Nursing, schools of, 135, 143
Nursing occupations
  training, cost of, 8

O

Observations, dispersion of
  measures of, 278
Output (*see also* Production)
  costs related to, 135–136, 137
  definition of, 102
  investment affecting, 159
Output, growth of, 210–211, 216
  computation of, 211–212
  formula of, 211
Output, hospital
  definition of, 144
  measure of, 144–147
Output, hospital optimal (*see* Output, optimal hospital)
Output, hospital terminal
  definition of, 146
Output, hospital total
  formula for, 148
  measure of, 149
Output, labor
  increases in, 211
Output, marginal, 111
Output, measure of, 131, 136–137, 139, 144 (*see also* Hospital costs, studies in)
  computation for, 142–143
  formulas for, 133–134, 140–142
  problems in, 133
  unit of, 135
Output, optimal hospital
  combinations for, feasible, 149
  determination of, 149
Output, service
  measure of, 132
  unit of
    formula for, 132

P

Paasche Index, 41
  construction of (table), 43
Paasche Index formula
  computation of, 42

Parameters
  value, determination of, 264
Patinet classifications
  discussion of, 156
Perfectly Competitive Market (*see* Market, Perfectly Competitive)
Physician efficiency
  reimbursement affecting, alternative, 251, 254–255, 257
Physician visits
  income affecting, distribution of, 30 (table), 31
  race affecting (table), 31
PI (*see* Income, personal)
Plan, rolling economic
  cost of, 225
  definition of, 225
  efficiency of, 225–226
Planning, economic, viii
  benefits of, potential, 222–224
  cost of, 224–225
  use of, effective, 222
  uses of, 221
Planning, economic health
  approaches to, 226–229
    limitations of, 229
  defense of, 226
  difficulties of, 226
Planning, formal economic
  definition of, 222
Planning, informal economic
  discussion of, 222
Planning, macro economic, 226
Planning, micro economic, 226
Planning models, economic health
  development of, 229
Planning-programming-budgeting studies
  approaches to, 171–172
  steps involved in, 172
  techniques of, 172
  uses of, 171
Poliomyelitis
  eradication of, benefits of, 182
    estimation of, 184
  eradication of, cost of, 176
  eradication of, economic benefits of, 175
  loss per case, mean economic, 184

Poliomyelitis (*Continued*)
  morbidity loss
    estimation of, 183
    measurement of, 192
  mortality loss
    estimation of, 182–183
    measurement of, 192
  prevention, estimation of, 184–185,
    187–188
  prevention, mean rate of, 184
Poliomyelitis research
  analysis of, 179
  application of, cost of, 193, 194
  awards for, monetary (table), 181,
    182
  benefit of, estimation of, 190
  benefit of, evaluation of, 180
  cost of, examination of, 193
  expenditures for, 189, 191
  rates of return on, internal, 179–180,
    186 (table), 187, 188, 189, 190–
    191, 192, 193, 194, 195
    formula for, 80
  vaccination costs affecting (table),
    184
  success, estimation of, 185
  treatment loss
    estimation of, 183
    measurement of, 192
Poliomyelitis vaccinations
  benefits, external, 191
  benefits, internal, 191
  cost of, implicit, 185, 186, 188–189
  cost of, total, 185–186, 188–189
  growth of, test tube, 190
Pollution, air
  affects of, economic, 27
Pollution, water
  affects of, economic, 27
Poor, the
  health care for, 4 (*see also* Health
    care industry)
Population, growth rate of, 221
Population explosion, 217
Population growth
  factors affecting, 216–217
  health affecting, 216
  mores affecting, cultural, 219
  rate of, 217

Population growth (*Continued*)
  rate for non-industrialized nations,
    218
Population growth, sustained, 216
Population growth rate
  health affecting, 219
PPB studies (*see* Planning-program-
    ming-budgeting studies)
Present discounted value (*see* Value,
    present)
Price, equilibrium, 64–65
Price, "shadow," 102
Price fixing, 102
Price indices, 18, 24
  comparisons between, 24–25
  uses of, 25–26
Probability
  definition of, 273
  discussion of, 273–274
  formula for, 274
Probability estimates
  validity, conditions for, 274
Production
  assignments of, 103
  concepts of, 110
  concepts of, economic, 101
  discussion of, 101
  factors of, 102
  output and, 102
  profit motive affecting, 101
Production, indirect methods of
  investment affecting, 159
Production costs
  determination of, 117–118
Production curve
  construction of, 117
  cost of, total (graph), 118, 119
Production efficiency
  computations of, 106
  computation of, geometric method
    for, 108
  computation of, mathematical, 108–
    109
  definition of, 105–106
  determination of, geometric (graph),
    107, 114–115 (graph), 115
  determination of, mathematical, 115–
    116
  formula for, 109

Production expansion path (graph), 117
Production function (table), 105, 117, 151, 212, 214
concept of, 103
formulas for, 104–105, 109, 110, 112, 120
limitations of, 106
representation of, geometric (graph), 106
Production function, Cobb-Douglas, 112
Production inputs
categories of, 102
combinations of, 103
costs of, 106
measurement of, monetary, 102
relationships of, technological, 104–105
formula for, 104–105
Production models
types of, 124–125
Production output
relationships of, technological, 104–105
formulas for, 104–105
Production patterns, 11
Production possibility curves, 113
Products, final
definition of, 19
Products, intermediate
definition of, 19
Profit, 102 (*see also* Wages)
Profit motive, 101
Profit rate, target, 20
Programming, linear, 101
Progress, disembodied technological
definition of, 214
Progress, embodied technological
definition of, 215
Progress, technological
definition of, 214
Public Health Service, 92
Public Law, 89–97, 234 (*see also* Medicare and Medicaid)

Q

Quantity
changes in, 60 (*see also* Demand, changes in)

R

Rate of return
determination of, geographic (graph), 171
Rate of return, internal, 159, 169
computation of, 169–170
computation, formula for, 170
Rate of return calculations, internal
use of, 173
Rate of return rule of investment, internal
limitations of, 170–171
Rate of return studies
techniques of, 172
Rationality, 11, 14
definition of, 11–12
Rationing
definition of, 64
Regression
discussion of, 280
Regression coefficient
error, standard, 288
Regression coefficient, partial
definition of, 286–287
Renal disease, chronic, 177
cost, total, 202
drug treatment, maintenance
cost of, 201
treatment of, 196–198 (*see also* specific treatments)
expenditures, federal, 197
treatment, cost of, 197, 200–201
Rent
definition of, 102
Requirement vectors
components of,
formula for, 155
estimation of, 155
Requirement vectors, average
formula for, 148
Requirement vectors, patient, 147, 148
components of, 147
Requirement vectors, total
formula for, 148
Research, empirical, 16
basis of, 15
National income accounts affecting, 28

Research, theoretical
basis of, 15
Residual factor
function of, 214
Resource, fixed
usage, formula for, 151
Returns, diminishing, 110–111, 112 (*see
also* Law of decreasing marginal returns)
Returns, negative marginal, 111
Returns to scale, 118, 120
definition of, 111–112
Returns to scale, constant, 112, 120, 151
Returns to scale, decreasing
definition of, 112
Returns to scale, diminishing, 118
Returns to scale, increasing
definition of, 112
Revenue, total
definition of, 60–61
price-quantity relationship affecting,
61
Risk aversion, 192

S

Sabin oral vaccine, 184, 186, 191
Salaries
definition of, 102
Salaries, nurses, 25 (table), 26
Salk vaccine, 191
Sample
definition of, 274
Sample, random
definition of, 274
discussion of, 274–275
Sample, stratified random
definition of, 275
Saskatchewan Department of Public
Health, 87
Saskatchewan Hospital Services Plan,
82, 83
Scale, diseconomics of, 112
Scale, economics of, 112
Scale, returns to (*see* Returns to scale)
"Service cost centers," 132
"Service cost centers, auxiliary," 133,
139
Service output
estimation, computation for, 136

Service units
cost, average (table), 134
cost, relative (table), 134
Service and goods
characteristics of, 158
Service and goods, consumer
definition of, 158
Service and goods, investment
definition of, 159
Significance
definition of, 288
Size, economics of
existence of, 123
Slope, 107, 108
definition of, 265
representation of (graph), 265
Smallpox vaccination, 217
Spearman's Rank Correlation, 236
Spearman's Rank Correlation coefficient,
238
Spearman's Rho
formula of, 284
Specialists visits, medical
income affecting, distribution of (table), 31
Standard cost (*see* Cost, standard)
Standard deviations (*see* Deviations,
standard)
Statistical Abstract of the United States,
5, 193, 196, 200, 233, 235, 236, 237,
238
Substitution effect
definition of, 58
Supply
definition of, 62
factors affecting, 62–63
price-quantity relationship affecting,
62–63
Supply, price elasticity of
demand compared with, price elasticity of, 62
Supply and demand relationship
discussion of, 63–65
Supply curve, 62 (diagram), 63
Supply schedule, 62
Survey of Consumer Expenditures, 45
Survey of Consumer Expenditures
1960–1961, 44

T

Tangency, 107, 108
Tangency point, 115
Tangent
  definition of, 265
Tangent
  representation of (graph), 265
Tangent
  slope, value of
    computation of, 266–269
Tax
  categorization of, 243
  restructuring of, 245
Tax, income
  elasticity of, 243
Tax, property
  elasticity of, 243–244
Tax, sales
  elasticity of, 243–244
Tax base, 244
  changing of, 245
  definition of, 243
Tax effort
  definition of, 33
Tax elasticity
  definition of, 243
Tax rate
  changes in, 245
  definition of, 243
Tax rate, property
  determination of, 244
Tax revenue
  discussion of, 241–245
  distribution of, 244
  sharing of, 245
Tax revenue, sources of
  distribution of (table), 242
Technological progress (see Progress,
    technological)
Technology
  definition of, 62
  utilization of, 210 (see also Supply,
    factors affecting)
Technology, advances in
  production techniques, affecting, 62–
    63
Tendency, central
  measures of, 276

Theory, economic
  definition of, 15–16
  judgment of, 15 (see also Research,
    theoretical)
Total revenue (see Revenue, total)
TR (see Revenue, total)
Trade, free, 210
Trade theory, international, 140
Transfer payments
  definition of, 21
Transformation, logarithmic, 73
Transformation curve, 115, 116 (graph),
  114
  concept of, 103
  construction of, 113–114
  formula for, 113
Transformation process, 151

U

United Hospital Fund of New York, 132,
  133, 135, 139, 141, 142
United States Bureau of Labor Statistics,
  126
United States Department of Com-
    merce, 20, 22, 44, 83
United States Department of Health,
    Education and Welfare, 30, 31, 87,
    88, 98, 184, 185, 188, 191, 196, 254
United States Department of Labor, 40,
    43, 45
United States Public Health Service: *Na-
    tional Health Survey*, 87, 88, 98
United States Senate, 87
United States Treasury bills, three
    month (graph), 162
Urban overcrowding
  affects, economic, 27
Uremia patients, chronic
  age, average, 204
Utilization, hospital, 124
  age affecting, 79, 81–82, 90–92
  "border crossing" affecting, 75
  choice, consumer, 98
  components of, 74
  definition of, 74
  demand relationships affecting, 88 (ta-
    ble), 89, 90 (table), 97, 98
  dwelling unit affecting, persons per,
    93, 98

Utilization, hospital (*Continued*)
  dwelling unit affecting, population
      per, 84
  education affecting, 79, 83–84, 86, 94–
      95
  estimation of, 79, 87
  estimation, development of, 92
  estimation, framework for, 75 (*see also*
      Demand model) factors, relating
      selection, criteria for, 79
  housing affecting, quality of, 83
  income affecting, distribution of, 79,
      83, 85, 86, 94–95, 98, 100
  insurance affecting, 79, 85–86, 95–96
  logarithm of, 100
  marital status affecting, 82, 84, 93, 98
  measures of (table), 80
  price of service affecting, 84–85
  race affecting, 79, 83, 94
  sex affecting, 82, 93
  urbanization affecting, 83, 94
  variables affecting, economic (table),
      91
  variables affecting, insurance, 100
  variables affecting, price, 95–96
  variables affecting, sociodemographic
      (table), 91, 92
  variables affecting, time (table), 97,
      98
  variations in, 90

V

Value, current, 164
Value, present, 159, 172 (*see also* Future
      Payments)
  characteristics of, 165
  definition of, 163–164
  formula for, 164
  interest rate affecting, 165
  time span affecting, 165
Value, probability, 166–167
Value calculation, present
  interest rate affecting, choice of, 167
Variables
  classifications of, 260–261
  definition of, 260
  description of, 80
  discussion of, 78–79
  examination of, 87

Variables (*Continued*)
  limitations of, 77
  mean of (table), 80, 81
  ranges of (table), 80, 81
  selection of, 77–78
  selection, reasons for, 78
Variables, dependent, 77, 78, 80, 88, 97,
      260–261
Variables, dummy
  definition of, 289
  discussion of, 289–290
Variables, economic (table), 80
Variables, endogenous
  definition of, 261
Variables, exogenous
  definition of, 261
Variables, implicit price, 84
Variables, income, 85
Variables, independent (table), 80, 88,
      97, 260–261
  logarithm of, 100
Variables, policy
  definition of, 261
Variables, price, 72
Variables, sociodemographic, 72 (table),
      80, 85, 90
Variables, target, 261
  definition of, 262
Variables, time, 96–97
Variance
  computation of, 278
  formula for, 278
Vector, patient requirement (*see* Re-
      quirement vectors, patient)
Veterans payments, 21

W

Wage earners, urban, 43 (*see also* Con-
      sumer Price Index)
Wage index, 140
Wage patterns, 11
Wages
  definition of, 102
  education affecting, investments in,
      173
  manpower training affecting, invest-
      ments in, 173
Wages, actual
  definition of, 39

Wages, adjusted starting hospital (table), 130

Wages, hospital
  differentials in, 134, 138, 139–140
  differentials in, fringe benefit, 129
  differentials, regional (table), 126, 139
  rural and urban
    differentials between, 126–128
  union organization affecting, 128

Wages, nurses
  differentials, regional, 127

Wages, real
  definition of, 39

Wages, starting hospital (table), 127
  (table), 128, 129

Water resources
  rate of return, internal, 180

Wealth
  definition of, 23

Welfare, social, 21, 245

Welfare, total social
  health care expenditures, per centage
    of (table), 235

Wholesale Price Index, 24 (*see also*
  Price indices)

Worker's compensation, 21